Recent Results in Cancer Research

Volume 196

Managing Editors

P. M. Schlag, Berlin, Germany
H. -J. Senn, St. Gallen, Switzerland

Associate Editors

P. Kleihues, Zürich, Switzerland
F. Stiefel, Lausanne, Switzerland
B. Groner, Frankfurt, Germany
A. Wallgren, Göteborg, Sweden

Founding Editor

P. Rentchnik, Geneva, Switzerland

For further volumes:
http://www.springer.com/series/392

Florian Otto · Manfred P. Lutz
Editors

Early Gastrointestinal Cancers

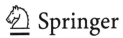
Springer

Editors
Florian Otto
Tumor- und Brustzentrum ZeTuP
St. Gallen
Switzerland

Manfred P. Lutz
Saarbrücken
Germany

ISSN 0080-0015
ISBN 978-3-642-31628-9   ISBN 978-3-642-31629-6   (eBook)
DOI 10.1007/978-3-642-31629-6
Springer Heidelberg New York Dordrecht London

Library of Congress Control Number: 2012949069

© Springer-Verlag Berlin Heidelberg 2012
This work is subject to copyright. All rights are reserved by the Publisher, whether the whole or part of the material is concerned, specifically the rights of translation, reprinting, reuse of illustrations, recitation, broadcasting, reproduction on microfilms or in any other physical way, and transmission or information storage and retrieval, electronic adaptation, computer software, or by similar or dissimilar methodology now known or hereafter developed. Exempted from this legal reservation are brief excerpts in connection with reviews or scholarly analysis or material supplied specifically for the purpose of being entered and executed on a computer system, for exclusive use by the purchaser of the work. Duplication of this publication or parts thereof is permitted only under the provisions of the Copyright Law of the Publisher's location, in its current version, and permission for use must always be obtained from Springer. Permissions for use may be obtained through RightsLink at the Copyright Clearance Center. Violations are liable to prosecution under the respective Copyright Law.
The use of general descriptive names, registered names, trademarks, service marks, etc. in this publication does not imply, even in the absence of a specific statement, that such names are exempt from the relevant protective laws and regulations and therefore free for general use.
While the advice and information in this book are believed to be true and accurate at the date of publication, neither the authors nor the editors nor the publisher can accept any legal responsibility for any errors or omissions that may be made. The publisher makes no warranty, express or implied, with respect to the material contained herein.

Printed on acid-free paper

Springer is part of Springer Science+Business Media (www.springer.com)

Contents

Part I   Multimodal Approach to Colorectal Cancer

Clinically Relevant Study End Points in Rectal Cancer   3
1   Introduction   4
2   End Points in Phase I Trials   6
3   End Points in Phase II Neoadjuvant Rectal Cancer Trials   7
   3.1   Pathological Parameters of Response   8
   3.2   Imaging Response   12
4   Endpoints in Phase III Trials   13
   4.1   Disease-Free Survival and Local Recurrence   15
   4.2   The Need for Long-Term Follow-Up   15
5   Discussion   16
References   16

Neoadjuvant Treatment in Rectal Cancer: Do We Always
Need Radiotherapy or Can We Risk Assess Locally Advanced
Rectal Cancer Better?   21
1   Introduction   22
2   Late Effects of Radiotherapy   23
3   Local Recurrence   24
   3.1   Is Neoadjuvant Chemotherapy an Alternative?   26
   3.2   Can Radiotherapy be Omitted?   26
   3.3   Are There Clearly Distinguishable Groups Who Do
        Not Need RT?   26
4   Conclusion   32
References   33

Treatment Dilemmas in Patients with Synchronous Colorectal Liver Metastases 37
1   Introduction... 38
2   Patients with Asymptomatic Cancer of the Colon
and Unresectable Synchronous Liver Metastases 38
    2.1   Results of Initial Treatment with Chemotherapy........... 39
    2.2   Results of Initial Resection of the Primary Tumor 40
    2.3   The Effect of Treatment Strategy on Overall Survival....... 42
3   Patients Presenting with Resectable Synchronous Liver Metastases
and Rectal Cancer 43
    3.1   Results of Staged or Simultaneous Rectal
and Liver Resection Combined with Perioperative
Radiotherapy and Chemotherapy 44
    3.2   Enhancing Efficacy of Perioperative Radiotherapy
and Chemotherapy 44
    3.3   Results of the Liver-First Approach 45
References... 46

Part II   Improving Treatment of Pancreatic Cancer

Pancreatic Surgery: Beyond the Traditional Limits 53
1   Introduction... 54
2   Portal/Mesenteric Vein Resection........................... 55
3   Arterial Resection 56
4   Extended Lymphadenectomy................................ 57
5   Multivisceral Resection.................................... 58
6   Resection for M1 PDAC.................................... 58
7   Surgery for Recurrent PDAC................................ 59
8   Pancreatic Parenchyma Sparing Procedures.................... 59
9   Conclusion 60
References... 61

Adjuvant Therapy for Pancreatic Cancer........................ 65
1   Introduction... 67
2   Rationale for Adjuvant Therapy............................. 67
3   Evidence for Adjuvant Chemotherapy 68
    3.1   Systemic Chemotherapy 68
    3.2   Regional Chemotherapy 72
4   Evidence for Adjuvant Chemoradiotherapy 73
    4.1   Intraoperative Radiotherapy.......................... 73
    4.2   Postoperative Chemoradiotherapy...................... 73
    4.3   Chemoradiotherapy, and Follow on Chemotherapy......... 74

Contents

5   Evidence for Neoadjuvant Therapy 79
     5.1   Published Studies 79
     5.2   Ongoing Studies 80
6   Evidence from Meta-Analyses 80
     6.1   Adjuvant Therapy 80
     6.2   Neoadjuvant Therapy 81
7   Conclusions 82
8   Future Directions 82
References 82

Radiotherapy of the Pancreas: State of the Art in 2012 89
1   The Role of Radiotherapy in the Therapeutic Management
     of Pancreatic Cancer 90
     1.1   Adjuvant Approach 90
     1.2   Neoadjuvant Approach 92
     1.3   Approach of Unresectable Pancreatic Tumors 93
2   Techniques of Radiation Therapy Planning and Delivery 94
     2.1   Radiation Dose Escalation 95
     2.2   Intensity-Modulated Radiation Therapy 95
     2.3   Image-Guided Radiation Therapy and Stereotactic
         Body Radiation Therapy 97
3   Conclusions 99
References 99

Part III   Different Cancer Types in the Oesophagus and Stomach

Adenocarcinoma of the GEJ: Gastric or Oesophageal Cancer? 107
1   Introduction 108
2   Challenges of the Current Barrett's Concept 108
     2.1   Evidence of Two Pathways 108
     2.2   Evidence of Different Targets for Therapy 110
     2.3   Evidence for Surveillance Recommendations 111
References 112

Why is There a Change in Patterns of GE Cancer? 115
1   Introduction 117
2   An Ageing Population 118
     2.1   Factors Leading to Improved Life Expectancy 118
     2.2   Implications of an Ageing Population on Management
         of Upper GI Cancers 118

3	Colonisation with Helicobacter Pylori.		119
	3.1	Mechanisms of Oncogenesis	119
	3.2	H. pylori Eradication and Decline in Prevalence	119
	3.3	Association Between H. pylori and Oesophageal Cancers	120
4	The Role of Obesity.		120
5	Bile Acids and Dietary Fat		122
6	Tobacco and Alcohol		123
	6.1	Smoking and Gastric Cancer	123
	6.2	Alcohol, GORD and Oesophageal Cancers	123
7	Gastric Polyps		124
	7.1	Epidemiology of Gastric polyps	124
	7.2	Adenomatous Polyps and Risk of Malignancy	124
	7.3	Hereditary Polyposis Syndromes	125
8	Other Medical Conditions		125
	8.1	Pernicious Anaemia	125
	8.2	Partial Gastrectomy.	126
	8.3	Plummer-Vinson Syndrome	126
	8.4	Coeliac Disease	127
	8.5	Oesophageal Achalasia	127
	8.6	Hereditary Tylosis (Familial Palmoplantar Keratosis)	128
9	Anti-Inflammatory Drugs		128
10	Family History		129
	10.1	Sporadic Gastric cancer.	129
	10.2	Inherited Cancer Syndromes	130
11	Having Other Cancers		130
12	Radiation Exposure		131
13	Reduced Immunity.		131
14	Work Chemicals		132
15	Hormone Replacement Therapy.		132
16	Physical Activity		133
17	Conclusion		133
References			135

Part IV Choosing the Best Treatment for Oesophageal Cancer

Endoscopic Treatment for Esophageal Squamous Cell Carcinoma.. . . . 143

1	Introduction.		143
2	Indications of Endoscopic Resection for Esophageal SCC.		144
	2.1	Absolute Indication.	144
	2.2	Relative Indications	144
3	Endoscopic Mucosal Resection		145
	3.1	Procedures.	145
	3.2	Advantage and Disadvantage of EMR.	145

Contents ix

4 Endoscopic Submucosal Dissection (ESD) 145
   4.1 Procedure 145
   4.2 Marking and Submucosal Injection. 146
   4.3 Mucosal incision 146
   4.3 Submucosal Dissection 148
   4.5 Hemostasis 150
   4.6 Prevention of Bleeding 150
5 Complications of Esophageal EMR/ESD. 151
References. 153

Open or Minimally Invasive Resection for Oesophageal Cancer? 155
1 Introduction. 156
2 MIO Techniques 157
3 Results 158
4 MIO Learning Curve 163
5 Comments and Future. 164
References. 165

Choosing the Best Treatment for Esophageal Cancer 169
1 Introduction. 170
2 Postoperative Mortality. 170
3 R0-Resection. 171
4 Lymphadenectomy. 171
5 Multimodal Treatment 172
6 Adjuvant Therapy 172
7 Neoadjuvant Radiotherapy 172
8 Neoadjuvant Chemotherapy or Radiochemotherapy 173
9 Response Prediction. 174
10 Targeted Drugs in Multimodal Therapy 174
References. 175

Part V Multimodal Therapy of GEJ Cancer

**Multimodal Therapy of GEJ Cancer: When is the
Definitive Radiochemotherapy the Treatment of Choice?** 181
1 Introduction. 182
2 Standard Treatment Options in Localized Disease 182
   2.1 Perioperative Therapy. 182
   2.2 Definitive Chemoradiotherapy 182
3 Conclusion 184
References. 184

Radiotherapy of Gastroesophageal Junction Cancer 187

1 Background. 188
2 Diagnostic Workup 189
3 Early Stage Disease 189
4 Locally Advanced Disease 189
5 Neoadjuvant Therapy. 190
6 Response-Guided Therapy. 191
7 Definitive Chemoirradiation 193
8 Adjuvant Therapy 193
9 Salvage Radiotherapy. 194
10 Palliative Radiotherapy. 195
11 New Radiation Technologies. 195
12 New Combination Possibilities 196
13 Conclusions. 197
References. 197

Optimizing Neoadjuvant Chemotherapy Through the Use of Early Response Evaluation by Positron Emission Tomography. 201

1 Introduction. 202
2 PET Tracers 203
3 PET for Staging. 203
4 PET and Prognosis. 204
5 PET and Treatment Response 205
    5.1 Post-Therapeutic Response Assessment. 205
    5.2 Pre-Therapeutic Assessment. 206
    5.3 Early Metabolic Response 207
6 Conclusions. 208
References. 209

Part VI Gastric Cancer

Optimal Surgery for Gastric Cancer: Is More Always Better? 215

1 Introduction. 216
2 Surgical Anatomy 216
3 Characteristics of the Primary Tumour 218
    3.1 T1 Disease. 219
    3.2 T2 and T3 Disease 221
    3.3 T4 Disease. 222
    3.4 Extended Lymphadenectomy 223
    3.5 Metastatic Disease 224
4 Patient Factors. 225
5 Conclusions. 225
References. 226

Contents

Can Adjuvant Chemoradiotherapy Replace Extended Lymph Node Dissection in Gastric Cancer? 229
1   Introduction. 230
2   Surgery. 230
3   Chemotherapy 231
4   Chemoradiotherapy 233
5   R1-Resection. 235
6   Conclusion 236
References. 237

Predicting the Response to Chemotherapy in Gastric Adenocarcinoma: Who Benefits from Neoadjuvant Chemotherapy? 241
1   Introduction. 242
2   Histological Response Evaluation 243
3   Histological Tumour Characteristics as a Predictive Marker of Chemotherapy Response. 243
    3.1   Efficacy of Neoadjuvant Treatment in SRC Gastric Cancer. . . 244
    3.2   Chemoresistance SRC Gastric Cancer: Postulated Mechanisms 245
4   Imaging as a Predictive Biomarker of Chemotherapy Response. 245
    4.1   Response Evaluation: EUS and CT. 246
    4.2   18-F-Fluoro-2-deoxyglucose Positron Emission Tomography: FDG-PET 246
    4.3   Is Response Prediction Improved with Other Radiotracers? FLT-PET. 249
5   Molecular Markers: Predicting Response to Chemotherapy and Targeting Treatment. 250
    5.1   Thymidylate Synthase. 250
    5.2   Thymidine Phosphorylase and Dihydropyrimidine Dehydrogenase. 252
    5.3   Glutathione S-Transferase 253
    5.4   p53. 255
    5.5   Bcl-2. 255
    5.6   Survivin 257
    5.7   Microsatellite Instability 257
    5.8   Inhibition of Angiogenesis: Vascular Endothelial Derived Growth Factor 258
6   Targeted Therapies in Gastric Cancer: Signs of Future Promise. 258
    6.1   Tyrosine Kinase Inhibitors. 258
    6.2   Monoclonal Antibodies Against VEGF 259
    6.3   HER Family 259
7   Conclusions and Future Directions. 261
References. 262

Prediction of Response and Prognosis by a Score Including only Pretherapeutic Parameters in 410 Neoadjuvant Treated Gastric Cancer Patients 269

1   Chapter 1 270
     1.1   Background 270
     1.2   Prognostic Biomarkers in Gastric Cancer. 271
     1.3   Aims of the Study 272
2   Chapter 2 272
     2.1   Patients 272
     2.2   Clinical Staging 273
     2.3   Surgery 273
     2.4   Histopathological Work-Up and Response Evaluation 273
     2.5   Statistical Analysis 274
3   Chapter 3 274
     3.1   Results 274
     3.2   Prognostic Index and Risk Groups 278
4   Chapter 4 280
     4.1   Conclusions 280
     4.2   Future Directions 284
References 285

Adjuvant Chemotherapy: An Option for Asian Patients Only? 291

1   Introduction 292
2   Surgery 293
     2.1   Extent of Lymphadenectomy 293
     2.2   Epidemiology 296
     2.3   Maruyama Index 296
3   Post/Perioperative Therapy 297
     3.1   Adjuvant Chemotherapy 297
     3.2   Postoperative Chemoradiotherapy 301
     3.3   Perioperative Chemotherapy 302
4   Conclusions 303
References 304

Selecting the Best Treatment for an Individual Patient 307

1   Introduction 308
2   Treatment of Early Gastric Cancer 309
     2.1   Adjuvant Setting 309
     2.2   Peri-Operative Setting 311
3   Pharmacogenomics 314
     3.1   Adjuvant Setting 314
     3.2   Peri-Operative Setting 315
4   Conclusions 316
References 316

Part I
Multimodal Approach to Colorectal Cancer

Clinically Relevant Study End Points in Rectal Cancer

Carlos Fernandez-Martos, Angel Guerrero and Bruce Minsky

Abstract

In rectal cancer currently there are no clearly validated early end points which can serve as surrogates for long-term clinical outcome such as local control and survival. However, the use of a variety of response rates (i.e. pathological complete response, downsizing the primary tumor, tumor regression grade (TRG), radiological response) as endpoints in early (phase II) clinical trials is common since objective response to therapy is an early indication of activity. Disease-free survival (DFS) has been proposed as the most appropriate end point in adjuvant trials and is one of the most frequently used in newer rectal cancer trials. Due to the devastating nature of local recurrence in locally advanced rectal cancer, local control (which is itself a subset of the overall DFS endpoint) is still considered an important endpoint. Recently, circumferential resection margin (CRM) has been proposed as novel early end point because the CRM status can account for effects on DFS and overall survival after chemoradiation, radiation (RT), or surgery alone. Consensus is needed to define the most appropriate end points in both early and phase III trials in locally advanced cancer.

C. Fernandez-Martos (✉)
Gastointestinal Oncology Unit, Medical Oncology Department,
Fundacion Instituto Valenciano de Oncologia,
Calle Gregorio Gea 31, 46009 Valencia, Spain
e-mail: cfmartos@fivo.org

A. Guerrero
Medical Oncology Department, Fundacion Instituto Valenciano de Oncologia,
Calle Gregorio Gea 31, 46009 Valencia, Spain

B. Minsky
Department of Radiation Oncology, MD Anderson Cancer Center,
1515 Holcombe Blvd, Houston, TX 77030, USA

F. Otto and M. P. Lutz (eds.), *Early Gastrointestinal Cancers*,
Recent Results in Cancer Research 196, DOI: 10.1007/978-3-642-31629-6_1,
© Springer-Verlag Berlin Heidelberg 2012

Contents

1	Introduction	4
2	End Points in Phase I Trials	6
3	End Points in Phase II Neoadjuvant Rectal Cancer Trials	7
	3.1 Pathological Parameters of Response	8
	3.2 Imaging Response	12
4	Endpoints in Phase III trials	13
	4.1 Disease-Free Survival and Local Recurrence	15
	4.2 The Need for Long-Term Follow-Up	15
5	Discussion	16
	References	16

1 Introduction

In locally advanced resectable rectal cancer (T3/4 and/or any N+) preoperative therapy followed by total mesorectal excision (TME) is now the standard approach in Europe and USA. The main evidence supporting this strategy is the significant benefit in local control observed in phase III trials when comparing preoperative versus postoperative therapy (Sauer et al. 2004), or preoperative radiation (RT) and TME versus surgery alone (Kapiteijn et al. 2001). Furthermore, preoperative chemoradiation increased the pathological complete response (pCR) rate over radiotherapy alone (Bosset et al. 2005; Gerard et al. 2006).

Unfortunately, except in the Swedish trial which was performed in the pre TME era (Swedish rectal cancer trial 97), these benefits did not translate into improved disease-free survival (DFS) or overall survival (Table 1). To date, no randomized study has shown that delivery of adjuvant chemotherapy in patients undergoing preoperative chemoradiation improves outcome as compared with observation. The 5-year cumulative rate of local relapse rates are less than 10 % in modern series but 5-year cumulative rates of distant metastases are about 35 % and currently represent the greatest threat to these patients.

Currently, many clinically relevant questions including modification of RT, surgery, and systemic therapy remain unanswered in the treatment of locally advanced rectal cancer. Surgery is the cornerstone of locally advanced rectal cancer treatment. However, in patients who experience a complete clinical response to preoperative combined therapy some investigators suggest that it may not be necessary (Habr-Gama et al. 2004; Maas et al. 2011).

The controversy regarding the merits of short-course RT and long-course chemoradiation is ongoing. Two phase III trials have shown no differences in local recurrence or DFS between both strategies (Bujko et al. 2005; Ngan et al. 2010). The difficulty of combining concurrent chemotherapy with the short-course RT as well as the lack of downsizing, have been used as arguments against its use in patients with cT3–4 and or N+ disease who have a higher risk of local recurrence

Clinically Relevant Study End Points in Rectal Cancer

Table 1 Primary and some secondary end points of landmark clinical trials in preoperative treatment in rectal cancer

Trial	Randomization	1° End Point	pCR	5y LR	5y DFS	OS
Swedish rectal cancer trial	S alone (n = 557) SCPRT-S (n = 553)	OS	0 % 0 %	27 % 11 % $p < 0.001$	NS	48 % 58 % $p = 0.004$
CKVO 95-04	S alone (n = 908) SCPRT-S (n = 897)	OS	0 % 0 %	10.9 %* 5.6 % $p < 0.001$	NS	63 %* 64 % $p = 0.902$
Polish trial	SCRT-S CRT-S	SPS	1 % 16 %	9 % 14 % $p = 0.170$	58 % 55 % $p = 0.82$	67 % 66 % $p = 0.96$
CAO-ARO-AIO 94	S-CRT-CT (n = 421) CRT-S-CT (n = 4Q2)	OS	0 % 8 %	13 % 6 % $p = 0.006$	65 % 68 % $p = 0.32$	74 % 76 % $p = 0.80$
FFCD 9203	RT-S-CT (n = 367) CRT-S-CT (n = 375)	OS	3.6 % 11.4 %	16.5 % 8.1 % $p = 0.004$	55 % 59 % $p = $ nd	67 % 67 % $p = 0.684$
EORTC 22921	1. -RT-S (n = 252) 2. -CRT-S (n = 253) 4. -CRT-S-CT (n = 253) 3. -RT-S-CT (n = 253)	OS	5.3 % $(1 + 3)^a$ V 13.7(2 + 4)A	17.1 % 8.7 % 9.6 % 7.6 % $p = 0.002$	52 % (1 + 2) v 58 %(3 + 4) $p = 0.13$	63 %(1 + 2) v 67 %(3 + 4) $p = 0.12$

SCPRT short-course preoperative radiotherapy; *S* surgery; *SPS* sphincter preserving surgery; *CRT* chemoradiation; *CT* chemotherapy; *LR* local recurrence; *OS* overall survival; *DFS* disease-free survival; * at 4 year; [a] pTQ

and distant metastasis. To address this, consolidative chemotherapy after short-course RT is being studied in two phase III trials.

Retrospective studies suggest that RT therapy may not be necessary in all patients with locally advanced rectal cancer (Gunderson et al. 2004). Recent phase I/II experience with preoperative chemotherapy alone have shown, in selected patients who did not require an APR, a rate of pCR similar to that observed with chemoradiation (Schrag et al. 2010; Fernandez-Martos et al. 2012).

The integration of new agents in the long-course radiation platform is attractive to improve both local and systemic efficacy. The Oxaliplatin-Fluoropyrimidine-radiation combination significantly increased the pCR in one phase III trial (Roedel et al. 2011) however, this was not confirmed in 3 others (Gérard et al. 2010; Aschele et al. 2011; Roh et al. 2011).

Adjuvant chemotherapy in locally advanced rectal cancer is recommended in most clinical guidelines, however, adjuvant chemotherapy after chemoradiation and surgery has not shown benefit in two phase III trials (Bujko et al. 2010).

Locally advanced rectal cancer represents a challenging disease for the design of clinical trials and for reporting of end points. In this review we discuss clinically relevant end points both in early Phase I and II as well as in definitive phase III trials.

2   End Points in Phase I Trials

Since neoadjuvant radiochemotherapy followed by surgery is considered the standard treatment of locally advanced rectal cancer, novel drugs for this pathology are usually tested in multimodality preoperative trials with the aim of enhancing RT effect. Ideally, in vitro and in vivo studies with human tumors models should precede the design of trials combining RT with anticancer agents in order to obtain preclinical data about the efficacious and lack of overlapping toxicities (Tepper et al. 2010). The primary end points of a combined modality phase I study are similar to a single agent study: to determine the maximally tolerated dose (MTD) and to establish the recommended dose and schedule for phase II trials. The most common design is a fix standard RT dose with escalation of the drug being tested. The schedule and dose to be explored will depend on the known characteristics of the agent and might vary from those assessed for the new drug alone. If the goal is radiosensitization, continuous dosing during RT is desirable (Seiwert et al. 2007). The conventional "3 + 3" cohort expansion design is typical for these studies. The phase II recommend dose is based on a certain frequency of toxic effects that by nature of their severity limit further dose escalation (dose-limiting toxicity (DLT)). DLT is usually defined using the NCI CTCAE grading scales as grade IV hematological toxicity and grade III non-hematological toxicity, assessed during the RT course. Other toxicities end points employed are RT treatment breaks and surgical complications (Clavien grading system). There is a concern about the enhancement of delayed RT toxicities and how to predict them in early clinical trials. Currently there are no clearly validated early predictive biomarkers of late RT toxicity that could be used to assess the MTD (Madelon et al. 2010).

For cytotoxic agents, phase I trials seek to determine the optimal dose that corresponds to the highest dose associated with an acceptable level of toxicity. However, molecular targeted agents may not emulate the standard efficacy-toxicity model of cytotoxics agents. They may show a plateau on the dose-efficacy curve, suggesting that higher doses will not improve the benefit of the drug. The dose that results in a relevant level of target modulation and clinical activity may differ greatly from the MTD, and using toxicity as an endpoint may be unnecessary or unachievable in trials investigating targeted agents. For these agents alternative end points to toxicity have been proposed (Eisenhauer 1998):

1. measuring inhibition of a target in tumor samples
2. plasma drug levels that are biologically relevant
3. biomarkers of activity in non-tumoral tissues.

Although biomarkers have been incorporated into clinical trials with increasing frequency, they have had a minimal contribution to dose and schedule selection for phase II studies. Toxicity and evidence for antitumor effect remain the main end points used for decisions to proceed or not with further drug development (Table 2) (Bernardo et al. 2007). The use of biomarkers is associated with several challenges that limits its use in dose escalation decision in a phase I trial (Biomarkers definition working group 2001; Dancey et al. 2010):

1. a reliable assay for measurement of the drug effect must be available in real time for conduct of the trial
2. the appropriate measure of achieved target effects for a specific drug must be defined
3. the optimal level of "target inhibition" with clinical benefit must be known.

Phase I clinical trials translate laboratory findings into clinical practice. Hopefully, the incorporation of biomarkers into the early phase of the drug development will improve understanding of how new drugs work, in conjunction with RT, and allow for more accurate identification of patients who will benefit from those therapies.

3 End Points in Phase II Neoadjuvant Rectal Cancer Trials

The preoperative treatment platform is the most common strategy used in small, non-randomized phase II trials. The use of some measure of response as the primary end point is common since objective response to therapy is a clear early indication of activity. The most popular primary end point in these trials is the rate of pCR (Table 3). Other measures of early efficacy have been suggested. These include pathological (downstaging, tumor regression grade (TRG), circumferential resection margin (CRM), R0 resection rate) as well as radiological response and functional imaging changes. These end points might seem appropriate, particularly with radiotherapy-based studies, since the irradiated area is easily evaluated.

Table 2 Selected ongoing and recently finished phase 1 trials in resectable rectal cancer

NCT	RT	CT	MTA	1° END POINT	2° END POINT
01282502	Fixed	5-FU (fixed)	Midostaurin (escalated)	MTD	Tumor regression surgical complications tumor biomarkers
01407107	Fixed	5-FU (fixed) nitroglycerin (escalated)	None	MTD	pCR
01397305	None	Pemetrexed (fixed) mudofolin (escalated)	None	MTD	pCR polymorphisms
00869570	Fixed	Capecitabine (escalated)	Sorafenib (fixed)	MTD	pCR
01160926	Fixed	Capecitabine (fixed)	Cediranib (escalated)	MTD	Tissue biomarkers imaging biomarkers
01376453	Fixed	5-FU (fixed)	Sorafenib (escalated)	MTD	pCR
01395667	Escalated	FOLFOX (fixed)	Bevacizumab (fixed)	MTD	pCR
00307736	Fixed	5-FU (fixed)	Bevacizumab (fixed) erlotinib (escalated)	MTD	Local control
00280176	Fixed	5-FU (fixed)	Bortezomib (escalated)	MTD	Tumor biomarkers pCR
00704600	Fixed	Capecitabine (fixed)	Nefilnavir (escalated)	MTD	pCR
00409994	Fixed	None	Rapamycin (escalated)	Surgical complications	pCR

NCT clinicaltrials.gov identifier; *RT* radiotherapy; *CT* chemotherapy; *MTA* molecular targeted agent; *MTD* maximally tolerated dose; *pCR* pathologic complete response

3.1 Pathological Parameters of Response

Pathological parameters are an early indication of the effect of the preoperative treatment. The results are variable and may reflect the lack of standard definitions among pathologists of how to handle the specimen, number of sections taken, correlation with pre- and post-operative radiological imaging, and the regression grading schema employed (Chetty et al. 2012).

3.1.1 Pathological Complete Response

The pCR rate is the most commonly used end point in on-going phase II trials of preoperative chemoradiation. Is usually defined as the absence of any residual

Clinically Relevant Study End Points in Rectal Cancer

Table 3 Primary end points of open and recruiting phase II trials in Europe and America registered in clinicaltrials.gov (December 2011)

End point	Intervention	ClinicalTrials.gov identifier
Pathological complete response	Pani/RT-Surg	NCT01574962
	Pani/CRT-Surg	NCT01443377 NCT00967655
	Cet/CRT-Surg	NCT00611858 NCT00686166
	CRT ± CT-Surg	NCT00335816
	CT-CRT-CT-Surg	NCT01489332
	CT-CRT-Surg	NCT01363843
	Beva/CT-Surg	NCT01426074
	CT-Surg-CT	NCT00831181 NCT00832299
	CRT ± beva-Surg	NCT00828672*
Radiological response	CT-selective RT-Surg CRT-TEM or TME	NCT00909987 NCT01273051
Downstaging	SCPRT-CT-Surg	NCTQ1Q6QQQ7
Local Recurrence	CRT-TEM or obs**	NCT00939666
R0 Resection Rate	CT-good R-Surg or CAP50-Surg CT-bad R-CAP50 v CAP60-Surg	NCT01333709*
PET sensibility/specificity for tumor response	PET-CRT-PET	NCT00254683
PET to detect hipoxia	PET-CT/RT	NCT00574353
Bowel Quality of Life	IMRT/SCRT-Surg	NCT01148056
CT Compliance	CT-CRT-Surg CRT-Surg-CT	NCT01274962*
Termination of therapy	Beva/CT-CRT-Surg	NCT01434147*
% of patients who commence neo CT and RT undergo surgical resection	CT ± pani-SCPRT-Surg	NCT01160926

Pani panitumumab; *RT* radiation; *CRT* chemoradiation; *Surg* surgery; *Cet* cetuximab; *CT* chemotherapy; *Beva* bevacizumab; *TME* total mesorectal escision; *TEM* transanal endoscopic microsurgery; *SCPRT* short-course preoperative radiotherapy; *Obs* observation; *R* response; *CAP*50 capecitabine and radiation to a total dose of 50 grays; *CAP*60 capecitabine and radiation to a total dose of 60 grays; *PET* positron emission tomography; *IMRT* intensity modulated radiation *Phase II randomized; **In clinical complete or very good response

cancer cells within the resected surgical specimen (ypT0N0) although there are currently different ways to define a complete pathological response. These include ypT0, ypT0 plus ypTmic, or ypT0N0 (Glynne-Jones and Anyamene 2006).

Whether improvement in pCR in early clinical trials is a valid predictor to select treatments that are likely to result in improved survival is unclear.

Several analyses have been performed to determine if patients who achieve a pCR have improved DFS and overall survival. Many are retrospective and most data are from non-randomized trials. Some suggest better outcomes for those who achieve a pCR (Maas et al. 2010; Chari et al. 1995; Capirci et al. 2008), while others do not (Onaitis et al. 2001).

Three phase III European trials published in the last decade comparing preoperative RT versus preoperative 5-FU-based chemoradiation in patients with resectable locally advanced rectal cancer failed to demonstrate any difference in long-term results despite the fact that a significant increase in pCR was observed in the chemoradiation arm (Bosset et al. 2005; Gerard et al. 2006; Bujko et al. 2006).

Methy and colleagues, using single trial validation methods, explored the surrogacy of pCR and other pathological parameters based in the FFCD 9203 trial (Methy et al. 2010). In this trial, pCR was not a surrogate for overall survival. More recently Bonnetain and colleagues pooled two large phase III trials [EORTC 22921 (1,011 pts) and FFCD 9203 (756 pts) trials] to assess, with increased statistical power, the benefit of preoperative chemoradiation versus RT alone on progression-free and overall survival. Using meta-analysis, they explored whether pCR was an early surrogate endpoint for progression-free or overall survival. The analysis failed to demonstrate pCR as a surrogate for long-term outcomes (Bonnetain et al. 2011).

Based on these and other data, pCR remains an unvalidated surrogate endpoint to determine outcome in terms of cancer DFS and overall survival.

3.1.2 Downstaging/Downsizing

Downstaging refers to a decrease in postoperative pathological versus preoperative radiological T and/or N stages. The definition varies across studies: some define downstaging when the tumor regressed by one TNM stage while others refer to a decrease in preoperative radiological T status compared with postoperative pathologic T status. In many small phase II trials and retrospective studies, DFS and overall survival were significantly increased in patients with downstaging compared with patients without downstaging (Valentini et al. 2002; Fernandez-Martos et al. 2004; Liersch et al. 2006).

Preoperative staging techniques, such as endorectal ultrasound (ERUS), computed tomography (CT), or magnetic resonance imaging (MRI), are limited in their ability to provide accurate staging information. Thus, assessment of response comparing the preoperative ERUS stage with the pathologic stage overestimates the rate of tumor downstaging caused by preoperative chemoradiation (Glynne-Jones et al. 2006). In the Methy study, downstaging was not a surrogate for local control or overall survival (Methy et al. 2010).

3.1.3 Tumor Regression Grade

An alternative method to assess treatment response is achieved by grading the histologic changes in the resected specimen that are a result of preoperative chemoradiation. Tumor regression after preoperative therapy is assessed by examining the residual neoplastic cells and scoring the degree of both cytological and stromal changes. On the basis of the combination of these changes, tumor regression is classified according to a grade system. To asses TRG several similar classifications have been proposed (Veccio et al. 2005; Wheeler et al. 2002; Dworak et al. 1997 Bouzourene et al. 2002). The strongest correlation between long-term outcomes and TRG was obtained when TRG is grouped in either three (complete vs. intermediate vs. no/poor response) (Rodel et al. 2005) or two categories (responders vs. no responders) (Veccio et al. 2005; Bouzourene et al. 2002). In the analysis by Rodel et al. 5-year DFS after curative resection and chemoradiation was significantly higher in patients with complete versus intermediate versus poor response. ($p = 0.006$). In the analysis from Vecchio and colleagues and Bouzourene and colleagues the responders were found to be predictive of long-term outcomes.

In the analysis from Methy et al. TRG did not fulfill the Prentice criteria for surrogacy. However, given the proportion of treatment effect was 12.1 %, the TRG did explain the highest proportion of the treatment effect observed on local control.

3.1.4 Circumferential Resection Margin

Usually the Circumferential Resection Margin (CRM) involvement is considered positive when the tumor is <1 mm from the inked margin of the surgical specimen. An alternative cutoff is 2 mm (Nagtegaal and Quirke 2008). The relation of the tumor with the mesorectal fascia can be predicted reliably before treatment starts, and the impact of different treatment modalities (surgery, chemotherapy, and radiotherapy) can be assessed by the CRM status. Initially, CRM was introduced as a prognostic factor in surgical series for local recurrence (Quirke et al. 1986). Further retrospective analysis of larger series of surgery alone showed that in addition, patients with CRM +ve after TME had an increased risk for distant metastases (37.6 vs 12.7 %, $p < 0.0001$) as well as decreased survival (Nagtegaal and Marijnen 2002).

Subsequent analysis performed after neoadjuvant therapy (RT or chemoradiation) has shown a strong correlation with late outcome parameters, such as local recurrence, distant metastases, and DFS. Nagtegaal and Quirke reviewed previously published data which included 17,538 rectal cancer patients in order to evaluate the prognostic value of the CRM in relation to the changes in treatment and after neoadjuvant radiotherapy and chemoradiation. They reported that the predictive value of the CRM for local recurrence is significantly higher than when no preoperative therapy had been delivered (hazard ratio [HR] = 6.3 v 2.0, respectively; $p = 0.05$).

Based on these and other data, CRM has been proposed as reliable early end point in neoadjuvant rectal cancer trials.

In some European countries neoadjuvant rectal cancer treatment depends on preoperative MRI assessment of the CRM. However, this approach is not standard in other European countries or North America. Phase III trials comparing two neoadjuvant therapies published in the last decade (Bosset et al. 2005; Gerard et al. 2006; Bujko et al. 2006), or recently completed trials (Gérard et al. 2010; Aschele et al. 2011; Roh et al. 2011; Roedel et al. 2011 and PETTAC 6) did not use CRM to select patients. In this population the expected rate of CRM +ve after neoadjuvant therapy is low. In the trial from Bosset et al. the incidence was 9 %, however, only 35 % of patients underwent TME (Bosset et al. 2005). The phase III German CARO/ CAO/AIO 04 trial randomized patients preoperatively to receive chemoradiation with either 5FU/RT or 5FU/oxaliplatin/RT. Surgery quality control was performed and 75 % of patients underwent a good quality TME. Following surgery, the incidence of CRM +ve was 6 versus 5 %, respectively (Roedel et al. 2011). Therefore, given the low incidence of CRM +ve, the use of CRM as an early end point needs a large sample size. Furthermore, although the Polish trial reported a reduction in CRM +ve rates from 13 % with preoperative short-course RT to 4 % with long-course chemoradiation ($p = 0.017$),there were no differences in 4-year DFS or overall survival.

The ongoing British ARISTOTLE trial (ISRCTN09351447) is comparing the combination of capecitabine/RT versus capecitabine/irinotecan/RT in patients with mesorectal fascia involved or threatened defined by MRI or distal third rectal carcinoma. The histopathologically confirmed CRM—resection rate is a secondary end point. Hopefully, this trial will define the role of the CRM as an early surrogate end point in this high-risk population.

3.2 Imaging Response

The wait and see policy in patients with a clinically complete responders after preoperative chemoradiation (Maas et al. 2011)) as well as new strategies with preoperative chemotherapy and selective RT for non-responding patients (Schrag et al. 2010; Fernandez-Martos et al. 2010), have encouraged the development of a noninvasive determination of response. Response assessment with 18F-deoxyglucose positron emission tomography (^{18}F-FDG-PET) and more recently MRI have been correlated with long-term outcomes.

3.2.1 ^{18}F-FDG-PET

Although the sensitivity of PET may be reduced after induction chemotherapy, a study from Memorial Sloan-Kettering Cancer Center demonstrated that ^{18}F-FDG-PET detected 100 % of patients with response to neoadjuvant therapy and accurately predict long-term outcomes (Guillem and Moore 2004).

A recent systematic review examined the role of 18F-FDG-PET in monitoring responses in rectal cancer (Geus-Oei et al. 2009). Although 19 studies addressing the role of PET were heterogeneous with respect to the methods applied for PET quantification, the evaluation interval, metabolic response criteria, and clinical

Table 4 Primary and some secondary end points of completed phase III trials comparing preoperative fluoropyrimidine combined with radiation versus fluoropyrimidine and oxaliplatin combined with radiation or versus capecitabine combined with radiation

TRIAL	N	Randomization	1° Endpoint	% ypT0N0	% Node+	DFS
Accord12/040 5-prodige 2	598	RT/CAPE RT/CAPOX	pCR	13.9 19.2 $p = 0.09$	30.5 28.5	69 %* 74 %
STAR-1	747	RT/FU RT + FOLFOX	OS	16 16 $p = 0.9$	26 29	ND
NSABP R-04	1608	RT/FU or CAPE RT/FOLFOX or CAPOX	3-y LRC	19.1 20.9 $p = 0.46$	29 29.6	ND
CAO/ARO/AIO 04	1265	RT/FU RT-FOLFOX	3-y DFS	12.8 16.5 $p = 0.045$	30 28	ND
Margit	161	RT/FU RT/CAPE	OS	5.4 13.2 $p = 0.16$		66 %** 75 %

RT radiotherapy; *CAPE* capecitabine; *CAPOX* capecitabine and oxaliplatin; *FOLFOX* fluorouracil, folinic acid and oxaliplatin; *pCR* pathologic complete response; *OS* overall survival; *LRC* locoregional control; *DFS* disease-free survival; *ND* no data *At 3 years **At 5 years in the overall population; $n = 401$ patients

endpoints (histology or survival), the majority of the studies showed that ^{18}F-FDG-PET is a significant predictor of therapy outcome.

3.2.2 Magnetic Resonance Imaging

High-resolution MRI has been used to assess tumor response prior to surgical resection using morphologic and volumetric criteria, and has an overall accuracy of 86 % (Barbaro et al. 2009). The relevance of post-treatment MRI assessment in predicting survival outcomes has been for the first time reported in a prospective cohort study of 111 patients undergoing preoperative chemoradiation or long-course radiotherapy (Patel et al. 2011). By multivariate analysis, the MRI assessed TRG (mrTRG) was significant for overall survival and post-treatment prediction of mrCRM was significant for local recurrence.

4 Endpoints in Phase III Trials

Although overall survival has been the standard endpoint of phase III adjuvant rectal trials, preoperative phase III trials have examined multiple endpoints. These have included local control, sphincter preservation, toxicity, DFS, and overall survival. As seen in Table 1, the primary endpoint of most of the landmark trials of

Table 5 Primary endpoints of ongoing phase III trials in locally advanced rectal cancer

Trial	N	Randomization	1° End Point	Status
PETACC6 EORTC	1090	CAPE/RT-Surgery-CAPE CAPOX/RT-Surgery-CAPOX	DFS	Open
ARISTOTLE UK	920	CAPE/RT-Surgery CAPIRI/RT-Surgery	DFS at planned four stages	Open
SCRIPT Dutch	840	SCPRT or CT/RT-Surgery-Obs SCPRT or CT/RT-Surgery-CAPE	OS	Open
RAPIDO Dutch/ Swedisch	885	SCRT-CT-Surgery CT/RT-Surg-CT optional	3-y DFS	Open
Polish NCT00833131	540	SCPRT-CCT-Surgery CRT-Surgery	R0 resection rates	Open
Stockholm 3	840	SCPRT-Surgery (within 1 w) SCPRT-Surgery (after 4–8 w) RT (50 Gy)-Surgery (after 4–8 w)	Time to recurrence	Open
Lituania NCT00597311	150	SCPRT-Surgery (after 6 w) CRT-Surgery-(after 6 w)	5-y DFS and OS	Open
IAEG NCT01459328	350	CRT-Surgery SCPRT-CT- Surgery	OS	Open
Brussel NCT01224392	156	CAPE/RT (46 Gy) RT(46 + 9.2 Gy boost)	Reduction in metabolic tumor activity	Open

Cape capecitabine; *RT* radiotherapy *CAPOX* capecitabine and oxaliplatin; *CRT* chemoradiation; *CT* chemotherapy; *SCPRT* short-course preoperative radiotherapy; *OS* overall survival; *DFS* disease-free survival; *CCT* consolidating chemotherapy, patients are permitted to receive up to 6 weeks of neoadjuvant chemotherapy before enrolling **68 % of pts received preoperative RT

preoperative therapy is overall survival. These include the Swedish Rectal Cancer Trial (1997), Dutch CKVO 95–04 (Kapiteijn et al. 2001), German CAO-ARO-AIO 94 (Sauer et al. 2004), NSABP R-03 (Roh et al. 2009), FFCD 9203 (Gerard et al. 2006), and the EORTC 22921 (Bosset et al. 2005). Other primary endpoints included local recurrence (MRC CR07) (Sebag-Montefiore et al. 2009) and sphincter preserving surgery (Polish Trial) (Bujko et al. 2006). More recently completed phase III trials have used more varied primary endpoints (Table 4). Two used overall survival STAR-1 (Aschele et al. 2011) and Margit (Hofheinz et al. 2011) whereas others have used pCR (Accord 12/0405-prodige 2) (Gérard et al. 2010), 3-year local recurrence (NSABP R-04) (Roh et al. 2011) and 3-year DFS (German CAO/ARO/AIO 04) (Roedel et al. 2011).

Likewise, most ongoing phase III trials do not use overall survival as the primary endpoint. As seen in Table 5 examples include R0 resection rates (Polish NCT00833131) and reduction in metabolic tumor activity (Brussel NCT 01224392).

4.1 Disease-Free Survival and Local Recurrence

Overall survival has long been the gold standard primary endpoint for adjuvant cancer trials. However, the long follow-up required to demonstrate a overall survival benefit as well as the effect of salvage therapies after relapse are clear reasons for the need of surrogate endpoints that can be assessed earlier. In adjuvant colon cancer DFS—defined as the time from randomization to any event, irrespective of cause—at 2 or 3 years have been validated as surrogate for overall survival. It is considered to be the most informative endpoint for assessing the effect of treatment and therefore the most relevant to clinical practice as recommended by the ACCENT group analysis (Sargent et al. 2005, 2011). A similar analysis was performed by Burzykowski and colleagues, and included three randomized adjuvant colorectal cancer trials performed by the Japanese Foundation for Multidisciplinary Treatment for Cancer (Burzykowski et al. 2008). A total of 5,233 patients (2,381 rectal cancer) were treated with oral fluoropyrimidines. Their analysis supports the conclusion of Sargent and colleagues that 2- or 3-year DFS is the best option for the prediction of overall survival at 5 years. More recently, a pooled analysis of EORTC 22921 and FFCD 9203 trials demonstrate that progression-free survival—defined as the time from randomization to any death and any local or distant relapse of cancer—was the only validated surrogate variable for overall survival (Bonnetain et al. 2011).

Due to the devastating impact of local recurrence in locally advanced rectal cancer, local recurrence (which is itself a subset of the overall DFS endpoint) is still an important endpoint. However, low rates of local relapses can be expected after chemoradiation and TME in unselected clinically staged II and III rectal cancer, requiring a large sample size if local recurrence is the primary end point. Quality of life assessment has been proposed to ensure's clinical patient benefit (Bonnetain et al. 2011). In trials including high-risk population or those testing chemotherapy alone before surgery, local recurrence is an appropriate co-primary end point.

4.2 The Need for Long-Term Follow-Up

Local recurrences can occur late in patients with rectal cancer. In contrast to the results reported in the trials of adjuvant treatment of colon cancer where 3-year and possibly 2-year DFS predicts for 5-year survival (Sargent et al. 2011), the INT 0114 postoperative rectal adjuvant trial confirmed that local control and survival continue to decrease beyond 5 years (Tepper et al. 2002). At 7 years the local recurrence rate was 17 % and the survival was 56 % compared with 14 and 64 %, respectively, at 5 years.

Limiting the analysis to trials where all patients underwent a TME, a similar detriment in outcomes was seen with long-term follow-up. In the German CAO/ARO/AIO 94 trial, patients who received preoperative chemoradiation had an increase in local recurrence (7 vs. 5 %) and decrease in survival (60 vs. 74 %) at 10 vs. 5 years, respectively (Sauer et al. 2011). The incidence of local recurrence for all patients in the preoperative RT arm of the Dutch CKVO trial of 5 Gy × 5 increased from 3 % at a median follow-up of 3.5 years to 6 % at a median follow-up of 6 years (Peeters et al. 2007). These data underscore the importance of long-term follow-up, regardless of which preoperative approach is used.

5 Discussion

The primary end points of a combined modality phase I study are similar to a single agent study: to determine the MTD and to establish the recommended dose and schedule for phase II trials. The neoadjuvant platform provides an sensible way to explore biomarkers in tumors tissue in pre and post-treatment samples.

Pathological parameters of response and more recently radiological imaging are commonly used end points in phase II neoadjuvant trials. The difference in definitions, interobserver variability as well as lack of consensus of how to process the surgical specimen are variables which can impact the results. Most of the data suggest a good correlation between any parameter of pathological response used in preoperative treatment and long-term results. However, this has been not enough to accept it use as a surrogate for disease-free or overall survival for any of the analysed parameters (Glynne-Jones et al. 2006). ^{18}F-FDG-PET and MRI may be helpful in shortening the duration of early clinical trials assessing new antineoplastic agents and strategies in the preoperative treatment of rectal cancer. Therapy response assessment with ^{18}F-FDG-PET and MRI remain an active areas of clinical investigation.

In summary, the use of DFS includes all clinically relevant events in adjuvant trials, and appears to be the best definitive end point in neoadjuvant rectal cancer trials. However, it must be emphasized because the well-described issue of late local recurrence and its associated devastating impact, the results of phase III adjuvant rectal cancer trials which use short-term endpoints (2- or 3-year DFS) will need to be interpreted with caution.

References

Aschele C, Cionini L, Lonardi S et al. (2011) Primary tumor response to preoperative chemoradiation with or without oxaliplatin in locally advanced rectal cancer: pathologic results of the STAR-01 randomized phase III trial. J Clin Oncol 29:2773–2780

Barbaro B, Fiorucci C, Tebala C et al (2009) Locally advanced rectal cancer: mr imaging in prediction of response after preoperative chemotherapy and radiation therapy. Radiology 250:730–739

Bernardo HL et al. (2007) Trends in the use and role of biomarkers in phase I oncology trials. Clin Cancer Res 13(22):6719 Nov 15

Biomarkers Definitions Working Group (2001) Biomarkers and surrogate endpoints: preferred definitions and conceptual framework. Clin Pharmacol Ther 69:89–95

Bonnetain F, Bosset J, Gerard J et al. (2011) An analysis of preoperative chemoradiotherapy with 5FU/leucovorin for T3-4 rectal cancer on survival in a pooled analysis of EORTC 22921 and FFCD 9203 trials: surrogacy in question? J Clin Oncol 29(suppl; abstr 3506)

Bosset JF, Calais J, Mineur L et al (2005) Enhanced tumorocidal effect of chemotherapy with preoperative radiotherapy for rectal cancer: preliminary results—EORTC 22921. J Clin Oncol 23:5620–5627

Bouzourene H, Bosman FT, Seelentag W (2002) Importance of tumor regression assessment in predicting the outcome in patients with locally advanced rectal carcinoma who are treated with preoperative radiotherapy. Cancer 94:1121–1130

Bujko K, Nowacki MP, Kepka L et al. (2005) Postoperative complications in patients irradiated pre-operatively for rectal cancer: report of a randomised trial. Comparing short-term radiotherapy vs chemoradiation. Colorectal Dis 7:410–416

Bujko K, Nowacki M, Nasierowska-Guttmejer A et al (2006) Long-term results of a randomized trial comparing preoperative short-course radiotherapy with preoperative conventionally fractionated chemoradiation for rectal cancer. Br J Surg 93:1215–1223

Bujko K, Glynne-Jones R, Bujko M (2010) Does adjuvant fluoropyrimidine-based chemotherapy provide a benefit for patients with resected rectal cancer who have already received neoadjuvant radiochemotherapy? A systematic review of randomised trials. Ann Oncol 21(9):1743–1750

Burzykowski T, Buyse M, Yothers G (2008) Exploring and validating surrogate endpoints in colorectal cáncer. Lifetime Data Anal 14:54–64

Capirci C, Valentini V, Cionini L et al (2008) Prognostic value of pathologic complete response after neoadjuvant therapy in locally advanced rectal cancer: long-term analysis of 566 ypCR patients. Int J Radiat Oncol Biol Phys 72:99–107

Chari RS, Tyler DS, Anscher MS et al (1995) Preoperative radiation and chemotherapy in the treatment of adenocarcinoma of the rectum. Ann Surg 221:778–786

Chetty R, Gill P, Govender D et al. (2012) A multi-centre pathologist survey on pathological processing and regression grading of colorectal cancer resection specimens treated by neoadjuvant chemoradiation. Virchows Arch Jan 13. [Epub ahead of print]

Dancey JE et al (2010) Biomarker studies in early clinical trials of novel agents guidelines for the development and incorporation of novel agents. Clin Cancer Res 16:1745–1755

Dworak O, Kelholz L, Hoffman A (1997) Pathological feature of rectal cancer after preoperative radiochemotherapy. Int J Colorectal Dis 12:19–23

Eisenhauer EA (1998) Phase I and II trials of novel anti-cancer agents: endpoints, efficacy and existentialism. The Michel clavel lecture, held at the 10th NCI-EORTC conference on new drugs in cancer therapy. Ann Oncol 9:1047–1052. Amsterdam, 16–19 Jun 1998

Fernandez-Martos C, Aparicio J, Bosch C Et al. (2004) Preoperative uracil, tegafur, and concomitant radiotherapy in operable rectal cancer: a phase II study with 3 years follow-up. J Clin Oncol

Fernandez-Martos C, Safont M, Feliu J et al. (2010) Induction chemotherapy with or without chemoradiation in intermediate-risk rectal cancer patients defined by magnetic resonance imaging (MRI): a GEMCAD study. Proc Am Soc Clin Oncol 28:Abstr TPS 196

Fernandez-Martos C, Estevan R, Salud A et al. (2012) Neoadjuvant capecitabine, oxaliplatin, and bevacizumab (CAPOX-B) in intermediate-risk rectal cancer (RC) patients defined by magnetic resonance (MR): GEMCAD 0801 trial. J Clin Oncol 30, 2012 (suppl; abstr 3586)

Gerard JP, Conroy T, Bonnetain F et al (2006) Preoperative radiotherapy with or without concurrent fluorouracil and leucovorin in T3–4 rectal cancers. Results of FFCD 9203. J Clin Oncol 24:4620–4625

Gérard JP, Azria D, Gourgou-Bourgade S et al. (2010) Comparison of two neoadjuvant chemoradiotherapy regimens for locally advanced rectal cancer: results of the phase III trial ACCORD 12/0405-Prodige 2.J ClinOncol 28:1638–1644

Geus-Oei L, Vriens L, van Laarhoven H et al (2009) Monitoring and predicting response to therapy with 18F-FDG PET in colorectal cancer: a systematic review. J Nucl Med 50:43–54

Glynne-Jones R, Anyamene N (2006) Just how useful an endpoint is complete pathological response after neoadjuvant chemoradiation in rectal cancer? Int J Radiat Oncol Biol Phys 66(2):319–320

Glynne-Jones R, Mawdsley S, Pearce T et al (2006) Alternative clinical end points in rectal cancer—are we getting closer? Ann Oncol 17:1239–1248

Guillem J, MD Moore H, Akhurst T et al (2004) Sequential preoperative fluorodeoxyglucose-positron emission tomography assessment of response to preoperative chemoradiation: a means for determining longterm outcomes of rectal cancer. J Am Coll Surg 199:1–7

Gunderson LL, Sargent DJ, Tepper JE et al (2004) Impact of T and N stage and treatment on survival and relapse in adjuvant rectal cancer: a pooled analysis. J Clin Oncol 22:1785–1796

Habr-Gama A, Perez RO, Nadalin W et al (2004) Operative versus nonoperative treatment for stage 0 distal rectal cancer following chemoradiation therapy: long-term results. Ann Surg 240:711–717

Hofheinz R, Wenz R, Post S et al. (2011) Capecitabine (Cape) versus 5-fluorouracil–based (neo)adjuvant chemoradiotherapy for locally advanced rectal cancer: long-term results of a randomized, phase III trial. J Clin Oncol 29 (suppl; abstr 3504)

Kapiteijn E, Marijnen CA, Nagtegaal ID et al (2001) Preoperative radiotherapy combined with total mesorectal excision for resectable rectal cancer. N Engl J Med 345:638–646

Liersch T, Langer C, Ghadimi M et al (2006) Lymph node status and TS gene expression are prognostic markers in stage II/III rectal cancer after neoadjuvant fluorouracil-based chemoradiotherapy. J Clin Oncol 24:4062–4068

Maas M, Nelemans P, Valentini V et al (2010) Long-term outcome in patients with a pathological complete response after chemoradiation for rectal cancer: a pooled analysis of individual patient data. Lancet Oncol 11:835–844

Maas M, Beets-Tan R, Lambregts D et al (2011) Wait-and-see policy for clinical complete responders after chemoradiation for rectal cancer. J Clin Oncol 29:4633–4640

Madelon PJ et al (2010) A systematic methodology review of phase I radiation dose escalation trials. Radiother Oncol 95:135–141

Methy N, Bedenne L, Conroy T et al (2010) Surrogate end points for overall survival and local control in neoadjuvant rectal cancer trials: statistical evaluation based on the FFCD 9203 trial. Ann Oncol 21:518–524

Nagtegaal I, Quirke P (2008) What is the role for the circumferential margin in the modern treatment of rectal cancer? J Clin Oncol 26:303–312

Nagtegaal ID, Marijnen CAM, Klein Kranenbarg E et al (2002) Circumferential margin is still an important predictor of local recurrence in rectal carcinoma: Not one millimeter but two millimeters is the limit. Am J Surg Pathol 26:350–357

Ngan S, Fisher R, Goldstein D et al (2010) TROG, AGITG, CSSANZ, and RACS. A randomized trial comparing local recurrence (LR) rates between short-course (SC) and long-course (LC) preoperative radiotherapy (RT) for clinical T3 rectal cancer: an intergroup trial (TROG, AGITG, CSSANZ, RACS) [abstract no. 3509]. J Clin Oncol 28(15 Suppl.):3509

Onaitis MW, Noone RB, Fields R et al (2001) Complete response to neoadjuvant chemoradiation for rectal cancer does not influence survival. Ann Surg Oncol 8:801–806

Patel U, Taylor F, Blomqvist L et al (2011) Magnetic resonance imaging–detected tumor response for locally advanced rectal cancer predicts survival outcomes: MERCURY experience. J Clin Oncol 29:3753–3760

Peeters KCMJ, Marijnen CAM, Nagtegaal ID et al (2007) The TME trial after a median follow-up of 6 years: increased local control but no survival benefit in irradiated patients with resectable rectal carcinoma. Ann Surg 246:693–701

Quirke P, Durdey P, Dixon MF et al (1986) Local recurrence of rectal adenocarcinoma due to inade- quate surgical resection: Histopathological study of lateral tumor spread and surgical excision. Lancet 2:996–999

Rodel C, Martus P, Papadoupolos T et al (2005) Prognostic significance of tumor regression after preoperative chemoradiotherapy for rectal cancer. J Clin Oncol 23:8688–8696

Roedel C et al. (2011) Preoperative chemoradiotherapy and postoperative chemotherapy with 5-fluorouracil and oxaliplatin versus 5-fluorouracil alone in locally advanced rectal cancer: first results of the German CAO/ARO/AIO-04 randomized phase III trial. ASCO annual meeting abstract no: LBA3505

Roh MS, Colangelo LH, O'Connell MJ et al (2009) Pre-operative multimodality therapy improves disease-free survival in patients with carcinoma of the rectum (NSABP-R-03). J Clin Oncol 27:5124–5130

Roh MS, Yothers GA, O'Connell MJ et al. (2011) The impact of capecitabine and oxaliplatin in the preoperative multimodality treatment in patients with carcinoma of the rectum: NSABP R-04. J Clin Oncol 29 (suppl; abstr 3503)

Sargent D, Wieand H, Haller D et al (2005) Disease-free survival versus overall survival as a primary end point for adjuvant colon cancer studies: individual patient data from 20,898 patients on 18 randomized trials. J Clin Oncol 23:8664–8670

Sargent D, Shi Q, Yothers G et al (2011) Two or three year disease-free survival (DFS) as a primary end-point in stage III adjuvant colon cancer trials with fluoropyrimidines with or without oxaliplatin or irinotecan: data from 12,676 patients from MOSAIC, X-ACT, PETACC-3, C-06, C-07 and C89803. Eur J Cancer 47(7):990–996

Sauer R, Becker H, Hohenberger W et al (2004) Preoperative versus postoperative chemora-diotherapy for rectal cancer. N Engl J Med 1731:351–402

Sauer R, Liersch T, Merkel S et al. (2011) Preoperative versus postoperative chemoradiotherapy for locally advanced rectal cancer: results of the German CAO/ARO/AIO-94 randomized phase III trial after a median follow-up of 11 years. Proc ASCO 29:225 s (abstr)

Schrag MR, Weiser KA, Goodman KA et al (2010) Neoadjuvant FOLFOX-bev, without radiation, for locally advanced rectal cancer [abstract no. 3511]. J Clin Oncol 28 (15 Suppl.):3511

Sebag-Montefiore D, Stephens RJ, Steele R et al (2009) Preoperative radiotherapy versus selective postoperative chemoradiotherapy in patients with rectal cancer (MRC CR07 and NCIC-CTG C016): a multicenter, randomised trial. Lancet 373:811–820

Seiwert TY, Salama JK, Vokes EE (2007) The concurrent chemoradiation paradigm–general principles. Nat Clin Pract Oncol 4:86–100

Tepper J, O'Connell M, Niedzwiecki D et al (2002) Adjuvant therapy in rectal cancer: analysis of stage, sex, and local control—final report of intergroup 0114. J Clin Oncol 20:1744–1750

Tepper J, Wang A (2010) Improving local control in rectal cancer: radiation sensitizers or radiation dose? J Clin Oncol 1:1623–1624

Valentini V, Coco C, Picciocchi A et al (2002) Does downstaging predict improved outcome after preoperative chemoradiation for extraperitoneal locally advanced rectal cancer? A long-term analysis of 165 patients. Int J Radiat Oncol Biol Phys 53(3):664–674

Vecchio F, Valentini V, Minsky B et al (2005) The relationship of pathologic tumor regression grade (trg) and outcomes after preoperative therapy in rectal cancer. Int J Radiat Oncol Biol Phys 62(3):752–760

Wheeler JM, Warren BF, Mortensen NJ et al (2002) Quantification of histologic regression of rectal cancer after irradiation. Dis Colon Rectum 45:1051–1056

Neoadjuvant Treatment in Rectal Cancer: Do We Always Need Radiotherapy–or Can We Risk Assess Locally Advanced Rectal Cancer Better?

Rob Glynne-Jones

Abstract

There is good quality evidence that preoperative radiotherapy reduces local recurrence but there is little impact on overall survival. This is not completely unexpected as radiotherapy is a localised treatment and local control may not prevent systemic failure. Optimal quality-controlled surgery for patients with operable rectal cancer in the trial setting can be associated with local recurrence rates of less than 10 % whether patients receive radiotherapy or not (Quirke et al. 2009). However, despite the reassuring results of randomised trials, concerns remain that radiotherapy increases surgical morbidity (Horisberger et al. 2008; Stelzmueller et al. 2009; Swellengrebel et al. 2011), which can compromise the delivery of postoperative adjuvant chemotherapy. There are also significant late effects from pelvic radiotherapy (Peeters et al. 2005; Lange et al. 2007) and a risk of second malignancies (Birgisson et al. 2005; van Gijn et al. 2011). If preoperative radiotherapy does not impact on survival, can it be omitted in selected cases? The answer is yes—with the proviso that we are using good quality magnetic resonance imaging and good quality TME surgery within the mesorectal plane and the predicted risk of subsequent metastatic disease justifies its use. In this case, the concept of neoadjuvant chemotherapy (NACT) is a potentially attractive alternative strategy which might have less early and long-term side effects compared to preoperative radiotherapy— particularly where the MRI predicts a high risk of metastatic disease in the context of a modest risk of local recurrence. This chapter discusses a more precise method of risk categorisation for locally advanced rectal cancer, and discusses possible options for neoadjuvant chemotherapy (NACT).

R. Glynne-Jones (✉)
Centre for Cancer Treatment, Mount Vernon Hospital,
Rickmansworth Road, Northwood, Middlesex HA6 2RN, UK
e-mail: Rob.glynnejones@nhs.net

F. Otto and M. P. Lutz (eds.), *Early Gastrointestinal Cancers*,
Recent Results in Cancer Research 196, DOI: 10.1007/978-3-642-31629-6_2,
© Springer-Verlag Berlin Heidelberg 2012

Contents

1 Introduction 22
2 Late Effects of Radiotherapy 23
3 Local Recurrence 24
   3.1 Is Neoadjuvant Chemotherapy an Alternative? 26
   3.2 Can Radiotherapy be Omitted? 26
   3.3 Are There Clearly Distinguishable Groups Who Do Not Need RT? 26
4 Conclusion 32
References 33

1 Introduction

Preoperative chemoradiation (CRT) has been the standard of care in the United States for all patients with clinical stage II and III rectal cancer because of the low rates of local recurrence achieved, acceptable levels of acute and late toxicity, and the potential for sphincter preservation compared to postoperative chemoradiation. In parts of Northern Europe, a blanket approach to short course preoperative radiotherapy (SCPRT) using 25 Gy over 5 days followed by immediate surgery within 2–5 days, with the predominant aim of reducing the risk of pelvic recurrence has gained widespread acceptance. Recent improvements in the quality of surgery, magnetic resonance imaging and pathical reporting of the operative specimen, mean the time has come to question both these approaches.

The majority of the rectum lies below the peritoneal reflection and has no serosa, allowing tumour growth to extend deeply into peri-rectal fat. Historically, high rates of local pelvic recurrence following radical surgery were described. However, surgical practice has evolved, and the technique of meticulous mesorectal dissection where the surgeon removes all of the surrounding mesorectal fat using sharp dissection in a neat anatomical package is associated with much lower rates of local recurrence and improved survival. With expert total mesorectal excision (TME) consistently performed in specialist centres, metastatic disease is now the predominant problem (Cecil et al. 2004), reflecting the likely presence of distant micrometastases at diagnosis, rather than inadequate surgery. It is true that old meta-analyses have shown that preoperative adjuvant radiotherapy reduces local recurrence rates by almost 50 % and overall mortality by 2–10 %. However,the local recurrence rates were very high in the region of 15–30 %, and importantly the trials included in these meta-analyses all use patient data from long before the introduction of total mesorectal excision (TME) surgery, which questions their current relevance.

Conventional therapies for patients with locally advanced rectal cancer appear to have reached a therapeutic plateau, as none of the recent phase III studies investigating the use of radiotherapy or chemoradiation have improved overall survival (OS). This may also reflect the difficulty of performing large-scale multicentre studies, where the quality assurance is inevitably more variable.

In addition to the risk of a local recurrence, 10–40 % of patients require extensive surgical procedures, which lead to a permanent stoma. Surgeons will strive to preserve the anal sphincter, but it has been reported that in the United Kingdom there is a wide variation in the proportion of patients undergoing an abdomino-perineal excision of the rectum (APER) (Morris et al. 2008)—which may either reflect skills and training or the variability in the use of radiotherapy and concerns regarding function after the combination of preoperative radiotherapy and ultra low anterior resection.

In general, we have focussed on avoiding local recurrence and facilitating sphincter sparing in our phase III trials, hoping that improvements in survival would automically follow if the primary endpoints were achieved. Sadly this has not been the case. Trials suggest that in resectable cancers, where the preoperative magnetic resonance imaging (MRI) predicts the circumferential resection margin (CRM) is not potentially involved, then SCPRT and CRT are equivalent in terms of outcomes such as local recurrence, DFS, and OS (Bujko et al. 2006; Ngan et al. 2010). However, none of the trials of radiotherapy alone (Peeters et al. 2007; Sebag-Montefiore et al. 2009) or chemoradiation published in the last decade have impacted on DFS or OS (Sauer et al. 2004; Bosset et al. 2006, Gerard et al. 2006; Roh et al. 2009). Local recurrence is now sufficiently low that (unlike in breast cancer) it fails to impact on overall survival. Alternatively, either the populations in these trials are too low risk to benefit or the inadequacy of the systemic therapy within current chemoradiation schedules may help to explain this finding.

In contrast, for more advanced cases, where the CRM is breached or threatened according to the MRI, the integration of more active chemotherapy and biological agents into chemoradiation, is an attractive strategy. There is an obvious need to improve response to downsize the tumour to achieve a curative resection, and there is a high risk of metastases. In patients where even technically optimised surgery is unlikely to achieve a curative resection—5FU-based chemoradiation has been shown to have a statistically significant effect on resectability and relapse-free survival (Frykholm et al. 2001; Braendengen et al. 2008). However, these trials have been underpowered to show a benefit in terms of overall survival. At the time of diagnosis between 20 and 25 % of patients with rectal cancer will be found to have overt metastatic disease, and a further 30–40 % will subsequently develop metastases.

2 Late Effects of Radiotherapy

Pelvic radiotherapy is associated with significant risks of permanent morbidity—with about 5–10 % of experiencing grade 3 or 4 late morbidity. Small bowel tolerance is the main dose-limiting factor. Effects on sexual functioning (Marijnen et al. 2005), urinary incontinence (Pollack et al. 2006), faecal incontinence (Lange et al. 2007) have been documented after SCPRT. These complications depend on the size of the radiation field, shielding, the overall treatment time, the fraction size and total dose. Mature results of the Swedish Rectal Cancer Trial confirm problems after RT particularly bowel obstruction and abdominal pain (Birgisson et al. 2006). There are also unexplained late cardiac effects (Pollack et al. 2006), and insufficiency fractures in the pelvis (Herman et al. 2009). In addition in the Dutch TME study the deaths from second malignancy were higher in the RT arm than the TME arm alone (13.7 % versus 9.4 %) (van Gijn et al. 2011). Given this finding is seen after only 11.6 years of follow-up—this difference is highly likely to widen at 15–25 years. As follow-up in the majority of studies is generally short, the risks of these late effects are likely to be underestimated over decades. It is true that to develop these side effects and second malignancies one has to survive the cancer, but unlike many other disease sites, radiotherapy does not impact on survival. It is unclear how much these effects are highlighted in the consent process for radiotherapy. In contrast to radiotherapy, the side effects of chemotherapy are usually short term, although the neuropathy from oxaliplatin may be permanent.

Because of the high risk of metastatic disease, integrating more active chemotherapy is attractive, and enthusiasm has been stimulated by the efficacy of oxaliplatin in dealing with distant micro-metastases in the adjuvant setting in colon cancer (Kuebler et al. 2007; André et al. 2009) although patients with rectal cancer were excluded as ineligible. The possible options for systemic chemotherapy option have expanded, but postoperative adjuvant chemotherapy remains only partially effective, and toxicity (particularly with oxaliplatin) is substantial. The current therapeutic challenge is to optimise all our available non-operative strategies by effective cytotoxic chemotherapy at systemic doses. Incorporating new agents into current therapeutic regimens to reduce the burden of metastases is a priority for research. Trials integrating oxaliplatin into CRT have not increased the pathological complete response rate (pCR) but suggest the use of two drugs halves the positive CRM rate (Gerard et al. 2010; Aschele et al. 2011).

Compliance to postoperative chemotherapy following chemoradiation is poor. Neoadjuvant chemotherapy (NACT) offers an alternative strategy. At least 20–25 % of patients in whom chemotherapy with 5FU might be considered may not be sufficiently fit or decline treatment (Sauer et al. 2004; Bosset et al. 2006; Gerard et al. 2006). Compliance to additional postoperative oxaliplatin appears even worse (Rödel et al. 2007).

3   Local Recurrence

One reason that local recurrence occurs after potentially curative resection is explained by the work of Quirke and colleagues in 1986. The presence of microscopic tumour cells within one millimetre of the radial or circumferential resection margin (CRM) is clearly demonstrated to be associated with a very high rate of local recurrence and poor survival. High-resolution pelvic MRI using surface-phased array coils is now routinely applied in the UK and much of Europe as a preoperative staging and selection tool for the use of neoadjuvant radiation. MRI strongly predicts the likelihood of involvement of the circumferential resection margin (CRM) particularly in the mid-rectum, involvement of the levators in the low rectum and the extramural depth of invasion. The risks of local failure are much lower for cancers in the upper rectum. This MRI preoperative assessment can identify patients at risk of the surgeon being unable to achieve an R0 resection (Mercury 2007). The accuracy of predicting tumour extent beyond the muscularis propria was within 0.5 mm tolerance in the mid-/upper rectum, and suggests MRI can accurately predict ultimate outcome. MRI can also accurately measure the distance between the anorectal junction and/or and the distal part of the tumour and the luminal length of the tumour. However, MRI, multisclice CT and ERUS all remain inadequately accurate to detect involved or uninvolved lymph nodes despite specific imaging features such as size $> = 8$ mm/round/heterogenous/irregular in nodal border. Current studies have also failed to confirm that FDG-PET has improved the accuracy of nodal staging.

Location of the primary tumour (anterior and low confer more risk) and site within the rectum (upper, middle and lower) is also important. MRI is increasingly influencing both the rationale for neoadjuvant radiotherapy, and the design of current trials. Other pathological factors which increase the risk of recurrence include T4 tumours, nodal involvement, extramural vacular invasion, perineural invasion and extranodal deposits (Kusters et al. 2010). Some of these can be identified also on preoperative MRI. Other recognised clinical, individual or social factors that influence the development of recurrence include surgeon variability, grade and sex and BMI.

However, our sophistication in making decisions and our categorisation of risk for these tumours has not kept pace, since about 65–70 % of rectal cancers are classified as locally advanced rectal cancer (LARC).

The most recent update of the Dutch TME trial in rectal cancer (van Gijn et al. 2011) reported a 10-year local recurrence cumulative incidence of 5 % in the group assigned to short course preoperative radiotherapy (5×5 Gy) versus 11 % in the surgery alone group ($P < 0.001$). This 50 % reduction in local recurrence is maintained long-term, and in a non–protocolised subset analysis of 435 TNM stage III patients with a negative circumferential margin (CRM), i.e., 23 % of the total population, preoperative radiotherapy appears to improve 10-year overall survival from 40 to 50 % ($p = 0.032$). However, this finding does not take into account the quality of the mesorectal excision. Node positive patients with defects in the mesorectum are likely to be at high risk of local recurrence whereas complete mesorectal excision will lead to local recurrence overall in the range 7–8 % (Quirke et al. 2009).

Yet, for all groups the results of the Dutch trial do not show a difference in overall survival (van Gijn et al. 2011), which implies that either the result has arisen by chance as a type I error or some population groups within the trial (? node negative) are disadvantaged in terms of survival by radiotherapy.

3.1 Is Neoadjuvant Chemotherapy an Alternative?

There is clearly a high risk of metastatic disease in locally advanced rectal cancer, yet systemically active doses of chemotherapy are not delivered in CRT schedules, and compliance to postoperative adjuvant chemotherapy is generally poor. Extrapolating from positive studies in colon cancer, many oncologists are encouraged to use a FOLFOX regimen as postoperative chemotherapy for stage III patients after chemoradiation. The optimal number of cycles of such treatment has not been determined. Hence, some groups have exdtrapolated even further and added chemotherapy either prior to CRT, when compliance to chemotherapy is high (Fernández-Martos et al. 2010, 2011), or following chemoradiation to increase the response rate (Garcia-Aguilar et al. 2011). Some groups have suggested this strategy leads to excellent long-term results, but raise concerns for a high early death rate (Chua et al. 2010). Others have proposed neoadjuvant chemotherapy alone without radiation (Glynne-Jones et al. 2012).

3.2 Can Radiotherapy be Omitted?

Several groups have explored omitting radiotherapy when MRI suggests the tumour is easily resectable. This omission does not appear to have increased the local recurrence rate (Taylor et al. 2011, Frasson et al. 2011, Mathis et al. 2012). It seems clear that the surgeon needs to expect to be able to perform an optimal plane of surgery, i.e. to achieve a surgical specimen with an intact mesorectum displaying only minor irregularities over a smooth mesorectal surface; with no defect deeper than 5 mm; with no coning and with a smooth circumferential resection margin on slicing (Quirke et al. 2009) (Table 1).

Three feasibility/retrospective studies of neoadjuvant chemotherapy (NACT) alone without radiation (Cercek et al. 2010; Schrag et al. 2010; Ishii et al. 2010) used FOLFOX plus/minus bevacizumab (Table 2).The pCR rate after chemotherapy alone varied from to 7–35 %, but as small non-randomised studies are unable to show an impact on metastatic disease. The studies are too small and not sufficiently mature to assess the local recurrence rate. However, the proof of principle has given rise to many current studies exploring neoadjuvant chemiotherapy (Table 3).

3.3 Are There Clearly Distinguishable Groups Who Do Not Need RT?

Accurate information on primary tumour local extension, precise location, potential nodal-stage, potential CRM involvement and extra-mural venous invasion is essential for defining the optimum treatment strategy on an individual basis. Currently, the definition of locally advanced rectal cancer is variable from unit to unit. Currently, in the UK many MDTS categorise patients into "the good, the bad and the ugly", which allows definition of three different settings where preoperative neoadjuvant treatment may or may not be required. For clinically

Table 1 Histopathological grading of the quality and completeness of the mesorectum in a total mesorectal excision specimen

	Mesorectum	Defects	Coning	CRM
Complete	Intact, smooth	Not defects deeper than 5 mm	None	Smooth, regular
Nearly complete	Moderate bulk, but irregular	No visible muscularis propria	Moderate	Irregular
Incomplete	Little bulk and very irregular	Down to muscularis propria	Moderate–marked	Irregular

unresectable cancers or where MRI shows a threatened/breached CRM (10–15 % of cases), or in cancers which require surgical resection beyond the conventional total mesorectal excision (TME) plane, then radiation as a component of CRT is clearly necessary. In contrast, early cT1/T2 tumours are not usually treated with radiotherapy because of the low risk of local recurrence. The problem with these above systems is that the intermediate risk represents a wide spectrum, with variable behaviour and should be defined more accurately with further risk groupings. Since in the trials about 50 % of patients have low rectal cancer within 5 cms of the anal margin, probably more than 50 % are stage 2 and up to 30 % are T2 initially. A T3 subclassification has been proposed in 2001 by Merkel from the Erlangen group, who suggested the subdivision of T3 into T3a < 5 mm and T3b > 5 mm (Merkel et al. 2001). The Mercury Study Group extended this subclassification further into four groups: "a" (<1 mm outside the wall), "b" (1–5 mm), "c" (5–15 mm) and "d" (>15 mm) (MERCURY 2007; Smith and Brown 2008a). Distinction between cT2 and cT3a remains difficult, but may be less relevant to outcome because the Erlangen data suggests prognosis is not significantltly different for these two groups. MRI can define macroscopic extra-mural vascular invasion (EMVI), which occurs in about 40 % of patients (Smith and Brown 2008b). This feature predicts for systemic failure with good concordance between MRI EMVI and eventual pathology EMVI prognostic outcome (Dirschmid et al. 1996; Sternberg et al. 2002), suggesting that patients with macroscopic EMVI have only a 30 % 3-year disease-free survival.

A structure which defines three risk groups within the broad intermediate risk category, with low risk of local recurrence/low risk of metastatic disease, low risk of local recurrence/high risk of metastatic disease, high risk of local recurrence/ low risk of metastatic disease, high risk of local recurrence/high risk of metastatic disease is therefore proposed (Table 4).

Chemotherapy prior to CRT or SCPRT does not compromise the delivery CRT, but has not increased pCR rates, R0-resection rate, improved DFS or reduced metastases. There is significant late morbidity from pelvic radiotherapy and a doubling of the risk of second malignancy. Hence, NACT alone without radiotherapy could be explored compared with SCPRT or CRT in selected patients with resectable rectal cancer showing adverse features (extramural vascular invasion etc.) in a future research programme.

Table 2 Phase I/II studies of neoadjuvant chemotherapy without radiation

	No of pts[a]	Eligibility	Induction chemotherapy	Toxicity	PCR[b]	T Mic[c]	R0	Late outcome
Ishii et al. 2010	26	cT3/T4 N0-2	Irinotecan (80 mg/m^2), FUFA days 1, 8, and 15 for 4 weeks	Not stated	1/15 (7 %)	Not stated	Not stated	5 year RFS 74 % OS 84 %
Schrag et al. 2010	31	Clinical stage II-III (but not T4)	FOLFOX-bevacizumab (6 cycles bev 1-4)	2 pts withdrawn (angina arrhythmia)	8/29 (27 %)	Not stated	29/29 (100 %)	No data
Cercek et al. 2010	20	RT contraindicated or presence of synchronous metastases	6 pts FOLFOX14 pts FOLFOX + Bev	Not stated	7/20 (35 %) 2/6 (33 %) rectal cancer without metastases	Not stated	Not stated	No data

[a] number entering study
[b] number having had surgery
[c] using regression grading not yp

Table 3 Trials of Neoadjuvant chemotherapy in progress

STUDY (reference)	Pre-operative treatment	Entry criteria	Status	RT/CRT	Comments
Phase III trials					
GEMCAD (Fernández-Martos et al. 2010b) 41 patients	Capecitabine/oxaliplatin + bevacizumab 3 cycles then capox = total 4 cycles	MRI defined entry	Recruiting	Selective CRT according to response	Primary endpoint: Response rate (RECIST)
RAPIDO Phase III EudraCT number 2010-023957-12 885 patients	SCPRT (5x5 Gy) followed by Oxaliplatin/capecitabine 6 cycles vs Control Capecitabine +CRT	MRI defined entry	Yet to open	CRT 50.4 Gy/28# with capecitabine	Primary endpoint: 3 year DFS
Polish Study EGBRJ 0109 NCT00833131 540 patients	SCPRT (5 X 5 Gy) followed by FOLFOX (3 cycles) then surgery versus Versus 5FU/capecitabine CRT (50 Gy) as control	Unresectable rectal cancer	Recruiting	SCPRT versus CRT	Primary endpoint: the rate of R0 resection
Randomised Phase II trials					
BACCHUS NCRI Randomised phase II 60 patients	FOLFOX +bevacizumab for 5 courses,then final FOLFOX then surgery versus FOLFOXIRI bevacizumab for 5 courses,then final FOLFOXIRI then surgery	MRI defined entry	Yet to open	SCPRT or CRT only for progression/lack of response	Primary endpoint: pCR
randomised phase II GRECCAR 4 150 patients	FOLFIRINOX 4–8 weeks then reassess/randomised according to response. If good cap 50 Gy vs surgery. If poor cap 50 Gy vs cap 60 Gy	MRI defined entry	?started	If good cap 50 Gy vs surgery. If poor cap 50 Gy vs cap 60 Gy	Primary endpoint: %R0
French phase II NCT00865189 91 patients	FOLFOX +bevacizumab for 6 courses then CRT(with bevacizumab/5FU) versus CRT alone	Not MRI	Ongoing not recruiting		Primary endpoint: pCR
Chinese Randomised phase II NCT01211210 495 patients	FOLFOX (4 cycles) then surgery versus FOLFOX CRT Versus 5FU CRT (control)	Not MRI	Recruiting		Primary endpoint 3 year DFS
SWOG study NCT00070434 Up to 65 patients	Multiple regimens	T4 rectal cancer	Ongoing not recruiting	CRT with cape	Primary endpoint: Response

Table 4 Proposed mid-Rectal cancer risk categorisation based on MRI and clinical risk factors

Low risk	Intermediate risk		High risk	
Low risk local recurrence/ Low risk metastases	Low risk local recurrence/ moderate risk metastases	Moderate risk of local recurrence/high risk metastases	High risk of local recurrence/higher risk metastases	High risk local recurrence/High risk metastases
MRI cT2/T3a/T3b < 4 mm extension into muscularis propria. CRM not threatened (predicted ≥ 2 mm) cN0 CT M0	MRI cT3b > 4 mm extension into muscularis propria. CRM not threatened (predicted ≥2 mm) cN1, CT M0	MRI cT3b > 4 mm cT3c, cN2, V2 CRM not threatened (predicted > 2 mm) CT M0	MRI cT3d, T4a (resectable) CRM not threatened (predicted ≥2 mm) CT M0	MRI cTany extension into muscularis propria, T4b CRM breached or threatened (predicted < 1 mm) CT M0 ? Mucinous
Clinical factors	Obesity			
	Male/with anterior tumours			
	Narrow pelvis Previous			
	pelvic surgery			
	Large bulky tumour			
	Sepsis/fistula/perforation			
NICE guidelines low risk +, but does not include T3b < 4 mm	*UK nice guidelines intermediate risk*			NICE guidelines high risk a threatened (< 1 mm) or breached resection margin or low tumours encroaching onto inter-sphincteric plane or levator involvement
	any cT3b or greater, in which the potential surgical margin is not threatened **or**			
	any suspicious lymph node not threatening the surgical resection margin **or**			
	the presence of extramural vascular invasion			

(continued)

Table 4 (continued)

	Low risk	Intermediate risk	High risk
NICE	do not give RT	*Nice guidelines (UK)* SCPRT or CRT	NICE CRT recommended
Potential mri directed recommendations	No requirement for preop radiotherapy Immediate surgery	If surgeon convinced able to perform R0 resection and good quality in mesorectal plane could omit RT / SCPRT or CRT depending on whether shrinkage of tumour required or Neoadjuvant chemotherapy alone	Requires chemoradiation (CRT) / SCPRT or CRT depending on whether shrinkage of tumour required or Neoadjuvant chemotherapy alone

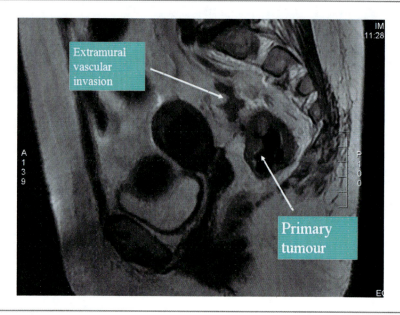

4 Conclusion

Preoperative chemoradiotherapy is an important component of the multimodality treatment of rectal cancer if the CRM is threatened. To achieve pelvic control the surgeon needs an R0 resection. Pelvic failure gives rise to awful and debilitating symptoms, including intractable pain and intestinal obstruction, and a very poor quality of life. However, for less advanced cases, an R0 resection may be more straightforward, and the risk of metastatic disease now predominates over the risk of local recurrence. Modern MRI can define patients with a high risk of metastases (EMVI, T3c andT3d)—particularly in the mid-rectum. This high risk of metastatic disease means that the use of chemotherapy at systemically effective doses would seem essential if we are to improve survival in patients with locally advanced rectal cancer. The use of radiotherapy has compromised the integration of full sysytemic doses into chemoradiation schedules and the uptake of postoperative chemotherapy. In contrast NACT has been shown to allow full delivery of chemotherapy in systemic doses and an appropriate intensity without compromising surgery.

Rectal cancer trials using radiotherapy or chemoradiation in locally advanced rectal cancer are notoriously difficult to recruit, and may require decades to accrue sufficient appropriate patients. Patients with stage II have comprised the majority in these trials (and in some up to 30 % have been stage I). Their outcome would have been good anyway, and to demonstrate an improvement in a randomised trial would have required many thousands of patients. So to date, Phase III trials have been consistently underpowered and taken too long to perform to provide meaningful results. We still lack data to confirm that by intensifying treatment, the outcome will necessarily be better. Quality assurance is increasingly important in terms of imaging for patient selection, surgery, the delivery of radiotherapy and histopathology. Key components of quality control for radiotherapy trials should include mandated MRI-defined entry criteria, and the inclusion of patients at high risk of loco-regional failure.

The current term of 'locally advanced rectal cancer' or 'T3/T4' rectal cancer includes a large proportion of patients who either do not need radiotherapy or equally are not going to benefit in a significant way from chemotherapy, using analogies of the benefit of chemotherapy in low risk stage II colon cancer. We need a new description/term for locally advanced rectal cancer, which provides an effective risk categorisation. What is the predominant risk? Local recurrence or metastatic disease? A proposal is tabled in this chapter.

Patients should be categorised according to clinical stage TNM, site in the rectum, quadrant and accurate localisation in respect to the mesorectal fascia and levators. Other factors, such as cN-stage and vascular and nerve invasion are important histologically although the prediction of nodal involvement is poor at present and only macroscopic/gross vascular invasion can be imaged at present. Let us work together to achieve a common language and framework to marry MRI and pathological reporting.

So can we do without radiotherapy if the CRM is not threatened? This proposal may be more easily accepted in the upper and mid-rectal cancers than in low cancers. But if we still cling to the notion that RT is needed in all cases because of issues of quality assurance, then have we simply turned full circle and are back to advocating preoperative radiotherapy to compensate for poor surgical technique? Or can we accept that if we see the surgeon performing good quality surgery in 80–90 % of his specimens within the mesorectal plane and the MRI suggests clear margins that the benefit from CRT is marginal.

However, large well-conducted carefully imaged randomised phase III trials with excellent quality assurance will be required comparing chemotherapy alone with the current standard of SCPRT or CRT and long-term follow-up if we are to provide the definitive answers.

References

André T, Boni C, Navarro M et al (2009) Improved overall survival with oxaliplatin, fluorouracil, and leucovorin as adjuvant treatment in stage II or III colon cancer in the MOSAIC trial. J Clin Oncol 27(19):3109–3116

Aschele C, Cionini L, Lonardi S et al (2011) Primary tumor response to preoperative chemoradiation with or without oxaliplatin in locally advanced rectal cancer: pathologic results of the STAR-01 randomized phase III trial. J Clin Oncol 29(20):2773–2780

Birgisson H, Pahlman L, Gunnarsson U, Glimelius B (2005) Occurrence of second cancers in patients treated with radiotherapy for rectal cancer. J Clin Oncol 23:6126–6131

Birgisson H, Pahlman L, Glimelius B (2006) Adverse effects of preoperative radiation therapy for rectal cancer: long-term follow-up of the Swedish rectal cancer trial. J Clin Oncol 23:8697–8705

Bosset JF, Collette L, Calais G et al (2006) Chemoradiotherapy with preoperative radiotherapy in rectal cancer. N Engl J Med 355:1114–1123

Braendengen M, Tveit KM, Berglund A et al (2008) Randomized phase III study comparing preoperative radiotherapy with chemoradiotherapy in nonresectable rectal cancer. J Clin Oncol 26(22):3687–3694

Bujko K, Nowacki MP, Nasierowska-Guttmejer A et al (2006) Long-term results of a randomized trial comparing preoperative short-course radiotherapy with preoperative conventionally fractionated chemoradiation for rectal cancer. Br J Surg 93(10):1215–1223

Cecil DT, Sexton R, Moran BJ, Heald RJ (2004) Total mesorectal excision results in low local recurrence rates in lymph node-positive rectal cancer. Dis Colon Rectum 47:1145–1150

Cercek A, Weiser MR, Goodman KA, et al., (2010) Complete pathological response in the primary of rectal or colon cancer treated with FOLFOX without radiation. J Clin Oncol 28:3649 (15S suppl (May 20 Supplement): 297s (abstract))

Chua YJ, Barbachano Y, Cunningham D et al (2010) Neoadjuvant capecitabine and oxaliplatin before chemoradiation and total mesorectal excision in MRI-defined poor-risk rectal cancer: a phase 2 trial. Lancet Oncol 11(3):241–248

Dirschmid K, Lang A, Mathis G et al (1996) Incidence of extramural venous invasion in colorectal carcinoma: findings with a new technique. Hum Pathol 27(11):1227–1230

Fernandez-Martos C, Pericay C, Salud A (2011) Three-year outcomes of GCR-3: a phase II randomized trial comparing conventional preoperative chemoradiation (CRT) followed by surgery and postoperative adjuvant chemotherapy (CT) with induction CT followed by CRT and surgery in locally advanced rectal cancer. J Clin Oncol 29:abstr 3552 (Suppl)

Fernández-Martos C, Pericay C, Aparicio J et al (2010) Phase II, Randomized study of concomitant chemoradiation followed by surgery and adjuvant capecitabine plus oxaliplatin (CAPOX) compared with induction CAPOX followed by concomitant chemoradiation and surgery in magnetic resonance imaging-defined, locally advanced rectal cancer: grupo cancer de recto 3 study. J Clin Oncol 28(5):859–865

Frasson M, Garcia-Granero E, Roda D, et al (2011) Preoperative chemoradiation may not always be needed for patients with T3 and T2 N + rectal cancer. Cancer 117(14): 3118–3125. doi: 10.1002/cncr.25866

Frykholm GJ, Pahlman L, Glimerlius B (2001) Combined chemo- and radiotherapy vs radiotherapy alone in the treatment of primary, nonresectable adenocarcinoma of the rectum. Int J Radiat Oncol Biol Phys 50(2):427–434

Garcia-Aguilar J, Smith DD, Avila K et al (2011) Timing of rectal cancer response to chemoradiation consortium. optimal timing of surgery after chemoradiation for advanced rectal cancer: preliminary results of a multicenter, nonrandomized phase II prospective trial. Ann Surg 254(1):97–102

Gerard JP, Conroy T, Bonnetain F et al (2006) Preoperative radiotherapy with or without concurrent fluorouracil and leucovorin in T3–T4 rectal cancers: results of FFCD 9203. J Clin Oncol 24:4620–4625

Gerard JP, Azria D, Gourgou-Bourgade S et al (2010) Comparison of two neoadjuvant chemoradiotherapy regimens for locally advanced rectal cancer: results of the phase III trial ACCORD 12/0405-Prodige 2. J Clin Oncol 28:1638–1644

Glynne-Jones R, Anyamene N, Moran B, Harrison M (2012) Neoadjuvant chemotherapy in MRI-staged high-risk rectal cancer in addition to or as an alternative to preoperative chemoradiation? Ann Oncol [Epub ahead of print]

Herman MP, Kopetz S, Bhosale PR, Eng C, Skibber JM, Rodriguez-Bigas MA, Feig BW, Chang GJ, Delclos ME, Krishnan S, Crane CH, Das P (2009) Sacral insufficiency fractures after preoperative chemoradiation for rectal cancer: incidence, risk factors, and clinical course. Int J Radiat Oncol Biol Phys 74(3):818–823

Horisberger K, Hofheinz RD, Palma P et al (2008) Tumor response to neoadjuvant chemoradiation in rectal cancer: predictor for surgical morbidity? Int J Colorectal Dis 23(3):257–264

Ishii Y, Hasegawa H, Endo T et al (2010) Medium-termresults of neoadjuvant systemic chemotherapy using irinotecan, 5-fluorouracil, and leucovorin in patients with locally advanced rectal cancer. Eur J Surg Oncol 36(11):1061–1065

Kuebler JP, Wieand HS, O'Connell MJ et al (2007) Oxaliplatin combined with weekly bolus fluorouracil and leucovorin as surgical adjuvant chemotherapy for stage II and III colon cancer: results from NSABP C-07. J Clin Oncol 25(16):2198–2204

Kusters M, Marijnen CA, van de Velde CJ et al (2010) Patterns of local recurrence in rectal cancer; a study of the Dutch TME trial. Eur J Surg Oncol 36(5):470–476

Lange MM, den Dulk M, Bossema ER et al (2007) Risk factors for faecal incontinence after rectal cancer treatment. Cooperative clinical investigators of the Dutch total mesorectal excision trial. Br J Surg 94(10):1278–1284

Marijnen CA, van de Velde CJ, Putter H et al (2005) Impact of short-term preoperative radiotherapy on health-related quality of life and sexual functioning in primary rectal cancer: report of a multicenter randomized trial. J Clin Oncol 23(9):1847–1858

Mathis KL, Larson DW, Dozois EJ et al (2012) Outcomes following surgery without radiotherapy for rectal cancer. Br J Surg 99(1):137–143

MERCURY Study Group (2007) Extramural depth of tumour invasion at thin section MR in patients with rectal cancer. Results of the MERCURY Study. Radiology 243:132–139

Merkel S, Mansmann U, Siassi M, Papadopoulus T, Hohenberger W, Heranek P (2001) The prognostic inhomogeneity in pT3 rectal carcinomas. Int J Colorectal Dis 16:298–304

Morris E, Quirke P, Thomas JD et al (2008) Unacceptable variation in abdominoperineal excision rates for rectal cancer: time to intervene? Gut 57(12):1690–1697

Ngan S, Fisher R, Goldstein D et al., (2010) TROG, AGITG, CSSANZ, and RACS.A randomized trial comparing local recurrence (LR) rates between short-course (SC) and long-course (LC) preoperative radiotherapy (RT) for clinical T3 rectal cancer: an intergroup trial (TROG, AGITG, CSSANZ, RACS). J Clin Oncol 2010 28:(15):3509 (abstract)

Peeters KC, van de Velde CJ, Leer JW et al (2005) Late side effects of short-course preoperative radiotherapy combined with total mesorectal excision for rectal cancer: increased bowel dysfunction in irradiated patients—a Dutch colorectal cancer group study. J Clin Oncol 23(25):6199–6206

Peeters KC, Marijnen CA, Nagtegaal ID, For the Dutch Colorectal Cancer Group et al (2007) The TME Trial after a Median Follow-up of 6 Years: Increased local control but no survival benefit in irradiated patients with resectable rectal carcinoma. Ann Surg 246(5):693–701

Pollack J, Holm T, Cedermark B et al (2006) Long-term effect of preoperative radiation therapy on anorectal function. Dis Colon Rectum 49(3):345–352

Quirke P, Steele R, Monson J et al (2009) MRC CR07/NCIC-CTG CO16 trial investigators; NCRI colorectal cancer study group. Effect of the plane of surgery achieved on local recurrence in patients with operable rectal cancer: a prospective study using data from the MRC CR07 and NCIC-CTG CO16 randomised clinical trial. Lancet 373(9666):821–828

Rödel C, Liersch T, Hermann R et al (2007) Multicenter phase II trial of chemoradiation with oxaliplatin for rectal cancer. J Clin Oncol 25:668–674

Roh MS, Colangelo LH, O'Connell MJ et al (2009) Preoperative multimodality therapy improves disease-free survival in patients with carcinoma of the rectum: NSABP-R03. J Clin Oncol 27:5124–5130

Sauer R, Becker H, Hohenberger W, German Rectal Cancer Study Group et al (2004) Preoperative versus postoperative chemoradiotherapy for rectal cancer. N Engl J Med 351:1731–1740

Schrag D, Weiser MR, Goodman KA, et al., Neoadjuvant FOLFOX-bev, without radiation for locally advanced rectal cancer. J Clin Oncol 2010;28:3511 (15S_suppl (May 20 Supplement) 263s (abstract))

Sebag-Montefiore D, Stephens RJ, Steele R et al (2009) Preoperative radiotherapy versus selective postoperative chemoradiotherapy in patients with rectal cancer (MRC CR07 and NCIC-CTG C016): a multicentre, randomised trial. Lancet 373(9666):811–820

Smith N, Brown G (2008) Preoperative staging of rectal cancer. Acta Oncol 47(1):20–31

Stelzmueller I, Zitt M, Aigner F et al (2009) Postoperative morbidity following chemoradiation for locally advanced low rectal cancer. J Gastrointest Surg 13(4):657–667

Sternberg A, Amar M, Alfici R, Groisman G (2002) Conclusions from a study of venous invasion in stage IV colorectal adenocarcinoma. J Clin Pathol 55(1):17–21

Swellengrebel HA, Marijnen CA, Verwaal VJ et al (2011) Toxicity and complications of preoperative chemoradiotherapy for locally advanced rectal cancer. Br J Surg 98(3):418–426

Taylor FG, Quirke P, Heald RJ, For the MERCURY study group et al (2011) Preoperative high-resolution magnetic resonance imaging can identify good prognosis stage I, II, and III rectal cancer best managed by surgery alone: a prospective, multicenter, european study that recruited consecutive patients with rectal cancer. Ann Surg 253(4):711–719

van Gijn W, Marijnen CA, Nagtegaal ID et al (2011) Dutch Colorectal Cancer Group. Preoperative radiotherapy combined with total mesorectal excision for resectable rectal cancer: 12 year follow-up of the multicentre, randomised controlled TME trial. Lancet Oncol 12(6):575–582

Author Biography

Rob Glynne-Jones has received honoraria for lectures and advisory boards and has been supported in attending international meetings in the last 5 years by Merck, Pfizer, Sanofi-Aventis and Roche. He has also in the past received unrestricted grants for research from Merck-Serono, Sanofi-Aventis and Roche. He is principal investigator of a randomised phase II neoadjuvant chemotherapy study in the UK called 'BACCHUS'.

Treatment Dilemmas in Patients with Synchronous Colorectal Liver Metastases

T. J. M. Ruers and J. Hagendoorn

Abstract

Approximately 20 % of patients with colorectal cancer have synchronous liver metastases at the time of diagnosis. In some instances it is difficult to determine the best treatment strategy in these patients. For example, should the primary tumor be removed in those patients with unresectable liver metastases and who do not have any symptoms of the primary tumor? Or which operation should be performed first in patients with rectal cancer and synchronous resectable liver metastases? Unfortunately, there are no clear answers to these questions from prospective randomized trials. In the present article retrospective studies are analyzed in order to define the best possible treatment strategy for patients with synchronous colorectal liver metastases.

Contents

1	Introduction	38
2	Patients with Asymptomatic Cancer of the Colon and Unresectable Synchronous Liver Metastases	38
	2.1 Results of Initial Treatment with Chemotherapy	39
	2.2 Results of Initial Resection of the Primary Tumor	40
	2.3 The Effect of Treatment Strategy on Overall Survival	42
3	Patients Presenting with Resectable Synchronous Liver Metastases and Rectal Cancer	43
	3.1 Results of Staged or Simultaneous Rectal and Liver Resection Combined with Perioperative Radiotherapy and Chemotherapy	44
	3.2 Enhancing Efficacy of Perioperative Radiotherapy and Chemotherapy	44
	3.3 Results of the Liver-First Approach	45
References		46

T. J. M. Ruers (✉) · J. Hagendoorn
Department of Surgery, The Netherlands Cancer Institute,
Plesmanlaan 121, 1066 CX Amsterdam, The Netherlands
e-mail: t.ruers@nki.nl

F. Otto and M. P. Lutz (eds.), *Early Gastrointestinal Cancers*,
Recent Results in Cancer Research 196, DOI: 10.1007/978-3-642-31629-6_3,
© Springer-Verlag Berlin Heidelberg 2012

1 Introduction

About 20 % of patients with colorectal cancer present with liver metastasis at time of diagnosis (Mella et al. 1997). Only a selected group (20–30 %) of these patients is suitable for resection of hepatic metastases. In patients who present with synchronous liver metastases, several treatment options are available. For patients with resectable liver metastases and cancer of the colon, resection of the primary tumor followed by hepatic resection is generally the preferred treatment strategy. In several cases, even combined resection may be performed. In patients with rectal cancer and resectable liver metastases or patients with colorectal cancer and unresectable liver metastases, treatment decisions may be more complex.

For patients with synchronous liver metastases and rectal cancer, several treatment options may be considered. Treatment may start with (radio) chemotherapy followed by resection of the rectal cancer and at a later stage resection of the liver metastases. Alternatively, resection of the liver metastases may be planned first followed by treatment for the rectal cancer—the so-called liver-first approach.

Another treatment dilemma occurs in patients who present with unresectabe colorectal liver metastases while there are no signs or symptoms of the primary colorectal tumor. In these patients, a decision has to be made on whether the primary tumor has to be resected or whether chemotherapy can be started with the primary tumor still in situ. In the following sections, these treatments dilemmas will be further discussed.

2 Patients with Asymptomatic Cancer of the Colon and Unresectable Synchronous Liver Metastases

For most patients with stage IV colorectal cancer and unresectable colorectal liver metastases, the principal goal of treatment is palliation in terms of prolonged survival and quality of life (Millikan et al. 1997). The most common treatment strategy is to perform a palliative colorectal resection in order to prevent complications of the primary tumor such as intestinal obstruction, perforation, or hemorrhage. The SEER data registry showed that approximately 50 % of all patients with stage IV disease undergo resection of the primary tumor.

After resection of the primary tumor, systemic chemotherapy is administered for further treatment of metastatic disease. Resection of the primary colorectal tumor, however, is associated with a high overall morbidity of up to 21 % (Michel et al. 2004). In case of severe postoperative complications, systemic chemotherapy may have to be delayed, compromising any beneficial effects. Morbidity may be related to tumor load as well as to more complex surgical procedures in case of symptomatic disease. Moreover, patients often show weight loss and malnutrition together with a deterioration in overall condition. Reported mortality after resection of the primary tumor in patients with stage IV disease ranges from 1.3–16 %,

Treatment Dilemmas in Patients with Synchronous Colorectal Liver Metastases 39

which is significantly higher than resection for colorectal cancer in general (Eisenberger et al. 2008; Evans et al. 2009).

For this reason, there is a tendency toward a more conservative approach, especially in asymptomatic patients. In such patients, systemic chemotherapy may be the treatment of choice, reserving tumor resection for patients who develop symptomatic disease.

In patients with unresectable metastatic colorectal cancer, systemic therapy may result in response rates of up to 50 % (Kopetz et al. 2009; O'Connell et al. 2004; Sanoff et al. 2008; Grothey and Sargent 2005). Besides the effect of systemic treatment on the liver metastases, further growth of the primary tumor may be inhibited as well, thus reducing the probability of complications, such as bleeding, obstruction, and perforation. In addition, it has been suggested that patients with stage IV colorectal cancer and minimal symptoms from the primary tumor are likely to die from progressive systemic disease before they develop complications related to the primary tumor such as obstruction or bleeding (Sarela and O'Riordain 2001).

In patients with asymptomatic unresectable synchronous liver metastases both strategies—initial resection of the primary tumor or initial systemic therapy—are practiced, without clear evidence on which approach is best. There are no data from prospective randomized trials comparing resection of the primary tumor with a more conservative approach consisting of systemic therapy only. Retrospective analyses are often biased by patient selection in that patients with good performance status were more likely to be elected for surgery than patients in poor health.

2.1 Results of Initial Treatment with Chemotherapy

Intestinal obstruction is the most frequently occurring tumor-related complication in those patients initially treated with systemic therapy (Michel et al. 2004; Benoist et al. 2005; Scoggins et al. 1999; Ruo et al. 2003; Tebbutt et al. 2003; Muratore et al. 2007). The rate of this complication ranged from 5.6 % in a study by Muratore to 29 % in a study by Ruo (Ruo et al. 2003; Muratore et al. 2007). In the latter study, a high percentage (72 %) of left-sided or rectal carcinoma was included. Scheer et al. published a review on 7 series reporting on patients with stage IV colorectal cancer undergoing surgery for the primary tumor or systemic therapy. In their analysis, the pooled proportion of patients treated by systemic therapy that developed bowel obstruction was 13.9 % (9.6–18.8 %).

Across the studies analyzed by Scheer, the number of patients who experienced bleeding from the primary tumor was 3.0 % (95 % C.I. 0.95–6.0 %,); only two studies reported on peritonitis and fistula due to the unresected tumor (Scheer et al. 2008).

In a meta-analysis by Stillwell, including 8 retrospective studies, the pooled proportion of patients that needed surgery for bowel obstruction is reported at

18.3 % (Stillwell et al. 2010). As may be expected, this number was higher in rectal tumors than in right-sided tumors. The percentage of patients with bleeding from the primary tumor varied from 3.7 to 4.7 %. In this analysis, the pooled complication rate due to the presence of the primary tumor was 22.2 %, with percentages varying between the different studies from 13.1 to 30.4 %.

Nevertheless, a number of studies showed that systemic treatment with chemotherapy and targeted agents is safe in stage IV patients with their primary tumor in situ (Benoist et al. 2005; Karoui et al. 2008). Karoui et al. reported that 70 % of these patients showed significant response of the primary tumor, although overall survival may have been lower than generally reported for patients with metastatic colorectal cancer (Karoui et al. 2008). In a recent series by Poultside, 233 consecutive patients were described, all treated with systemic treatment for synchronous metastatic colorectal cancer and an unresected primary tumor (Poultsides et al. 2009). A total of 26 patients (11 %) developed a complication of the primary tumor, 16 of whom (7 %) underwent surgery, while 10 (4 %) patients were managed by a stent or radiotherapy. Of the 217 patients who never required emergency surgery (93 %), 47 (20 %) eventually underwent elective resection of the primary tumor and metastatic disease. The median time to surgery for this group was 8 months (5–32 months).

From the studies mentioned above, it can be concluded that the number of asymptomatic patients who have started with chemotherapy and will ultimately have to undergo intervention for the primary tumor because of complications, seems to vary between 11 and 22 %. For this reason, several authors question the need for initial resection of the primary tumor in those patients with neither obstruction nor bleeding from the primary colorectal tumor (Poultsides et al. 2009; Damjanov et al. 2009; Schmidt 2009).

2.2 Results of Initial Resection of the Primary Tumor

The main argument for initial resection of the primary tumor would be the prevention of complications of the primary tumor during systemic treatment. On the other hand, any survival benefit of resection has not been demonstrated and morbidity and mortality associated with surgery may be substantial.

In the meta-analysis by Scheer et al., five out of seven studies described the results of primary tumor resection (Scheer et al. 2008). In four of these studies, postoperative morbidity and mortality were described (Benoist et al. 2005; Scoggins et al. 1999; Ruo et al. 2003; Tebbutt et al. 2003).

Postoperative mortality ranged from 0 % in a study by Benoist to 4.6 % in a study by Scoggins (Benoist et al. 2005; Scoggins et al. 1999). Meta-analysis of these four studies showed a mortality rate of 2.7 %.

Postoperative morbidity ranged from 18.8 to 47.0 %, with an average of 11.8 % for major complications, such as obstruction (13.2 %), hemorrhage (1.5–3.9 %), and sepsis (2.3–10.6 %). Minor complications, such as wound infections

Table 1 Data on resection versus non-resection of the primary tumor in asymptomatic patients with unresectable metastatic colorectal cancer

Study	Number of patients		Median survival (months)		p-value
	Resection	Non-resection	Resection	Non-resection	
Scoggins et al. (1999)	66	23	14.5	16.6	Ns
Tebbutt et al. (2003)	280	82	14	8.2	Ns
Ruo et al. (2003)	127	103	16	9	<0.001
Michel et al. (2004)	31	23	21	14	Ns
Benoist et al. (2005)	32	27	23	22	Ns.
Galizia et al. (2008)	42	23	15.2	12.3	0.03
Bajwa et al. (2009)	32	35	14	6	0.005

(5.5–10.6 %) and urinary tract infection (2.4–6.1 %), were encountered in 20.6 % of the cases (Benoist et al. 2005; Scoggins et al. 1999; Ruo et al. 2003). A meta-analysis by Stillwell covers 8 studies including a total of 299 patients who were managed by primary resection of the tumor. In the pooled analysis, mortality was 1.7 % (0.7–3.9 %), while pooled morbidity was 22.2 % (16.6–29.0 %). Wound infection was the most frequently occurring complication. Severe complications (cardiopulmonary events, anastomotic leakage, sepsis, and prolonged ileus) were observed in 11 % of the cases.

Another argument against initial resection of the primary tumor arises from pre-clinical data showing that resection of the primary tumor may have a stimulating effect on the growth of distant metastases (Peeters et al. 2004). In 1994, it was demonstrated by the group of Folkman that in mice with Lewis lung carcinoma a circulating anti-angiogenic factor, produced by the primary tumor, was responsible for lack of angiogenesis, a high incidence of apoptosis, and hence a state of dormancy of its distant metastases. Within 3 days after resection of the primary tumor, distant metastases started to grow rapidly because of a sudden decline of the levels of these anti-angiogenic factors.

In humans, studies of primary tumor-induced growth suppression of distant metastases are scarce. In one study, tissue samples of metastatic colorectal liver lesions taken from patients with the primary tumor in situ were compared with those taken from patients who had undergone prior resection of the primary tumor. It was demonstrated that after surgical resection of the primary tumor, vascular density in the liver metastases was significantly higher (Peeters et al. 2004). These findings were in line with an increase in metastatic growth rate as demonstrated by immunohistochemical evaluation of the percentage of cells undergoing apoptosis and the percentage of cells in proliferation (Peeters et al. 2006). As a further indicator of tumor growth, metabolic activity was analyzed by FDG PET imaging of the liver metastases before and after resection of the primary tumor. In a control group, two subsequent PET scans were performed with a similar time interval, but without any surgical intervention having been carried out. A significant increase in metabolic activity of the liver metastases could be demonstrated after resection of the primary tumor, in which observation was not made in the control group (Peeters et al. 2005). However, these data should be interpreted with extreme caution and further research is needed to demonstrate whether such mechanism indeed exists in human.

2.3 The Effect of Treatment Strategy on Overall Survival

Table 1 lists the studies comparing both treatment strategies with regard to overall survival. It should be noted that these are all retrospective studies with inherent limitations. Hardly any information is provided on the selection criteria used for initial therapy choice. This selection bias makes comparison of results impossible.

Treatment decisions are likely to be influenced by performance status and tumor load at the time of diagnosis, thereby potentially effecting more favorable results in the resection group.

For patients who underwent resection of the primary tumor as initial treatment, median overall survival ranged from 14 to 23 months. For patients with systemic therapy as first treatment, median overall survival ranged from 6 to 22 months. In 6 of the 7 studies mentioned in Table 1, overall survival was superior in the resection group. Three studies reported statistically significant differences in overall survival between resected and non-resected patients. The study by Ruo reported a significant difference in median survival between the two groups: 16 versus 9 months for the resection ($n = 127$) and non-resection ($n = 103$) groups, respectively (Ruo et al. 2003). Patients in the resection group had a higher frequency of right-sided colon cancers ($p = 0.03$) and metastatic disease restricted to the liver ($p = 0.02$). From a univariate analysis, it was concluded that the number of distant sites involved, metastatic disease confined to the liver, and the volume of hepatic replacement by the tumor were significant prognostic variables, while resection status was not significantly associated with survival. In multivariate analyses, only the extent of liver involvement remained significant. Compared to literature, a high number of patients ($n = 30$, 29 %) in the chemotherapy group had to undergo subsequent surgical intervention for palliation of obstruction.

In a smaller series by Galizia, 42 symptom-free patients underwent resection, while 23 patients initially started with chemotherapy (Galizia et al. 2008). Median overall survival in the resection group was 15 months versus 12 months in the chemotherapy group ($p = 0.03$). On multivariate analysis, performance status, extent of liver involvement, and type of treatment were shown to be the only covariates that were independently associated with overall survival.

In the series of Bajwa, all analyzed patients ($n = 67$) received systemic treatment (Bajwa et al. 2009). Surgery was performed for bowel obstruction, bleeding, or stable disease in 32 cases. Overall survival after surgery was 14 months in the group that underwent resection compared to 6 months for patients treated with chemotherapy alone. Surgery (OR 0.26; $p = 0.00013$) and clinical response of the primary tumor (OR 0.53; $p = 0.012$) were independently associated with prolonged survival.

Altogether, the meta-analysis by Stilwell, which included 8 studies, calculated an estimated survival advantage of 6 months for patients undergoing resection (Stillwell et al. 2010). Four studies conducted a multivariate analysis of factors related to overall survival. Two studies, by Ruo et al. and Galizia et al., observed that liver tumor burden was significantly related to overall survival, while in the series of Bajwa et al. and Galizia et al. the type of treatment (resection) was related to superior survival (Ruo et al. 2003; Galizia et al. 2008; Bajwa et al. 2009). The studies by Gallizia et al. and Tebbutt et al. indicated that better performance status was related to improved survival (Tebbutt et al. 2003; Galizia et al. 2008).

Furthermore, the percentage of patients undergoing curative hepatic resection after downsizing of initially unresectable liver metastases was comparable between both treatment strategies (Stillwell et al. 2010). Analysis of four studies showed that curative resection rates ranged from 1.2 to 22 % in the chemotherapy groups. Comparable figures were noted in the resection groups (1.8–18.8 %). Quantitative analysis of these studies showed that there was no difference in likelihood of curative hepatic resection.

3 Patients Presenting with Resectable Synchronous Liver Metastases and Rectal Cancer

For patients with rectal cancer and (potentially) resectable metastases confined to the liver, resection of all malignant lesions with the intention of cure is the principal treatment target. At this time, however, there is no standardized treatment regimen validated in randomized clinical studies for patients presenting with rectal cancer and synchronous resectable liver metastases. Treatment of rectal cancer per se consists of short-course radiation therapy followed by surgery or long course chemoradiation therapy followed by surgery after an interval of a number of weeks. In the case of synchronous liver metastases, this would result in under-treatment of the metastatic disease during a substantial time interval, which may yet be prolonged by postoperative complications. Treatment of liver metastases consists of radical resection and/or local ablative therapy, such as radiofrequency ablation, combined with adjuvant chemotherapy (Lo et al. 2011). Several questions arise about the optimal application and sequence, when these therapies need to be combined. First, what strategy is the most efficacious at achieving radical treatment of all tumor? Second, what strategy minimizes the risk of formation or growth of metastases during treatment? Third, do we need to stratify patient categories—for instance, early versus advanced rectal cancer, extent of liver involvement, et cetera? Fourth, how do these data translate to (long-term) disease-free survival and overall survival? These questions will be addressed in the light of three possible clinical regimens: staged or simultaneous surgery combined with conventional chemotherapy and radiotherapy, surgery after novel chemoradiation regimens, and the liver-first approach.

3.1 Results of Staged or Simultaneous Rectal and Liver Resection Combined with Perioperative Radiotherapy and Chemotherapy

Older clinical case series show that the median overall survival of patients with stage IV colorectal cancer averages around 6 months, when treatment is limited to palliative resection of the primary tumor and/or palliative chemotherapy (5-fluorouracil) (Giacchi et al. 1988; Wagner et al. 1984; Bengtsson et al. 1981; Wood et al. 1976). Novel systemic therapeutic regimens, which include oxaliplatin, irinotecan, capecitabine, and molecular targeted therapy, may prolong median survival to more than 20 months (Scheithauer et al. 2003; Borner et al. 2002; Shields et al. 2004; Hurwitz et al. 2004; Kabbinavar et al. 2005). However, more recent data suggest that resection of all (primary and metastatic) disease, in a selected sub-group where this is feasible, may yield considerable survival benefit with a 5-year overall survival around 30 % (reviewed in (Simmonds et al. 2006).

Given the feasibility and good prognosis of resection of colorectal liver metastases in general, the currently most used approach is staged resection of the rectal tumor followed by liver resection, combined with perioperative chemoradiotherapy. For rectal cancer, no randomized data are available with respect to the sequence of these modalities. However, several studies compared classical staged resections with simultaneous resections. Some studies showed that simultaneous colorectal and liver resection can be carried out safely with 5-year overall survival rates that equal those in resections of metachronous metastases (i.e., ± 30 %) (Vassiliou et al. 2007; Weber et al. 2003; Thelen et al. 2007; Lyass et al. 2001). Others have emphasized that simultaneous resections carry an increased risk of morbidity (Reddy et al. 2007; Adam 2007), suggesting that patients need to be carefully selected according to the extent of the surgery needed. Turrini et al. showed in a cohort of 120 colorectal cancer patients with simultaneous, resectable liver metastases that there is no significant difference in median overall survival between staged resections (40 months) and simultaneous resections (46 months). However, more patients in the simultaneous cohort were able to complete their chemotherapy and receive an R0 resection (89 versus 67 %). The authors speculate that this may be due to complications after the first (rectal) procedure in the staged treatment regimen and that this may lead to more liver recurrence in the longer term (Turrini et al. 2007).

3.2 Enhancing Efficacy of Perioperative Radiotherapy and Chemotherapy

Conceptually, it is attractive to design a combined schedule of preoperative radiation therapy and chemotherapy, so that the primary and metastatic tumors are treated at the same time. This has two clinical-strategic benefits with respect to the liver disease. First, response of liver metastases to chemotherapy may be monitored, which is an indicator of long-term survival (Adam et al. 2004; Blazer et al. 2008).

However, this strategy may carry the risk of complete radiologic, but not pathologic, response (Benoist et al. 2006). Second, downsizing of the hepatic lesions may increase R0 resection rates and lead to more parenchyma-sparing surgery. Although it is clear that downsizing may increase resectability rates, it is debated whether neoadjuvant chemotherapy per se affects long-term survival in metastatic liver disease, while it can induce hepatotoxicity and postoperative morbidity and mortality (Lehmann et al. 2012). It is also unclear how rescue treatment with hepatic arterial infusion chemotherapy and cetuximab, after failure of standard chemotherapy (Blazer et al.2008; Boige et al. 2008), would fit into a scenario of synchronous liver metastases.

Preliminary data from a Dutch phase II trial address the issue of more efficacious scheduling of radiation- and chemotherapy in patients with rectal cancer and liver metastases (Van Dijk et al. 2010). In this study, patients with primary rectal cancer and resectable metastases confined to no more than two organs underwent sequential short-course (5x 5 Gy) radiation therapy and bevacizumab, capecitabine, and oxaliplatin in a neoadjuvant setting. Most patients were staged T3N1. Primary endpoint was the number of patients able to undergo an R0 resection. 50 Patients were included, 41 were operated upon and in 33 of these, radical resection of all disease was achieved. This study shows that short-course radiation therapy combined with chemotherapy and targeted antibodies may lead to adequate and effective treatment of all disease, also in case of T3-4 rectal tumors.

It remains to be determined how these data translate to long-term survival. In addition, the scheduling of surgery as well as the potential for downsizing initially unresectable metastases are factors that warrent further investigation. Furthermore, the combination of radiation therapy and vascular targeted agents may enhance antitumor efficacy due to "vascular normalization" (Jain 2005), a process of temporary improvement in the function of tumor microvascular function that may result in better oxygenation (and, hence, more radiation injury) and drug penetration. Interestingly, there is evidence suggesting that this process takes place in human rectal cancer in response to bevacizumab (Willett et al. 2004). At the same time, we speculate that combining these therapies might also counterbalance hypoxia-induced metastasis formation (De Bock et al. 2011). Further experimental and clinical randomized data are needed to validate the optimum neoadjuvant treatment schedule for rectal cancer with resectable metastases.

3.3 Results of the Liver-First Approach

Since long-term survival is mostly determined by the liver metastases, it could be argued that a liver-first approach is clinically advantageous. In this case, liver metastases are resected first, after which radiation therapy is applied to the rectum and further rectal surgery is planned. Although, theoretically, both the primary tumor and metastases can metastasize, this strategy's potential downside is that the primary tumor, when untreated, may keep 'shedding' tumor cells in the circulation. Clinically, only a few non-randomized studies have described a liver-first approach in colorectal cancer.

Several studies show that a liver-first approach with neoadjuvant chemotherapy is feasible and can result in a median survival up to 44 months as shown by Mentha et al. (Mentha et al. 2008). Comparable results were described by de Jong et al., who observed a 3-year survival rate of 41 % (de Jong et al. 2011). Verhoef et al. described 22 patients who underwent subsequently chemotherapy, liver resection, long-course radiation therapy, and rectal surgery for locally advanced rectal cancer with synchronous liver metastases. Of these patients, 73 % completed the full treatment protocol and were alive after a median period of 19 months after completion of treatment (Verhoef et al. 2009). The authors argue that a 'patient-tailored' approach is warranted for optimal scheduling, taking into account the extent of metastatic liver disease and the stage of rectal cancer (van der Pool et al. 2010). Altogether, these studies demonstrate the clinical feasibility of a liver-first approach in metastatic rectal cancer. It is unknown, however, what patient categories benefit most from this approach and what the best scheduling of perioperative chemotherapy and radiation therapy is.

In conclusion, the present literature suggests a trend toward a comprehensive treatment approach of rectal cancer with synchronous liver metastases, in which the optimum treatments for both disease sites are combined efficiently and efficaciously. Such treatment approach may include revised schedules of preoperative chemotherapy and radiation therapy, as well as upfront liver resection. Further research needs to determine what approach is warranted in each individual patient, and, ultimately, how these strategies affect morbidity, mortality, radicality of resections, quality of life, and overall survival.

References

Adam R (2007) Colorectal cancer with synchronous liver metastases. Br J Surg 94:129–131

Adam R, Pascal G, Castaing D, Azoulay D, Delvart V, Paule B, Levi F, Bismuth H (2004) Tumor progression while on chemotherapy: a contraindication to liver resection for multiple colorectal metastases? Ann Surg 240:1052–1061

Adam R, Aloia T, Lévi F, Wicherts DA, de Haas RJ, Paule B, Bralet MP, Bouchahda M, Machover D, Ducreux M, Castagne V, Azoulay D, Castaing D (2007) Hepatic resection after rescue cetuximab treatment for colorectal liver metastases previously refractory to conventional systemic therapy. J Clin Oncol 25:4593–4602

Bajwa A, Blunt N, Vyas S, Suliman I, Bridgewater J, Hochhauser D, Ledermann JA, O'Bichere A (2009) Primary tumour resection and survival in the palliative management of metastatic colorectal cancer. Eur J Surg Oncol 35(2):164–167

Bengtsson G, Carlsson G, Hafstrom L, Jonsson PE (1981) Natural history of untreated patients with liver metastases from colorectal cancer. Am J Surg 141:586–589

Benoist S, Pautrat K, Mitry E et al (2005) Treatment strategy for patients with colorectal cancer and synchronous irresectable liver metastases. Br J Surg 92:1155–1160

Benoist S, Brouquet A, Penna C, Julié C, El Hajjam M, Chagnon S, Mitry E, Rougier P, Nordlinger B (2006) Complete response of colorectal liver metastases after chemotherapy: does it mean cure? J Clin Oncol 24:3939–3945

Blazer DG 3rd, Kishi Y, Maru DM, Kopetz S, Chun YS, Overman MJ, Fogelman D, Eng C, Chang DZ, Wang H, Zorzi D, Ribero D, Ellis LM, Glover KY, Wolff RA, Curley SA, Abdalla EK, Vauthey JN (2008) Pathologic response to preoperative chemotherapy: a new outcome end point after resection of hepatic colorectal metastases. J Clin Oncol 26:5344–5351

Borner MM, Dietrich D, Stupp R, Morant R, Honegger H, Wernli M et al (2002) Phase II study of capecitabine and oxaliplatin in first- and second-line treatment of advanced or metastatic colorectal cancer. J Clin Oncol 20:1759–1766

Boige V, Malka D, Elias D, Castaing M, De Baere T, Goere D, Dromain C, Pocard M, Ducreux M (2008) Hepatic arterial infusion of oxaliplatin and intravenous LV5FU2 in unresectable liver metastases from colorectal cancer after systemic chemotherapy failure. Ann Surg Oncol 15:219–226

Damjanov N, Weiss J, Haller DG (2009) Resection of the primary colorectal cancer is not necessary in nonobstructed patients with metastatic disease. Oncologist 14:963–969

De Bock K, Mazzone M, Carmeliet P (2011) Antiangiogenic therapy, hypoxia, and metastasis: risky liaisons, or not? Nat Rev Clin Oncol 8:393–404

de Jong MC, van Dam RM, Maas M, Bemelmans MH, Olde Damink SW, Beets GL, Dejong CH (2011) The liver-first approach for synchronous colorectal liver metastasis: a 5 year single-centre experience. HPB (Oxford) 13:745–52

Eisenberger A, Whelan RL, Neugut AI (2008) Survival and symptomatic benefit from palliative primary tumor resection in patients with metastatic colorectal cancer: a review. Int J Colorectal Dis 23:559–568

Evans MD, Escofet X, Karandikar SS, Stamatakis JD (2009) Outcomes of resection and non-resection strategies in management of patients with advanced colorectal cancer. World J Surg Oncol 7:28

Galizia G, Lieto E, Orditura M, Castellano P, Imperatore V, Pinto M et al (2008) First-line chemotherapy vs bowel tumor resection plus chemotherapy for patients with unresectable synchronous colorectal hepatic metastases. Arch Surg 143:352–358

Giacchi R, Sebastiani M, Lungarotti F (1988) Natural history of synchronous hepatic metastases from a non-treated colorectal cancer. J Chir 125:419–423

Grothey A, Sargent D (2005) Overall survival of patients with advanced colorectal cancer correlates with availability of fluorouracil, irinotecan, and oxaliplatin regardless of whether doublet or single-agent therapy is used first line. J Clin Oncol %20;23:9441–42

Hurwitz H, Fehrenbacher L, Novotny W, Cartwright T, Hainsworth J, Heim W et al (2004) Bevacizumab plus irinotecan, fluorouracil, and leucovorin for metastatic colorectal cancer. N Engl J Med 350:2335–2342

Jain RK (2005) Normalization of tumor vasculature: an emerging concept in antiangiogenic therapy. Science 307:58–62

Kabbinavar FF, Hambleton J, Mass RD, Hurwitz HI, Bergsland E, Sarkar S (2005) Combined analysis of efficacy: the addition of bevacizumab to fluorouracil/leucovorin improves survival for patients with metastatic colorectal cancer. J Clin Oncol 23:3706–3712

Karoui M, Koubaa W, Delbaldo C, Charachon A, Laurent A, Piedbois P et al (2008) Chemotherapy has also an effect on primary tumor in colon carcinoma. Ann Surg Oncol 15:3440–3446

Kopetz S, Chang GJ, Overman MJ, Eng C, Sargent DJ, Larson DW et al (2009) Improved survival in metastatic colorectal cancer is associated with adoption of hepatic resection and improved chemotherapy. J Clin Oncol 27:3677–3683

Lehmann K, Rickenbacher A, Weber A, Pestalozzi BC, Clavien PA (2012) Chemotherapy before liver resection of colorectal metastases: friend or foe? Ann Surg 255:237–247

Lo SS, Moffatt-Bruce S, Dawson LA, Schwarz RE, The BS, Mayr NA, Lu JJ, Grecula JC, Olencki TE, Timmerman RD (2011) The role of local therapy in the management of lung and liver oligometastases. Nat Rev Clin Oncol 8:405–416

Lyass S, Zamir G, Matot I, Goitein D, Eid A, Jurim O (2001) Combined colon and hepatic resection for synchronous colorectal liver metastases. J Surg Oncol 78:17–21

Mella J, Biffin A, Radcliffe AG et al (1997) Population-based audit of colorectal cancer management in two UK health regions. Colorectal cancer working group, Royal college of surgeons of England clinical epidemiology and audit unit. Br J Surg 84:1731–1736

Mentha G, Roth AD, Terraz S, Giostra E, Gervaz P, Andres A, Morel P, Rubbia-Brandt L, Majno PE (2008) 'Liver first' approach in the treatment of colorectal cancer with synchronous liver metastases. Dig Surg 25:430–435

Michel P, Roque I, Di FF et al (2004) Colorectal cancer with non-resectable synchronous metastases: should the primary tumor be resected? Gastroenterol Clin Biol 28:434–437

Millikan KW, Staren ED, Doolas A (1997) Invasive therapy of metastatic colorectal cancer to the liver. Surg Clin North Am 77:27–48

Muratore A, Zorzi D, Bouzari H et al (2007) Asymptomatic colorectal cancer with un-resectable liver metastases: immediate colorectal resection or up-front systemic chemotherapy? Ann Surg Oncol 14:766–770

O'Connell JB, Maggard MA, Ko CY (2004) Colon cancer survival rates with the new American joint committee on cancer sixth edition staging. J Natl Cancer Inst 96:1420–1425

Peeters CF, Westphal JR, de Waal RM, Ruiter DJ, Wobbes T, Ruers TJ (2004) Vascular density in colorectal liver metastases increases after removal of the primary tumor in human cancer patients. Int J Cancer 112:554–559

Peeters CF et al (2005) Decrease in circulating anti-angiogenic factors (angiostatin and endostatin) after surgical removal of primary colorectal carcinoma coincides with increased metabolic activity of liver metastases. Surgery 137:246–249

Peeters CF, De Waal RM, Wobbes T, Westphal JR, Ruers TJ (2006) Outgrowth of human liver metastases after resection of the primary colorectal tumor: a shift in the balance between apoptosis and proliferation. Int J Cancer 119:1249–1253

Poultsides GA, Servais EL, Saltz LB, Patil S, Kemeny NE, Guillem JG et al (2009) Outcome of primary tumor in patients with synchronous stage IV colorectal cancer receiving combination chemotherapy without surgery as initial treatment. J Clin Oncol 27:3379–3384

Reddy SK, Pawlik TM, Zorzi D, Gleisner AL, Ribero D, Assumpcao L, Barbas AS, Abdalla EK, Choti MA, Vauthey JN, Ludwig KA, Mantyh CR, Morse MA, Clary BM (2007) Simultaneous resections of colorectal cancer and synchronous liver metastases: a multi-institutional analysis. Ann Surg Oncol 14:3481–3491

Ruo L, Gougoutas C, Paty PB et al (2003) Elective bowel resection for incurable stage IV colorectal cancer: prognostic variables for asymptomatic patients. J Am Coll Surg 196:722–728

Sanoff HK, Sargent DJ, Campbell ME, Morton RF, Fuchs CS, Ramanathan RK et al (2008) Five-year data and prognostic factor analysis of oxaliplatin and irinotecan combinations for advanced colorectal cancer: N9741. J Clin Oncol 26:5721–5727

Sarela A, O'Riordain DS (2001) Rectal adenocarcinoma with liver metastases: management of the primary tumour. Br J Surg 88:163–164

Schmidt C (2009) Metastatic colorectal cancer: is surgery necessary? J Natl Cancer Inst 101:1113–1115

Scoggins CR, Meszoely IM, Blanke CD et al (1999) Nonoperative management of primary colorectal cancer in patients with stage IV disease. Ann Surg Oncol 6:651–657

Scheithauer W, Kornek GV, Raderer M, Schoell B, Schmid K, Kovats E, Schneeweiss B, Lang F, Lenauer A, Depisch D (2003) Randomized multicenter phase II trial of two different schedules of capecitabine plus oxaliplatin as first-line treatment in advanced colorectal cancer. J Clin Oncol 21:1307–1312

Scheer MG, Sloots CE, van der Wilt GJ, Ruers TJ (2008) Management of patients with asymptomatic colorectal cancer and synchronous irresectable metastases. Ann Oncol 19(11):1829–35. (Epub 28 Jul 2008, Review)

Shields AF, Zalupski MM, Marshall JL, Meropol NJ (2004) Treatment of advanced colorectal carcinoma with oxaliplatin and capecitabine: a phase II trial. Cancer 100:531–537

Simmonds PC, Primrose JN, Colquitt JL, Garden OJ, Poston GJ, Rees M (2006) Surgical resection of hepatic metastases from colorectal cancer: a systematic review of published studies. Br J Cancer 94:982–999

Stillwell AP, Buettner PG, Ho YH (2010) Meta-analysis of survival of patients with stage IV colorectal cancer managed with surgical resection versus chemotherapy alone. World J Surg 34(4):797–807

Tebbutt NC, Norman AR, Cunningham D et al (2003) Intestinal complications after chemotherapy for patients with unresected primary colorectal cancer and synchronous metastases. Gut 52:568–573

Thelen A, Jonas S, Benckert C, Spinelli A, Lopez-Hänninen E, Rudolph B, Neumann U, Neuhaus P (2007) Simultaneous versus staged liver resection of synchronous liver metastases from colorectal cancer. Int J Colorectal Dis 22:1269–1276

Turrini O, Viret F, Guiramand J, Lelong B, Bège T, Delpero JR (2007) Strategies for the treatment of synchronous liver metastasis. Eur J Surg Oncol 33:735–740

van der Pool AE, de Wilt JH, Lalmahomed ZS, Eggermont AM, Ijzermans JN, Verhoef C (2010) Optimizing the outcome of surgery in patients with rectal cancer and synchronous liver metastases. Br J Surg 97:383–390

Van Dijk TH, Havenga K, Beukema J, Beets GL, Gelderblom H, de Jong KP, Rutten HJ, Van De Velde CJ, Wiggers T, Hospers G (2010) Short-course radiation therapy, neoadjuvant bevacizumab, capecitabine and oxaliplatin, and radical resection of primary tumor and metastases in primary stage IV rectal cancer: a phase II multicenter study of the Dutch colorectal cancer group. ASCO Meeting Abstract: J Clin Oncol 28:15s (suppl; abstr 3638)

Vassiliou I, Arkadopoulos N, Theodosopoulos T, Fragulidis G, Marinis A, Kondi-Paphiti A, Samanides L, Polydorou A, Gennatas C, Voros D, Smyrniotis V (2007) Surgical approaches of resectable synchronous colorectal liver metastases: timing considerations. World J Gastroenterol 13:1431–1434

Verhoef C, van der Pool AE, Nuyttens JJ, Planting AS, Eggermont AM, de Wilt JH (2009) The "liver-first approach" for patients with locally advanced rectal cancer and synchronous liver metastases. Dis Colon Rectum 52:23–30

Wagner JS, Adson MA, Van Heerden JA, Adson MH, Ilson DM (1984) The natural history of hepatic metastases from colorectal cancer. Ann Surg 199:205–208

Weber JC, Bachellier P, Oussoultzoglou E, Jaeck D (2003) Simultaneous resection of colorectal primary tumour and synchronous liver metastases. Br J Surg 90:956–962

Willett CG, Boucher Y, di Tomaso E, Duda DG, Munn LL, Tong RT, Chung DC, Sahani DV, Kalva SP, Kozin SV, Mino M, Cohen KS, Scadden DT, Hartford AC, Fischman AJ, Clark JW, Ryan DP, Zhu AX, Blaszkowsky LS, Chen HX, Shellito PC, Lauwers GY, Jain RK (2004) Direct evidence that the VEGF-specific antibody bevacizumab has antivascular effects in human rectal cancer. Nat Med 10:145–147

Wood CB, Gillis CR, Blumgart LH (1976) A retrospective study of the natural history of patients with liver metastases from colorectal cancer. Clin Oncol 2:285–288

Part II
Improving Treatment of Pancreatic Cancer

Pancreatic Surgery: Beyond the Traditional Limits

Sascha A. Müller, Ignazio Tarantino, David J. Martin and Bruno M. Schmied

Abstract

Pancreatic cancer is one of the five leading causes of cancer death for both males and females in the western world. More than 85 % pancreatic tumors are of ductal origin but the incidence of cystic tumors such as intrapapillary mucinous tumors (IPMN) or mucinous cystic tumors (MCN) and other rare tumors is rising. Complete surgical resection of the tumor is the mainstay of any curative therapeutic approach, however, up to 40 % of patients with potentially resectable pancreatic cancer are not offered surgery. This is despite 5-year survival rates of up to 40 % or even higher in selected patients depending on tumor stage and histology. Standard procedures for pancreatic tumors include the Kausch-Whipple- or pylorus-preserving Whipple procedure, and the left lateral pancreatic resection (often with splenectomy), and usually include regional lymphadenectomy. More radical or extended pancreatic operations are becoming increasingly utilised however and we examine the data available for their role. These operations include major venous and arterial resection, multivisceral resections and surgery for metastatic disease, or palliative pancreatic resection. Portal vein resection for local infiltration with or without replacement graft is now well established and does not deleteriously affect perioperative morbidity or mortality. Arterial resection, however, though often technically feasible, has questionable oncologic impact, is not without risk and

---

S. A. Müller · I. Tarantino · B. M. Schmied (✉)
Department of Surgery, Kantonsspital St. Gallen (KSSG),
Rorschacherstrasse 95, 9007 St. Gallen, Switzerland
e-mail: Bruno.schmied@kssg.ch

D. J. Martin
Concord and Royal Prince Alfred Hospitals, University of Sydney,
Sydney, Australia

F. Otto and M. P. Lutz (eds.), *Early Gastrointestinal Cancers*,
Recent Results in Cancer Research 196, DOI: 10.1007/978-3-642-31629-6_4,
© Springer-Verlag Berlin Heidelberg 2012

is usually reserved for isolated cases. The value of extended lymphadenectomy is frequently debated; the recent level I evidence demonstrates no advantage. Multivisceral resections, i.e. tumors, often in the tail of the pancreas, with invasion of the colon or stomach or other surrounding tissues, while associated with an increased morbidity and a longer hospital stay, do however show comparable mortality—and survival rates to those without such infiltration and therefore should be performed if technically feasible. Routine resection for metastatic disease however does not seem to show any advantage over palliative treatment but may be an option in selected patients with easily removable metastases. In conclusion pancreatic surgery beyond the traditional limits is established in tumors infiltration the venous system and may be a considered approach in selected patients with locally infiltrating pancreatic cancer or metastasis.

Contents

1	Introduction	54
2	Portal/Mesenteric Vein Resection	55
3	Arterial Resection	56
4	Extended Lymphadenectomy	57
5	Multivisceral Resection	58
6	Resection for M1 PDAC	58
7	Surgery for Recurrent PDAC	59
8	Pancreatic Parenchyma Sparing Procedures	59
9	Conclusion	60
	References	61

1   Introduction

Pancreatic Ductal Adenocarcinoma (PDAC) is a highly malignant carcinoma, making it one of the five leading causes of cancer-related death (Jemal et al. 2011). More than 85 % pancreatic tumors are of ductal origin but the incidence of cystic tumors such as intrapapillary mucinous tumors (IPMN) or mucinous cystic tumors (MCN) and other rare tumors is rising. Unfortunately, owing to late presentation of symptoms, only 10–20 % of patients suffering from PDAC are candidates for surgical resection, which remains the only theoretical chance for cure (Bold et al. 1999; Wagner et al. 2004). Factors contributing to the low resectability rate at presentation include liver metastases, extensive lymph node involvement, and invasion of retroperitoneal tissue, the superior mesenteric artery (SMA), the celiac axis, or the superior mesenteric-portal vein region. Preoperative evaluation of operability in locally advanced tumors is still a challenge regarding best prognosis and quality of life in patients with PDAC. Standard resections for curative tumour resection are the pancreaticoduodenectomy for pancreatic head tumors, distal pancreatic resection with splenectomy for pancreas tail tumours or total pancreatectomy (Diener et al.

2007; Tran et al. 2004; Müller et al. 2007). Improvements in surgical techniques, anesthetic protocols, and medical management, have significantly improved outcomes for patients undergoing pancreatic cancer surgery with mortality rates of <5 % (Koniaris et al. 2005; Büchler et al. 2003; Hartwig et al. 2011; Birkmeyer et al. 2007) and morbidity rates of 30–60 % (Büchler et al. 2003; Stojadinovic et al. 2003; Strasberg et al. 1997). Due to the improved mortality rates, pancreatic surgeons have explored more locally aggressive operations including additional venous and/or arterial vascular resection as well as extended lymphadenectomy or removal of adjacent vessels/organs in terms of multivisceral surgery and even metastatectomies (Glanemann et al. 2008; Shrikhande et al. 2010). In addition, over the last decade efforts have been directed toward the development of adjuvant and neoadjuvant therapy concepts to improve outcome leading to 5-year survival rates of merely 20–25 % (Cameron et al. 2006; Gillen et al. 2010; Werner and Büchler 2011). Whereas adjuvant chemotherapy has proven to be advantageous in terms of prolonging overall survival (Neoptolemos et al. 2004), neoadjuvant treatment regimens, and adjuvant chemoradiation are still controversially discussed, with large randomized controlled trials required for further evaluation (Kleeff et al. 2007a; Märten et al. 2009; Bickenbach et al. 2011). Habermehl et al. recently published data of 215 patients with locally advanced PDAC who received neoadjuvant gemcitabine-based chemoradiation (median dose 52.2 Gy) (Habermehl et al. 2012). In this study, 26 % of primary unresectable locally advanced PDAC were chosen to undergo secondary resection. A R0-resection could be achieved in 39.2 % of these patients. Importantly, patients with complete resection after chemoradiation had a significantly increased median overall survival with 22.1 compared to 11.9 months in non-resected patients (Habermehl et al. 2012). The aim of this report is to review pancreatic cancer surgery beyond the traditional limits addressing extended surgical resections and techniques.

2 Portal/Mesenteric Vein Resection

PV involvement with the tumor is very common in PDAC, because of its anatomical site and infiltrative characteristics (Horton and Fishman 2002; Buchs et al. 2010). It is not a predictor of aggressive tumor biology, but rather a reflection of tumor size and location (Cusack et al. 1994; Fuhrman et al. 1994; Shimada et al. 2006). Infiltration of major veins in locally resectable tumors is no longer considered to be a contraindication if the surgeon considers that venous resection and reconstruction results in a margin negative resection (Weitz et al. 2007; Siriwardana et al. 2006; Harrison et al. 1996; Shibata et al. 2001). Although venous resection has been reported in up to 20 % of pancreaticoduodenectomies at high-volume pancreatic surgery centers (Tseng et al. 2004; Yekebas et al. 2008; Müller et al. 2009), the belief in the usefulness of venous resection is still controversial reflected by remarkable differences between experienced US centers (range: 3–38 %) (Tseng et al. 2004; Bachellier et al. 2011). Limited venous ingrowth is generally treated with a tangential wedge resection with reconstruction completed by primary lateral venorrhaphy or a patch. In presence of more extensive venous ingrowth, a segmental resection is performed and reconstructed with a primary end-to-end anastomosis, or by using an autologous venous or prosthetic graft. Interestingly, up to 50 % of tumors thought to have vascular invasion intraoperatively have been found to have only peritumoral inflammation extending to the vessel wall after histologic examination (Müller et al. 2009; Riediger et al. 2006; Carrère et al. 2007). A review by Siriwardana et al. based on 52 studies with 1646 patients, revealed that while the procedure could be performed with reasonable morbidity (42 %) and mortality (6 %), the benefit in terms of overall survival was lacking (median survival of patients with venous resection was 13 months, and 1-, 3-, and 5-year survival rates were 50, 16, and 7 %, respectively) (Siriwardana et al. 2006). In addition, Fukuda et al. reported that a deeper portal invasion was associated with a poorer survival rate, similar to that of patients undergoing non-curative resection (Fukuda et al. 2007). Recently, we published a series with 110 patients undergoing pancreatoduodenectomy and venous resection (Müller et al. 2009). The median survival was 14.5 months (range: 7.3–24 months). The 1-, 2-, and 3-year survival rates were 55.2, 23.1, and 14.4 % respectively. No significant difference in survival was seen between patients who had venous resection with histologically confirmed tumor infiltration and patients who had venous resection with suspected tumor infiltration ($p = 0.65$). In conclusion, additional venous resection does not influence the general morbidity or mortality rates during pancreatoduodenectomy and can therefore successfully be performed in order to achieve tumor free margins.

3 Arterial Resection

A more controversial area concerns an infiltration of the hepatic artery, the superior mesenteric artery, and of the celiac trunk. Arterial resection has traditionally been considered as a contraindication to pancreatic resection for PDAC because arteries are closely related to the neural and lymphatic plexuses that imply that the disease is usually metastatic by the time the arteries are involved. In a systemic review including 1.646 patients from 52 studies, only 7.1 % of patients had adjacent arterial resection (common hepatic artery, superior mesenteric artery, and celiac axis as most common arterial resections) showing that the resistance to perform arterial resection is strong (Siriwardana et al. 2006). Nevertheless, pancreatic resections with major arterial resection have increasingly been reported for advanced tumors stages (Bockhorn et al. 2011; Stitzenberg et al. 2008; Wu et al. 2007; Hirano et al. 2007; Gagandeep et al. 2006). It comes not as a surprise that morbidity and mortality rates were higher compared to standard pancreatic resections, although all series were small and follow-up data were rarely available. In this context celiac or hepatic invasion, discovered intraoperatively, can be the object of a resection and a reconstruction, either by direct anastomosis, by interposition of an autologous arterial or venous graft or by using prosthesis. This is sustained by Hirano et al., who reported a high R0 resectability rate (91 %) with distal pancreatectomy and en bloc celiac axis resection. In his series a mortality rate of 0 %, and an estimated 5-year survival rate of 42 % was reported (Hirano et al. 2007). Yekebas et al. reported that patients with arterial resection had a similar median survival (15 months) to those without arterial resection, without increasing morbidity or mortality (Yekebas et al. 2008). Bachellier et al. could recently show that pancreatic resection with arterial resection for locally advanced PDAC can be performed safely with survival rates similar to those achieved for a comparable group of patients with locally advanced PDAC not requiring arterial resection (Bachellier et al. 2011). They conclude that arterial resection should not be considered by itself as a contraindication to pancreatic resection. Recently, Mollberg et al. published a meta-analysis including 26 studies with 366 and 2243 patients who underwent pancreatectomy with and without arterial resection (Mollberg et al. 2011). Pancreatectomy with concomitant arterial resection was associated with poor perioperative outcome and long-term survival confirming that arterial resection is generally a contraindication in pancreatic cancer surgery. The survival benefit offered by pancreatic resections with arterial resection compared to palliative therapy without tumor resection may, however, justify arterial resection in highly selected patients.

4   Extended Lymphadenectomy

Up to 30 % of patients with PDAC have retroperitoneal lymph node involvement that would not be resected by a standard pancreatoduodenectomy (Reddy et al. 2007). Because of the dismal prognosis of PDAC, extended radical lymphadenectomy for partial pancreaticoduodenectomy has been the subject of much discussion for decades (Fortner 1973; Rupp and Linehan 2009). The rationale for pancreatoduodenectomy with extended radical lymphadenectomy is based on the high incidence of intra- and extrapancreatic neural invasion (65 %) in PDAC, as well as the high incidence of lymphnode metastases (30–75 %) (Nakao et al. 1996). Many RCT evaluating extended versus standard lymphadenectomy were published and failed to show any survival benefit (Pedrazzoli et al. 1998; Yeo et al. 1999; Farnell et al. 2005; Reiser-Erkan et al. 2008; Nimura et al. 2011). Recently, there have been 2 meta-analyses published addressing this issue (Michalski et al. 2007; Iqbal et al. 2009). Michalski et al. included 3 randomized trials on standard ($n = 159$) and extended lymphadenectomy ($n = 160$) in pancreatic cancer. Overall, no significant differences in survival were found, whereas morbidity tended to be higher in the extended group (increased rates of delayed gastric emptying). The second meta-analysis confirmed these results showing that the extended procedure did not have an impact on overall survival.

5 Multivisceral Resection

To obtain complete removal of pancreatic cancer, surgeons have started to perform en bloc resections including the removal of adjacent organs, which are infiltrated by the pancreatic tumor (Hartwig et al. 2009; Nikfarjam et al. 2009). Not surprisingly, morbidity following such procedures has been shown to vary between 35–68 % while mortality ranged from 0–3 % (Hartwig et al. 2009; Nikfarjam et al. 2009; Sasson et al. 2002). 5-year overall survival rates have been shown to be between 16 and 22 % (Sasson et al. 2002; Shoup et al. 2003) with one study even reporting a 10-year disease-specific survival rate of 18 % (Shoup et al. 2003). In the largest series available to date ($n = 101$), Hartwig et al. showed a significantly increased surgical morbidity but not mortality rate in multivisceral resected patients (Hartwig et al. 2009). The evaluation of long-term survival showed a median survival of 19.8 months in patients with multivisceral resections, which was comparable to the survival after standard resections in the Heidelberg collective (Hartwig et al. 2009). The survival rates for 1-, 2-, and 3-years were 69.5, 42.7, and 37.2 %, respectively. Considering the high morbidity rate patients who qualify for multivisceral pancreatic resections should be well selected.

6 Resection for M1 PDAC

The presence of distant metastases in patients with PDAC has generally been an absolute contraindication for resection. There is only little information about outcomes after resection of metastatic PDAC (Shrikhande et al. 2007; Yamada et al. 2006). Shrikhande et al. reported of 29 patients who underwent pancreatic resection with resection of associated metastatic disease (interaortocaval lymph node dissection, liver resection, and/or multiorgan resections) (Shrikhande et al. 2007). The overall in-hospital mortality and morbidity of R0/R1 pancreatic resections for M1 disease ($n = 29$) was 0 and 24.1 %, compared with 4.2 and 35.2 % of R0/R1 pancreatic resections for M0 disease ($n = 287$). The median overall survival time was 13.8 months (95 % confidence interval [CI], 11.4–20.5), and the estimated 1-year overall survival rate was 58.9 % (95 % CI, 34.8–76.7) for patients with M1 disease. The median overall survival in those with metastatic interaortocaval lymph nodes was 27 months (95 % CI, 9.6–27.0), whereas it was 11.4 months (95 % CI, 7.8–16.5), and 12.9 months (95 % CI, 7.2–20.5) for those with liver and peritoneal metastases, respectively. A systematic review by Michalski et al. focussed on pancreatic cancer with associated liver metastasis resection (Michalski et al. 2008). Three case reports and 18 studies were included ($n = 103$ patients). Morbidity and mortality ranged from 24.1 to 26 % and from 0 to 4.3 %, respectively. Median overall survival ranged between 5.8 and 11.4 months. In summary, resection of liver metastasis for locally resectable pancreatic cancer might be performed in selected cases. Overall survival in patients with only one or few liver metastases that are concomitantly resected seems to be comparable to patients without evident metastasis.

7 Surgery for Recurrent PDAC

Local recurrence in the remnant pancreas, multiple liver metastases, and peritoneal dissemination frequently occur after curative resection (Hishinuma et al. 2006; Van den Brock et al. 2009). The high local recurrence rate is caused by the fact that even after macroscopically curative tumor resection, malignant cells are observed on the edge of resected specimens in up to 50 % of patients (Smeenk et al. 2005). Sperti et al. analyzed 78 patients after resection for PDAC (Sperti et al. 1997) and found that 72 % of all patients developed local recurrence and 62 % hepatic metastases. The chance for repeated pancreatectomy for PDAC developing in the remnant pancreas is quite low (Takamatsu et al. 2005; Kleeff et al. 2007a; Dalla Valle et al. 2006; Ogino et al. 2010). The largest series focussing on reoperation for recurrent disease was published by Kleeff et al. (2007a). In this study, 30 patients underwent radical resection with curative intent (R0/R1), R2 resection, palliative bypass, or only explorative laparotomy depending on the extent of the disease (Kleeff et al. 2007a). The median disease-free time (time span between the primary tumor resection and the operation for the recurrent tumor) was 12.0 months. Patients with late onset of recurrence (later than 9 months after initial resection) were more likely to benefit from re-resection with a median overall survival of 17.0 months compared with 7.4 months in patients with recurrence within <9 months ($p = 0.0038$). Furthermore, in patients younger than 65 years showed a tendency to benefit more from re-operation with a median overall survival of 11.6 months versus 7.8 months in patients older than 65 years ($p = 0.16$). In summary, resection for recurrent pancreatic cancer does not seem to substantially prolong overall survival. Nevertheless, repeated pancreatectomy may provide a chance of long-term survival if the recurrence of PDAC is limited to the remnant pancreas.

8 Pancreatic Parenchyma Sparing Procedures

Pancreatic pathologies localized in the pancreatic neck or body are usually removed by partial pancreatoduodenectomy or distal pancreatectomy. However, these procedures, despite low mortality, result in a significant loss of normal glandular tissue, potentially leading to endocrine and exocrine pancreatic dysfunction. The incidence of diabetes mellitus following pancreatoduodenectomy varies between 15 and 40 % (Martin et al. 1996; Beger and Büchler 1989). This rate is even higher in patients after distal pancreatectomy (up to 72 %) (Morrow et al. 1984). Benign tumors, including cystic lesions and endocrine tumors, do not necessarily require extensive pancreatic resections to achieve surgical cure (Talamini et al. 1998; Pitt et al. 2009). Therefore, parenchyma-sparing procedures such as enucleation or segmental pancreatectomy are more frequently performed in small benign or low-grade malignant tumors diseases (i.e. endocrine and cystic neoplasms of the pancreas such as branch-duct IPMN) (Sperti et al. 2010). Small

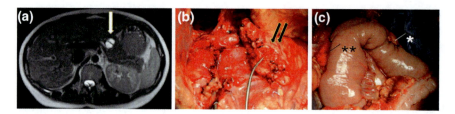

Fig. 1 Pancreatic neuroendocrine tumor in a 30-year-old woman with history of recurrent abdominal pain. **a** axial MRI shows a cystic tumor (*arrow*) at the pancreatic neck, near the superior mesenteric-splenic vein confluence. **b** Patient was treated with a segmental (*central*) pancreatectomy and regional lymphadenectomy (lymph node groups 8a, 9, 11, and 18 according to the Japanese Pancreas Society, 2009); probe intubates pancreatic tail duct (*double arrow*). **c** Reconstruction with a retrocolic Roux limb to the 2-layer, end-to-side pancreaticojejunostomy (*star*). Completed reconstruction with seromuscular patch of jejunum covering the stapled surface of the right pancreas (*double star*)

non-malignant tumors in particular can be treated with limited and parenchyma-sparing enucleations. Nevertheless, complications like pancreatic fistula (in up to 50 %), pseudocysts, or acute pancreatitis are common (Talamini et al. 1998; Pyke et al. 1992; Hackert et al. 2011). Neoplasms of the mid portion of the pancreas not suitable for enucleation because of the risk of injury to the main pancreatic duct can be treated with segmental pancreatectomy (Fig. 1). The rationale for this technique is to remove the neoplasm, preserve functional parenchyma, and avoid a major resection such as pancreatoduodenectomy or left splenopancreatectomy. Despite a higher incidence of pancreatic fistula, segmental pancreatectomy is a safe and an adequate operation in selected patients with centrally placed benign or even low-malignant-potential lesions of the pancreas (Talamini et al. 1998; Müller et al. 2006; Shah et al. 2009). The major advantage of segmental resection is the preservation of the exocrine and endocrine pancreatic function. Thus, parenchyma-sparing procedures should be performed whenever possible.

9 Conclusion

Available data on extended pancreatic resections for PDAC indicates that such major procedures are technically feasible and can be done with reasonable morbidity and mortality. However, the benefit of such surgery on more important variables such as overall survival and quality of life is often lacking. Extended resections beyond the traditional limits should only be performed in experienced pancreatic centers with a careful evaluation of each patients risk benefit ratio. Since no other appropriate treatment modalities are available to ameliorate the outcome of patients with advanced pancreatic disease, surgeons are asked to go beyond the traditional limits. Standard pancreatoduodenectomy and lymphadenectomy with venous resection when indicated is still the classic surgical procedure for PDAC in the pancreatic head. For those patients with small benign or

Pancreatic Surgery: Beyond the Traditional Limits

low-grade malignant lesions located in the pancreas, segmental resection or enucleation is emerging as a safe and effective option with acceptable morbidity and a low risk for development of exocrine and/or endocrine insufficiency.

References

Bachellier P, Rosso E, Lucescu I et al (2011) Is the need for an arterial resection a contraindication to pancreatic resection for locally advanced pancreatic adenocarcinoma? A case-matched controlled study. J Surg Oncol 103:75–84

Beger HG, Büchler M (1989) Chronic pancreatitis: indications and successes of surgical therapy. Z Gastroenterol Verh 24:107–110

Bickenbach KA, Gonen M, Tang LH et al. (2011) Downstaging in pancreatic cancer: a matched analysis of patients resected following systemic treatment of initially locally unresectable disease. Ann Surg Oncol Dec 1. [Epub ahead of print]

Birkmeyer JD, Sun Y, Wong SL et al (2007) Hospital volume and late survival after cancer surgery. Ann Surg 245:777–783

Bockhorn M, Burdelski C, Bogoevski D et al (2011) Arterial en bloc resection for pancreatic carcinoma. Br J Surg 98:86–92

Bold RJ, Charnsangavej C, Cleary KR (1999) Major vascular resection as part of pancreaticoduodenectomy for cancer: radiologic, intraoperative, and pathologic analysis. J Gastrointest Surg 3:233–243

Büchler MW, Wagner M, Schmied BM et al (2003) Changes in morbidity after pancreatic resection: toward the end of completion pancreatectomy. Arch Surg 138:1310–1314 discussion 1315

Buchs NC, Chilcott M, Poletti P-A et al (2010) Vascular invasion in pancreatic cancer: Imaging modalities, preoperative diagnosis and surgical management. World J Gastroenterol 21(16):818–831

Cameron JL, Riall TS, Coleman J et al (2006) One thousand consecutive pancreaticoduodenectomies. Ann Surg 244:10–15

Carrère N, Abid S, Julio CH et al (2007) Spleen-preserving distal pancreatectomy with excision of splenic artery and vein: a case-matched comparison with conventional distal pancreatectomy with splenectomy. World J Surg 31:375–382

Cusack JC Jr, Fuhrman GM, Lee JE et al (1994) Managing unsuspected tumor invasion of the superior mesenteric-portal venous confluence during pancreaticoduodenectomy. Am J Surg 168:352–354

Dalla Valle R, Mancini C, Crafa P et al (2006) Pancreatic carcinoma recurrence in the remnant pancreas after a pancreaticoduodenectomy. JOP 7:473–477

Diener MK, Knaebel H-P, Heukaufer C et al (2007) A systematic review and meta-analysis of pylorus-preserving versus classical pancreaticoduodenectomy for surgical treatment of periampullary and pancreatic carcinoma. Ann Surg 245:187–200

Farnell MB, Pearson RK, Sarr MG et al (2005) A prospective randomized trial comparing standard pancreatoduodenectomy with pancreatoduodenectomy with extended lymphadenectomy in resectable pancreatic head adenocarcinoma. Surgery 138:618–628 discussion 628–630

Fortner JG (1973) Regional resection of cancer of the pancreas: a new surgical approach. Surgery 73:307–320

Fukuda S, Oussoultzoglou E, Bachellier P et al (2007) Significance of the depth of portal vein wall invasion after curative resection for pancreatic adenocarcinoma. Arch Surg 142:172–179

Fuhrman GM, Charnsangavej C, Abbruzzese JL et al (1994) Thin-section contrast-enhanced computed tomography accurately predicts the resectability of malignant pancreatic neoplasms. Am J Surg 167:104–111 discussion 111–113

Gagandeep S, Artinyan A, Jabbour N et al (2006) Extended pancreatectomy with resection of the celiac axis: the modified Apple by operation. Am J Surg 192:330–335

Gillen S, Schuster T, Meyer ZBC et al (2010) Preoperative/neoadjuvant therapy in pancreatic cancer: a systematic review and meta-analysis of response and resection percentages. PLoS Med 7(4):e1000267

Glanemann M, Shi B, Liang F et al (2008) Surgical strategies for treatment of malignant pancreatic tumors: extended, standard or local surgery? World J Surg Oncol 6:123

Habermehl D, Kessel K, Welzel T et al (2012) Neoadjuvant chemoradiation with gemcitabine for locally advanced pancreatic cancer. Radiat Oncol 2(7):28

Hackert T, Hinz U, Fritz S et al (2011) Enucleation in pancreatic surgery: indications, technique, and outcome compared to standard pancreatic resections. Langenbecks Arch Surg 396:1197–1203

Harrison LE, Klimstra DS, Brennan MF (1996) Isolated portal vein involvement in pancreatic adenocarcinoma. A contraindication for resection? Ann Surg 224:342–347

Hartwig W, Hackert T, Hinz U et al (2009) Multivisceral resection for pancreatic malignancies: risk-analysis and long-term outcome. Ann Surg 250:81–87

Hartwig W, Hackert T, Hinz U et al (2011) Pancreatic cancer surgery in the new millennium: better prediction of outcome. Ann Surg 254:311–319

Hirano S, Kondo S, Hara T et al (2007) Distal pancreatectomy with en bloc celiac axis resection for locally advanced pancreatic body cancer: long-term results. Ann Surg 246:46–51

Hishinuma S, Ogata Y, Tomikawa M et al (2006) Patterns of recurrence after curative resection of pancreatic cancer, based on autopsy findings. J Gastrointest Surg 10:511–518

Horton KM, Fishman EK (2002) Multidetector CT angiography of pancreatic carcinoma: part 2, evaluation of venous involvement. AJR Am J Roentgenol 178:833–836

Iqbal N, Lovegrove RE, Tilney HS et al (2009) A comparison of pancreaticoduodenectomy with extended pancreaticoduodenectomy: a meta-analysis of 1909 patients. Eur J Surg Oncol 35:79–86

Jemal A, Bray F, Center MM et al (2011) Global cancer statistics. CA Cancer J Clin 61:69–90

Kleeff J, Michalski CW, Friess H et al (2007a) Surgical treatment of pancreatic cancer: the role of adjuvant and multimodal therapies. Eur J Surg Oncol 33:817–823

Kleeff J, Reiser C, Hinz U et al (2007b) Surgery for recurrent pancreatic ductal adenocarcinoma. Ann Surg 245:566–572

Koniaris LG, Staveley-O'Carroll KF, Zeh HJ et al (2005) Pancreaticoduodenectomy in the presence of superior mesenteric venous obstruction. J Gastrointest Surg 9:915–921

Märten A, Schmidt J, Ose J et al (2009) A randomized multicentre phase II trial comparing adjuvant therapy in patients with interferon alpha-2b and 5-FU alone or in combination with either external radiation treatment and cisplatin (CapRI) or radiation alone regarding event-free survival—CapRI-2. BMC Cancer 9:160

Martin RF, Rossi RL, Leslie KA (1996) Long-term results of pylorus-preserving pancreatoduodenectomy for chronic pancreatitis. Arch Surg 131:247–252

Michalski CW, Kleeff J, Wente MN et al (2007) Systematic review and meta-analysis of standard and extended lymphadenectomy in pancreaticoduodenectomy for pancreatic cancer. Br J Surg 94:265–273

Michalski CW, Erkan M, Hüser N et al (2008) Resection of primary pancreatic cancer and liver metastasis: a systematic review. Dig Surg 25:473–480

Mollberg N, Rahbari NN, Koch M et al (2011) Arterial resection during pancreatectomy for pancreatic cancer: a systematic review and meta-analysis. Ann Surg 254:882–893

Morrow CE, Cohen JI, Sutherland DE et al (1984) Chronic pancreatitis: long-term surgical results of pancreatic duct drainage, pancreatic resection, and near-total pancreatectomy and islet autotransplantation. Surgery 96:608–616

Müller MW, Friess H, Kleeff J et al (2006) Middle segmental pancreatic resection: an option to treat benign pancreatic body lesions. Ann Surg 244:909–918 discussion 918–920

Müller MW, Friess H, Kleeff J et al (2007) Is there still a role for total pancreatectomy? Ann Surg 246:966–974 discussion 974–975

Müller SA, Hartel M, Mehrabi A et al (2009) Vascular resection in pancreatic cancer surgery: survival determinants. J Gastrointest Surg 13:784–792

Nakao A, Harada A, Nonami T et al (1996) Clinical significance of carcinoma invasion of the extrapancreatic nerve plexus in pancreatic cancer. Pancreas 12:357–361

Neoptolemos JP, Stocken DD, Friess H et al (2004) A randomized trial of chemoradiotherapy and chemotherapy after resection of pancreatic cancer. N Engl J Med 18(350):1200–1210

Nikfarjam M, Sehmbey M, Kimchi ET et al (2009) Additional organ resection combined with pancreaticoduodenectomy does not increase postoperative morbidity and mortality. J Gastrointest Surg 13:915–921

Nimura Y, Nagino M, Takao S et al. (2011) Standard versus extended lymphadenectomy in radical pancreatoduodenectomy for ductal adenocarcinoma of the head of the pancreas: long-term results of a Japanese multicenter randomized controlled trial. J Hepatobiliary Pancreat Sci 2011 Oct 25. [Epub ahead of print]

Ogino T, Ueda J, Sato N et al (2010) Repeated pancreatectomy for recurrent pancreatic carcinoma after pylorus-preserving pancreatoduodenectomy: report of two patients. Case Rep Gastroenterol 4:429–434

Pedrazzoli S, DiCarlo V, Dionigi R et al (1998) Standard versus extended lymphadenectomy associated with pancreatoduodenectomy in the surgical treatment of adenocarcinoma of the head of the pancreas: a multicenter, prospective, randomized study. Lymphadenectomy Study Group. Ann Surg 228:508–517

Pitt SC, Pitt HA, Baker MS et al (2009) Small pancreatic and periampullary neuroendocrine tumors: resect or enucleate? J Gastrointest Surg 13:1692–1698

Pyke CM, van Heerden JA, Colby TV et al (1992) The spectrum of serous cystadenoma of the pancreas. Clinical, pathologic, and surgical aspects. Ann Surg 215:132–139

Reddy SK, Tyler DS, Pappas TN et al (2007) Extended resection for pancreatic adenocarcinoma. Oncologist 12:654–663

Reiser-Erkan C, Gaa J, Kleeff J (2008) T1 pancreatic cancer with lymph node metastasis and perineural invasion of the celiac trunk. Clin Gastroenterol Hepatol 6:e41–e42

Riediger H, Makowiec F, Fischer E et al (2006) Postoperative morbidity and long-term survival after pancreaticoduodenectomy with superior mesenterico-portal vein resection. J Gastrointest Surg 10:1106–1115

Rupp CC, Linehan DC (2009) Extended lymphadenectomy in the surgery of pancreatic adenocarcinoma and its relation to quality improvement issues. J Surg Oncol 15(99):207–214

Sasson AR, Hoffman JP, Ross EA et al (2002) En bloc resection for locally advanced cancer of the pancreas: is it worthwhile? J Gastrointest Surg 6:147–157 discussion 157–158

Shah OJ, Robbani I, Nazir P et al (2009) Central pancreatectomy: a new technique for resection of selected pancreatic tumors. HBPD INT 8:93–96

Shibata C, Kobari M, Tsuchiya T et al (2001) Pancreatectomy combined with superior mesenteric-portal vein resection for adenocarcinoma in pancreas. World J Surg 25:1002–1005

Shimada K, Sano T, Sakamoto Y et al (2006) Clinical implications of combined portal vein resection as a palliative procedure in patients undergoing pancreaticoduodenectomy for pancreatic head carcinoma. Ann Surg Oncol 13:1569–1578

Shoup M, Conlon KC, Klimstra D et al (2003) Is extended resection for adenocarcinoma of the body or tail of the pancreas justified? J Gastrointest Surg 7:946–952 discussion 952

Shrikhande SV, Barreto SG (2010) Extended pancreatic resections and lymphadenectomy: an appraisal of the current evidence. World J Gastrointest Surg 27(2):39–46

Shrikhande SV, Kleeff J, Reiser C et al (2007) Pancreatic resection for M1 pancreatic ductal adenocarcinoma. Ann Surg Oncol 14:118–127

Siriwardana HPP, Siriwardena AK (2006) Systematic review of outcome of synchronous portal-superior mesenteric vein resection during pancreatectomy for cancer. Br J Surg 93:662–673

Smeenk HG, Tran TCK, Erdmann J et al (2005) Survival after surgical management of pancreatic adenocarcinoma: does curative and radical surgery truly exist? Langenbecks Arch Surg 390:94–103

Sperti C, Beltrame V, Milanetto AC et al (2010) Parenchyma-sparing pancreatectomies for benign or border-line tumors of the pancreas. World J Gastrointest Oncol 2:272–281

Sperti C, Pasquali C, Piccoli A et al (1997) Recurrence after resection for ductal adenocarcinoma of the pancreas. World J Surg 21:195–200

Stitzenberg KB, Watson JC, Roberts A et al (2008) Survival after pancreatectomy with major arterial resection and reconstruction. Ann Surg Oncol 15:1399–1406

Stojadinovic A, Brooks A, Hoos A et al (2003) An evidence-based approach to the surgical management of resectable pancreatic adenocarcinoma. J Am Coll Surg 196:954–964

Strasberg SM, Drebin JA, Soper NJ (1997) Evolution and current status of the Whipple procedure: an update for gastroenterologists. Gastroenterology 113:983–994

Takamatsu S, Ban D, Irie T et al (2005) Resection of a cancer developing in the remnant pancreas after a pancreaticoduodenectomy for pancreas head cancer. J Gastrointest Surg 9:263–269

Talamini MA, Moesinger R, Yeo CJ et al (1998) Cystadenomas of the pancreas: is enucleation an adequate operation? Ann Surg 227:896–903

Tanaka M, Chari S, Adsay V et al (2006) International consensus guidelines for management of intraductal papillary mucinous neoplasms and mucinous cystic neoplasms of the pancreas. Pancreatology 6:17–32

Tran KTC, Smeenk HG, van Eijck CHJ et al (2004) Pylorus preserving pancreaticoduodenectomy versus standard whipple procedure: a prospective, randomized, multicenter analysis of 170 patients with pancreatic and periampullary tumors. Ann Surg 240:738–745

Tseng JF, Raut CP, Lee JE et al (2004) Pancreaticoduodenectomy with vascular resection: margin status and survival duration. J Gastrointest Surg 8:935–949 discussion 949–950

Van den Broeck A, Sergeant G, Ectors N et al (2009) Patterns of recurrence after curative resection of pancreatic ductal adenocarcinoma. Eur J Surg Oncol 35:600–604

Wagner M, Redaelli C, Lietz M et al (2004) Curative resection is the single most important factor determining outcome in patients with pancreatic adenocarcinoma. Br J Surg 91:586–594

Weitz J, Kienle P, Schmidt J et al (2007) Portal vein resection for advanced pancreatic head cancer. J Am Coll Surg 204:712–716

Werner J, Büchler MW (2011) Management of pancreatic cancer: recent advances. Dtsch Med Wochenschr 136:1807–1810

Werner J, Fritz S, Büchler MW (2012) Intraductal papillary mucinous neoplasms of the pancreas-a surgical disease. Nat Rev Gastroenterol Hepatol http://www.ncbi.nlm.nih.gov/pubmed/22392299

Wu YL, Yan HC, Chen LR et al (2007) Extended Appleby's operation for pancreatic cancer involving celiac axis. J Surg Oncol 96:442–446 discussion 447

Yamada H, Hirano S, Tanaka E et al (2006) Surgical treatment of liver metastases from pancreatic cancer. HPB (Oxford) 8:85–88

Yekebas EF, Bogoevski D, Cataldegirmen G et al (2008) En bloc vascular resection for locally advanced pancreatic malignancies infiltrating major blood vessels: perioperative outcome and long-term survival in 136 patients. Ann Surg 247:300–309

Yeo CJ, Cameron JL, Sohn TA et al (1999) Pancreaticoduodenectomy with or without extended retroperitoneal lymphadenectomy for periampullary adenocarcinoma: comparison of morbidity and mortality and short-term outcome. Ann Surg 229:613–622 discussion 622–624

Adjuvant Therapy for Pancreatic Cancer

Asma Sultana, Trevor Cox, Paula Ghaneh and John P. Neoptolemos

Abstract

Pancreatic cancer is a challenging malignancy to treat, as less than one-fifth of diagnosed cases are resectable, surgery is complex and postoperative recovery slow, treated patients tend to relapse and overall survival rates are low. It is one of the leading causes of cancer-related mortality. Adjuvant therapy has been employed in resectable disease, to target micrometastases and improve prognosis. Chemotherapy, chemoradiotherapy (chemoRT) and chemoradiotherapy (chemoRT) followed on by chemotherapy have been evaluated in randomised controlled trials. The European Study Group for Pancreatic Cancer (ESPAC)-1 and CONKO-001 trials clearly established the survival advantage of adjuvant chemotherapy with 5 fluorouracil (5FU) plus folinic acid and gemcitabine respectively over no chemotherapy. The ESPAC-3 (version 2) trial demonstrated equivalence between 5FU plus folinic acid and gemcitabine in terms of survival parameters, though gemcitabine had a better toxicity profile. The results of these key studies, together with smaller ones have been subjected to meta-analyses, with confirmation of improved survival with adjuvant systemic chemotherapy. The EORTC-40891 and ESPAC-1 trials found no survival advantage with adjuvant chemoRT compared to observation, and this has been reflected in a subsequent meta-analysis. The popularisation of chemoRT, with follow on chemotherapy (versus observation) was based on the small underpowered GITSG trial. The ESPAC-1 trial was unable to find a survival benefit for chemoRT, with follow on chemotherapy compared to

A. Sultana · T. Cox · P. Ghaneh · J. P. Neoptolemos (✉)
The Liverpool Cancer Research UK Trials Unit, and the Department of Molecular and Clinical Cancer Medicine Centre, University of Liverpool, Liverpool Cancer Research Centre, Royal Liverpool University Hospital, Daulby Street, Liverpool L69 3GA, UK
e-mail: j.p.neoptolemos@liverpool.ac.uk

F. Otto and M. P. Lutz (eds.), *Early Gastrointestinal Cancers*,
Recent Results in Cancer Research 196, DOI: 10.1007/978-3-642-31629-6_5,
© Springer-Verlag Berlin Heidelberg 2012

observation. The RTOG-9704 trial assessed chemoRT with follow on chemotherapy in both arms and found no difference between survival in the gemcitabine and 5FU arms. There has never been a published head-to-head randomised comparison of adjuvant chemotherapy to chemoRT, with follow on chemotherapy. Ongoing randomised trials are looking into adjuvant combination chemotherapy, chemotherapy with follow on chemoRT, and neoadjuvant therapy. Novel agents continue to be assessed in early phase trials with a major emphasis on predictive and prognostic biomarkers. Based on the available evidence, adjuvant chemotherapy with gemcitabine or 5FU/folinic acid is the current recommended gold standard in the management of resected pancreatic cancer.

Abbreviations

ChemoRT/CRT	Chemoradiotherapy
C.I.	Confidence interval
CT	Chemotherapy
EBRT	External beam radiotherapy
FA	Folinic acid
Gemcap	Gemcitabine + capecitabine
Gy	Gray
h ENT 1	Human equilibrative nucleoside transporter
HR	Hazard ratio
IORT	Intraoperative radiotherapy
IPD	Individual patient data
LNR	Lymph node ratio
PEXG	Cisplatin, epirubicin, capecitabine and gemcitabine
RCT	Randomised controlled trial
RFS	Recurrence-free survival
RT	Radiotherapy

Contents

1	Introduction	67
2	Rationale for Adjuvant Therapy	67
3	Evidence for Adjuvant Chemotherapy	68
	3.1 Systemic Chemotherapy	68
	3.2 Regional Chemotherapy	72
4	Evidence for Adjuvant Chemoradiotherapy	73
	4.1 Intraoperative Radiotherapy	73
	4.2 Postoperative Chemoradiotherapy	73
	4.3 Chemoradiotherapy, and Follow on Chemotherapy	74
5	Evidence for Neoadjuvant Therapy	79

5.1	Published Studies	79
5.2	Ongoing Studies	80
6	Evidence from Meta-Analyses	80
6.1	Adjuvant Therapy	80
6.2	Neoadjuvant Therapy	81
7	Conclusions	82
8	Future Directions	82
References		82

1 Introduction

Pancreatic cancer is the tenth most common cancer in the UK and USA in terms of incidence (Jemal et al. 2010; Office for National Statistics 2010), but is among the fourth or fifth leading causes of cancer death (Jemal et al. 2010; Office for National Statistics 2010). The only treatment with potential for cure is resection, but even in specialised centres just 10–15 % of diagnosed patients have resectable disease (Stathis and Moore 2010). In this select group, adjuvant chemotherapy has improved overall survival (Neoptolemos et al. 2010) or disease-free survival (Oettle et al. 2007), and more than doubled the 5 years survival rates from 10 % to nearly 25 % (Van Laethem et al. 2011).

Despite improvements, patients continue to succumb to locoregional recurrence and metastatic disease. Elucidation of cancer biology is continuing to evolve (Tuveson and Hanahan 2011; Pérez-Mancera et al. 2012), and recent research has revealed that metastases in pancreatic cancer occur much earlier than expected, providing a window of opportunity to direct treatment strategies sooner rather than later (Tuveson and Neoptolemos 2012). Increasingly efforts are being directed at early diagnosis, better treatment using combinations of existing chemotherapeutic agents (Costello and Neoptolemos 2011), searching for effective novel agents, and assessing individual patient risk and prognosis (Jamieson et al. 2011; Rizzato et al. 2011; Smith et al. 2011).

2 Rationale for Adjuvant Therapy

Pancreatectomy with standard lymphadenectomy is advocated for resectable disease. Meta-analyses of randomised controlled trials (RCT) comparing this against extended lymphadenectomy have failed to reveal any survival advantage for the latter (Michalski et al. 2007). Likewise there were no differences between morbidity, mortality and survival when meta-analyses were undertaken of RCTs examining classic whipple's resection versus pylorus preserving whipple's procedure (Diener et al. 2011).

This inability of radical surgery to improve results is owing to the tendency for the disease to recur either locoregionally or in the liver (Sperti et al. 1997; Abrams et al. 2001; Koshy et al. 2005; Hishinuma et al. 2006). Adjuvant treatment following curative resection acts by targeting micrometastatic disease (Chua and Cunningham 2005), thereby improving outcomes.

Randomised controlled trials of adjuvant chemotherapy, adjuvant chemoradiotherapy (chemoRT), adjuvant chemoRT with follow on chemotherapy and neoadjuvant therapy will be summarised, as also the results from both aggregate and individual patient data (IPD) meta-analyses.

3 Evidence for Adjuvant Chemotherapy

3.1 Systemic Chemotherapy

3.1.1 Published Trials

Bakkevold from Norway conducted the earliest randomised trial to compare chemotherapy to best supportive care (Table 1) following resection (Bakkevold et al. 1993). There was a statistically significant survival advantage for patients in the chemotherapy arm (5FU, doxorubicin and mitomycin C), with a median survival of 23 months compared to 11 months observed in the control group ($p = 0.04$). Limitations of this study are the fact that the regime was toxic, and the study pooled both pancreatic and periampullary tumours.

Takada et al. (Takada et al. 2002) enrolled 508 patients with pancreatic, gall bladder, bile duct and ampulla of Vater cancers, with data available on the subset of the 173 pancreatic cancer patients. Patients were assigned to either chemotherapy with mitomycin C and 5FU, or observation. No difference was seen between the two treatment arms for the endpoints of disease-free survival, time to recurrence and 5 years survival rates. A criticism of this trial was the use of oral 5FU, which has very poor efficacy because of its hepatic metabolism compared to intravenously administered 5FU or specially designed oral fluoropyrimidines (Shore et al. 2003).

The European Study Group for Pancreatic Cancer (ESPAC)-1 trial (Neoptolemos et al. 2001, 2004) was the first adequately powered, randomised study to evaluate adjuvant therapy in pancreatic cancer. This two-by-two factorial design trial accrued 541 patients over 6 years. Besides the two-by-two factorial design allocation (i.e. observation, chemoRT alone, chemotherapy alone and both), randomisation outside of the two-by-two factorial design, into one of the main treatment comparisons (i.e. chemotherapy versus no chemotherapy and chemoRT versus no chemoRT) was permitted.

The final analysis of the ESPAC-1 trial assessed the 289 patients randomised using the two-by-two factorial design, and followed up for a median of 47 months (Neoptolemos et al. 2004). There was significant survival advantage with chemotherapy, with the median survival being 20.1 months in the chemotherapy arm compared to the 15.5 months seen in the no chemotherapy arm ($p = 0.009$) (Fig. 1). Prognostic factors that impacted adversely on survival were the differentiation of tumours ($P < 0.001$), lymph nodal involvement ($P < 0.001$) and a

Table 1 Randomised controlled trials of adjuvant systemic chemotherapy

Series	Period	No of patients	Regimen	Median survival (months)	Actuarial survival (%) 1 year	Actuarial survival (%) 2 year	Actuarial survival (%) 3 year	Actuarial survival (%) 5 years
Bakkevold et al.(1993)	1984–	61	5-FU	23	70	–	27	4
	1987	31	/DOX/ /MMC –	11 ($p = 0.02$)	45	–	30	8
Takada et al.(2002) (pancreas)	1986– 1992	81 77	MMC/5-FU –	– –	– –	– –	– –	11.5 18 ($p = $ ns)
Kosuge et al.(2006)	1992– 2000	45 44	5FU+ Cisplatin –	12.5 15.8 ($p = 0.94$)	– –	– –	– –	26.4 14.9
ESPAC-1 Final (Neoptolemos et al. 2001)	1994– 2000	147 142	5-FU –	20.1 15.5 ($p = 0.009$)	– –	40 30	– –	21 8
Oettle et al.(2007) CONKO-001	1998– 2004	179 175	Gemcitabine –	22.1 20.2 ($p = 0.06$)	– –	– –	34 20.5	22.5 11.5
Ueno et al.(2009)	2002– 2005	58 60	Gemcitabine –	22.3 18.4 ($p = 0.19$)	77.6 75	48.5 40	– –	23.9 10.6
ESPAC-3 (version 2) (Neoptolemos et al. 2010)	2000– 2007	551 537	5FU/FA Gemcitabine	23 23.6 ($p = 0.39$)	78.5 80.1	48.1 49.1	– –	– –

DOX Doxorubicin, *MMC* mitomycin C, *CRT* chemoradiation, *5FU* 5 fluorouracil, *FA* folinic acid

maximum tumour size of >2 cm ($P = 0.003$), while resection margin status did not. In the 481 patients who had undergone either Kausch-Whipple (KW) or Pylorus Preserving KW (PPKW), post-operative complications did not dent the survival benefit seen with adjuvant chemotherapy (Bassi et al. 2005).

A small Japanese RCT by Kosuge et al. evaluated chemotherapy with 5FU and cisplatin versus observation in 89 patients with pancreas cancer, with R0 resection status (Kosuge et al. 2006). There was no survival advantage for chemotherapy (median survival 12.5 months) compared to observation (median survival 15.8 months). The criticisms of this study are the likelihood that it was under-powered, and the suboptimal duration of the chemotherapy as only 2 cycles were administered.

The CONKO-001 trial by Oettle et al. (Oettle et al. 2007) compared gemcitabine to best supportive care in 368 patients, and did not find a difference in overall survival between the 2 groups. Significantly improved disease-free survival was observed in the gemcitabine arm (13.4 versus 6.9 months in control arm; $p < 0.001$). Interestingly, the 5 years survival rate in the gemcitabine arm was nearly double that in the best supportive care group 22.5% versus 11.5 %. Subsequent analyses of their 5 years data (Neuhaus et al. 2008) showed a significantly improved median survival in the gemcitabine arm (22.8 months in the gemcitabine arm versus 20.2 months in the observation arm; $p = 0.005$).

Ueno et al. randomised 119 Japanese patients to receive either 3 cycles of adjuvant chemotherapy with gemcitabine or resection only (Ueno et al. 2009). Median disease-free survival was significantly improved, though not the overall survival, and toxicity profile was acceptable. Limitations of the trial are the sub-optimal duration of chemotherapy, the fact that 52 % of patients received intra-operative RT, and its underpowered nature.

Yoshitomi et al. (Yoshitomi et al. 2008) assigned 100 patients in a randomised phase 2 study to receive adjuvant gemcitabine or gemcitabine plus uracil/tegafur. The combination arm did not have an improved disease-free survival, and paradoxically a worse median survival, concluding there was no further role for the combination chemotherapy.

The most recent large RCT in this area, the ESPAC-3v2 trial randomised 1,088 patients over 7 years, with at least 2 years follow up (Neoptolemos et al. 2010). Patients were randomised to receive either 5FU + folinic acid, or gemcitabine, in version 2 of the trial (version 1 included an observation only arm which was closed once the results of ESPAC-1 trial conclusively demonstrated survival benefit for the chemotherapy arm). There was no significant overall survival difference (hazard ratio 0.94; 95 % CI 0.81–1.08) between the 5FU arm (median overall survival 23 months; 95 % CI 21–25 months) compared to the gemcitabine arm (median overall survival 23.6 months; 95 % CI 21.4–26.4 months) (Fig. 2). Likewise, there were no significant differences in progression-free survival and global quality of life scores between the two arms.

Toxicity profile on the other hand was significantly better in the gemcitabine arm compared to the 5FU arm (serious adverse events 7.5 versus 14 %; $p < 0.001$). This is reflected by the fact that median dose intensity was 79 % of the

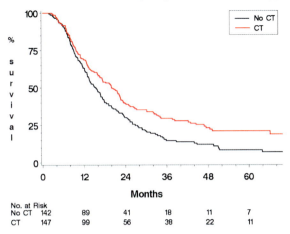

Fig. 1 Kaplan-Meier estimates of survival according to whether or not patients received chemotherapy in the ESPAC-1 trial final results

planned protocol for 5FU arm, compared to the improved 89 % for the gemcitabine arm. Independent prognostic factors of overall survival were tumour size and grade, nodal status, post-operative CA19-9 levels, performance status and smoking. As in ESPAC-1, resection margin status did not impact on overall survival on multivariate analysis.

This trial has credible external validity, as it is adequately powered, has a simple study design (in comparison to the criticism of the 2 × 2 factorial design of the ESPAC-1 trial), and recruited patients across Europe, Australasia, the Far East and North America.

Pooled data from 458 patients enrolled in the ESPAC-1, ESPAC-1 plus and ESPAC-3v1 trials were studied. There was 30 % reduction in risk of death following chemotherapy with 5FU/folinic acid (HR 0.70; 95 % CI 0.55–0.88; $p < 0.003$) compared to the control arm.

Bao et al. (Bao et al. 2011) in a phase 2 trial, studied a novel regime of fixed dose gemcitabine, which theoretically maximises cellular uptake of gemcitabine, plus erlotinib. 25 patients with R0 resection received the combination therapy for 4 months, followed by 8 months of erlotinib. Median recurrence-free survival (RFS) was 14 months in this small select group, similar to the results in ESPAC-3v2. Median overall survival was not reached, but was in excess of 2 years at the time of publication. In addition to the use of fixed-dose gemcitabine bi-weekly, the longer duration of maintenance therapy is a new feature. The authors do point out a potential possibility of overestimating RFS, as this was based on radiological progression with scans done at intervals of 6 months. Molecular analysis of Kras mutation, EGFR protein assessment and EGFR copy number did not influence RFS or recurrence patterns.

3.1.2 Ongoing Trials

The JASPAC-01 phase 3 trial currently recruiting in Japan aims to randomise 360 patients to receive either gemcitabine or S1, an orally active fluoropyrimidine (Maeda et al. 2008).

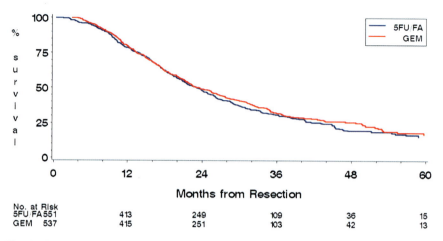

Fig. 2 Kaplan-Meier estimates of survival of the gemcitabine versus 5FU/folinic acid arms in the ESPAC-3v2 trial final results

The currently ongoing ESPAC-4 trial is taking the ESPAC-3v2 results forward, and comparing gemcitabine versus gemcitabine plus capecitabine (gemcap), an orally active fluoropyrimidine. It aims to recruit 1,080 patients, and commenced in 2008. In a recent trial of advanced pancreatic cancer, gemcap had significantly improved progression-free survival and response rate compared to single-agent gemcitabine, and revealed a trend towards improved overall survival (Cunningham et al. 2009). Meta-analyses of gemcap versus gemcitabine in the advanced cancer setting have shown significant overall survival benefit for gemcap over gemcitabine (Sultana et al. 2007). It will be interesting to see if similar results are reflected in the adjuvant situation as well.

The ESPAC-4 trial has a translational element which involves collecting blood, urine and tissue samples with a view to identifying expression profile in tumours that can predict response to treatment with gemcitabine and capecitabine.

3.2 Regional Chemotherapy

The rationale for regional chemotherapy was to direct treatment at the tumour, with the hope of reducing toxicity that accompanies systemically administered chemotherapy. Trials involving regional chemotherapy in the adjuvant setting were developed before results from the ESPAC-1 trial were published.

Based on a small study of 20 patients where a non-significant trend towards reduced liver metastases was seen in the regional chemotherapy arm (Hayashibe et al. 2007), an RCT of regional chemotherapy with 5FU, mitoxantrone and cis-platinum given via celiac axis infusion and 30×1.8 Gray (Gy) radiotherapy was conducted by Morak et al. (Morak et al. 2008). The observation arm of this study did not receive any chemotherapy, and once the ESPAC-1 data was in public domain, it was deemed unethical to continue to recruit to this arm, and the trial closed. In the 120 patients of pancreatic and periampullary tumours randomised, quality of life was improved in the treatment arm compared to the control arm (Morak et al. 2010). The downsides to this trial were that only 21 patients received treatment per protocol, and there was neither overall survival benefit, nor reduction in local/hepatic recurrences in the pancreatic cancer subgroup.

Currently there is insufficient evidence to support the use of regional chemotherapy.

4 Evidence for Adjuvant Chemoradiotherapy

Radiation treatment has been given with the idea of controlling any microscopic residual disease, since most recurrences following pancreaticoduodenectomy occur at the site of resection. Radiation has been given intraoperatively (IORT) or postoperatively and often with concurrent chemotherapy both for radiosensitisation and to address systemic micrometastases.

4.1 Intraoperative Radiotherapy

The irradiation of the upper abdomen by external beam radiotherapy (EBRT) causes considerable toxicity and IORT can reduce this, sparing normal tissues. The surrounding tissues can either be displaced or shielded, thereby allowing the delivery of larger RT doses in a single fraction to volumes harbouring tumour cells.

As most series on IORT are dogged by small numbers, inclusion of all stages of the disease and heterogenous treatment strategies, it is difficult to draw conclusions or make recommendations (Hiraoka et al. 1990; Zerbi et al. 1994; Fossati et al. 1995; Coquard et al. 1997; Reni et al. 2001). The one small randomised trial on IORT (Sindelar and Kinsella 1986) was published in abstract form and found no difference in survival between surgery only and IORT (median survival 12 months in both groups). At the present time there is little to support the use of adjuvant IORT, either alone or in combination with other forms of treatment.

4.2 Postoperative Chemoradiotherapy

Klinkenbijl et al. from Norway (EORTC-40891 trial) (Klinkenbijl et al. 1999) (Table 2) randomised 218 patients with both pancreatic and periampullary tumours to either observation or radiotherapy with split course RT (40 Gy) and concurrent 5FU as continuous infusion. In patients with pancreatic cancer, the trend was in favour of chemoradiation, with the overall survival being 12.6 months in the observation group and 17.1 months in the treatment group ($p = 0.099$). The long-term results of this trial, after a median follow up of 11.3 years maintained no difference in overall survival between the chemoRT and observation arms (death rate ratio 0.91; 95 % CI 0.68–1.23; $P = 0.54$) (Smeenk et al. 2007). The 10 years survival in the pancreatic head cancer subgroup was 8 %. The limitations of this study were the inclusion of pancreatic head and periampullary tumours, lack of maintenance chemotherapy and a questionable statistical design that limited its ability to detect a benefit for adjuvant chemoradiation (Garofalo et al. 2006).

In the ESPAC-1 trial (Neoptolemos et al. 2001), 70 patients were randomised to the chemoRT arm in the 2×2 factorial design, while a further 68 were randomly assigned to either chemoRT or no chemoRT. Radiation was administered as a split course, concurrent with 5FU. There was no difference in the median survival (15.5 months in chemoRT arm and 16.1 months in no chemoradiation arm; $p = 0.24$) and 2 year survival following chemoRT.

In the final results of the ESPAC-1 trial (Neoptolemos et al. 2004) the median survival was 15.9 months in the chemoRT arm and 17.9 months in the group who were not assigned to receive chemoRT ($p = 0.05$) (Fig. 3). The estimated 5-year survival was 10 % in the chemoRT arm compared to 20 % in those who did not receive chemoRT ($p = 0.05$). The lack of a survival advantage following chemoRT could be due to delays in administering radiation in patients who suffered post-operative complications. This reduces the potential benefit of chemotherapy that is derived by administering it as soon as possible after resection.

The EORTC 40013/FFCD/GERCOR phase 2 trial by Van Laethem et al. randomised 90 patients with R0 resection to either chemotherapy alone arm employing 4 cycles of gemcitabine, or chemoradiation arm, using 2 courses of gemcitabine followed by 50.4 Gy radiation concurrent with gemcitabine (Van Laethem et al. 2010). The primary endpoint was toxicity, and this was comparable in both arms (grade 4 toxicity 0 % in chemotherapy and 4.7 % in chemoRT arm). The good toxicity profile was felt to be due to the sequential concept used in the chemoRT arm, with initial chemotherapy followed on by chemoRT. There were no differences between the 2 groups for the secondary end points of overall survival (24 months in both arms), and disease-free survival (12 months in chemoRT arm and 11 months in chemotherapy alone arm).

4.3 Chemoradiotherapy, and Follow on Chemotherapy

4.3.1 Published Trials

The Gastrointestinal Tumour Study Group (GITSG) trial 9173 (Table 3) set the trend for the use of chemoRT followed by chemotherapy in resectable disease (Kalser and Ellenberg 1985). This trial randomised 43 patients to receive either chemotherapy or combined treatment (chemoRT followed by chemotherapy) in the form of split course EBRT (40 Gy) and concurrent 5FU, followed by 5FU for 2 year. The study was terminated prematurely both because of a low rate of accrual and because of an increasingly large difference in survival between the study arms. The median survival for the adjuvant treatment group was 20 months,

Table 2 Randomised controlled trials of adjuvant chemoradiotherapy

Series	Period	Number of patients	Regimen	Median survival (months)	Actuarial survival (%) 1 year	Actuarial survival (%) 2 year	Actuarial survival (%) 3 year	Actuarial survival (%) 5 years
(Klinkenbijl et al. 1999)	1987–1995	110	40 Gy + 5FU	24.5	41	–	–	10
		108	–	19 ($p = 0.208$)	51	–	–	20
ESPAC-1 final—2 × 2 factorial (Neoptolemos et al. 2004)	1994–2000	145	40 Gy + 5FU, with 5FU/FA maintenance	15.9	–	29	–	10
		144	–	17.9 ($p = 0.05$)	–	41	–	20
ESPAC-1 final—individual treatment groups (Neoptolemos et al. 2004)	1994–2000	69	Observation	16.9	–	–	–	11
		73	40 Gy + 5FU	13.9	–	–	–	7
Van Laethem et al. (phase 2)(2010)	2000–2007	45	Gem 4 cycles	24.4	–	50.2	–	–
		45	Gem 2 cycles, followed by Gem + 50.4 Gy	24.3	–	50.6	–	–

5FU 5- fluorouracil, *FA* folinic acid, *Gy* grey, *Gem* gemcitabine

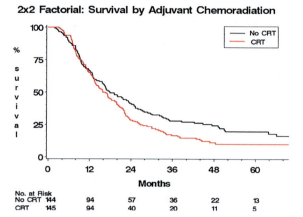

Fig. 3 Kaplan-Meier estimates of survival according to whether or not patients received chemoradiotherapy (*chemoRT*) in the ESPAC-1 trial final results

significantly longer than the 11 months in the no adjuvant treatment arm. Because there were so few cases, a further 30 patients were registered (not randomised) to the treatment arm and the median survival in this group was 18 months, with a 2 year survival rate of 46 % (Doughlass 1987). Owing to the small number of patients, the 95 % confidence intervals of the survival curves were so large as to overlap with survival curves in patients receiving no additional treatment. Thus, no convincing conclusion could be derived from this study, though it must be noted that the benefit from treatment could be due to the maintenance chemotherapy used in this study.

The Radiation Therapy Oncology Group Study 9704 (Regine et al. 2008) RCT compared gemcitabine versus 5FU administered pre- and post-5FU-based chemoradiation. Chemotherapy was given for 3 weeks before and 12 weeks after 50.4 Gy chemoRT. In the 451 patients randomised and eligible, there was no difference in overall survival between the 2 arms ($p = 0.34$). On subgroup analysis of the pancreatic head tumours, there was a trend towards improved survival in the gemcitabine arm (median survival 20.2 months) compared to the 5FU arm (median survival 16.9 months) but this was not statistically significant (HR 0.82; 95 % CI 0.65–1.03). Analysis of their 5 years data showed no changes to the original inferences drawn (Regine et al. 2011).

This was the first phase 3 trial to prospectively evaluate post-resectional CA19-9 levels (Berger et al. 2008). In Lewis antigen positive patients, post-resectional CA19-9 values of both >90 kU/L (HR 3.4; $p < 0.001$) and >180 kU/L (HR 3.53; $p < 0.001$) adversely impacted on survival. The prognostic value of nodal involvement is known, and the RTOG dataset was used to assess the influence of total examined nodes, number of positive nodes and lymph node ratio (LNR) on survival (Showalter et al. 2011). Total lymph nodes examined cut off of 15 was suggested to improve disease staging. Number of positive lymph nodes of >3 and LNR of 33 % were associated with worse overall and disease-free survival.

Immunohistochemistry for human equilibrative nucleoside transporter 1 (hENT1) protein, which transports gemcitabine into cells, was performed on tissue microarrays of 229 patients from the RTOG 9704 trial (Farrell et al. 2009). In both univariate and multivariate analyses, hENT1 expression was associated with improved overall and disease-free survival in the gemcitabine arm, but not the 5FU arm. Another secondary analysis in 141 patients suggested the RecQ1 A159C genotype had prognostic relevance in the chemoradiation arm (Li et al. 2011).

Review of the RT quality assurance in RTOG 9704 (Abrams et al. 2012) found that RT administration was nearly evenly split by per protocol versus less than per protocol (52 % versus 48%) administration. On post hoc analysis of overall survival, those patients who had received per protocol RT had significantly improved survival compared to the less than per protocol group (HR 0.75; 95 % CI 0.60–0.93). This is an interesting observation, but it must be interpreted against the backdrop that the RT quality assessment's impact on survival was not one of the a priori outcomes of the trial.

The ASOCOG Z05031 phase 2 trial evaluated cisplatin, 5FU and interferon-alfa-2b-based 3 dimensional conformal RT, followed on by 5FU chemotherapy (Picozzi et al. 2011). This study was closed to accrual before its target recruitment number of 93 was reached due to 95 % (80/89 patients) grade 3 or more all cause toxicity. Forty four percent of patients did not complete all phases of the treatment per protocol, and only 17 % were able to complete the chemoRT component without interruption. A previous phase 2 trial of interferon-based chemoRT, which differed from the ASOCOG Z05031 trial in using gemcitabine for follow on chemotherapy, also reported significant dose and treatment-limiting toxicities (Linehan et al. 2008).

The CAPRI trial evaluated chemotherapy with 5FU versus chemoradiation using cisplatin, interferon alpha-2b and 5FU, with follow on 5FU chemotherapy (Knaebel et al. 2005; Marten et al. 2009). The chemoradiation protocol was based on a phase II trial conducted by Picozzi et al. who reported an impressive 5 year survival of 55 % in 43 patients (Picozzi et al. 2003). In the 110 patients randomised, there was significantly reduced local recurrence in the chemoRT arm (29.3% versus 55.6 %; $p = 0.014$). This however did not translate into a survival benefit, as there was no significant difference in overall survival between the adjuvant 5FU/folinic acid arm (median overall survival 28.5 months) and the chemoRT arm (median overall survival 32.1 months) (Marten et al. 2010). There was greater grade 3/4 toxicity in the chemoRT arm (68 %) compared to the adjuvant chemotherapy group (16 %).

A phase 2 trial ECOG 2204 randomised 137 patients to receive one of 2 novel agents viz., cetuximab or bevacuzimab against a backdrop of capecitabine-based radiotherapy, with gemcitabine administered pre- and post-chemoRT (Berlin et al. 2010). The safety and toxicity profiles were acceptable, but as over 10 % of patients experienced recurrence, further development of this regime was felt to be futile.

4.3.2 Ongoing Trials

Algenpantucel-L (irradiated live allogenic human pancreatic cancer cells) in combination with gemcitabine chemotherapy plus 5FU-based radiotherapy (as in RTOG 9704) has been subjected to a phase 2 trial (NLG0205) (Hardacre et al. 2011).

Table 3 Randomised controlled trials of adjuvant chemoradiotherapy, followed on by chemotherapy

Series	Period	Number of patients	Regimen	Median survival (months)	Actuarial survival (%) 1 year	Actuarial Survival (%) 2 year	Actuarial Survival (%) 3 year	Actuarial Survival (%) 5 years
GITSG 9173(Kalser and Ellenberg 1985)	1987–1995	21	40 Gy + 5FU, with 5FU maintenance	21	–	43	–	19
		22	Observation	10.9 ($p = 0.03$)	–	18	–	5
ESPAC-1 final—individual treatment groups(Neoptolemos et al. 2004)	1994–2000	69	Observation	16.9	–	38.7	–	29
		72	40 Gy + 5FU, with 5FU/FA maintenance	19.9	–	35.5	–	13
RTOG-9704(Regine et al. 2008) All patients head of pancreas only eligible = 381	1998–2002	221	Gem preCRT, 50.4 Gy + 5FU, gem post CRT	–	–	–	–	–
		230	5FU preCRT, 50.4 Gy + 5FU, 5FU post CRT	– ($p = 0.34$)	–	–	–	–
		187	Gem preCRT, 50.4 Gy + 5FU, gem post CRT	20.5	–	–	31	–
		194	5FU preCRT, 50.4 Gy + 5FU, 5FU post CRT	16.9 ($p = 0.09$)	–	–	22	–

5FU 5- fluorouracil, *FA* folinic acid, *Gem* gemcitabine, *Gy* gray, *CRT* chemoradiation

In the 73 patients enrolled, toxicity was low, the median disease-free survival was 16 months (improved compared to the 11 months observed in the RTOG trial) and median overall survival had not been reached. These outcomes prompted the investigators to launch a phase 3 trial which commenced enrolment May 2010.

The CapRI-2 trial has been launched, with a view to randomise 135 patients to one of 3 arms (Marten et al. 2009). Two arms involve radiotherapy (3D conformal or intensity modulated), though the CapRI protocol has been de-escalated, while the third arm has adjuvant chemotherapy plus interferon alpha-2-b. It hypothesises that removal of the cisplatin and radiotherapy components are likely to reduce toxicity, with minimal impact on clinical response.

Another recently opened RCT, the EORTC/US Intergroup/RTOG 0848 trial aims to assess gemcitabine versus gemcitabine plus erlotinib given for 6 cycles, followed on by either 1 cycle of chemotherapy or 1 cycle of chemoRT (with 5FU or capecitabine, and employing intensity-modulated RT plus prospective central quality assurance of RT) in selected patients who do not progress on the initial chemotherapy (Regine et al. 2011). It remains to be seen if this trial will be adequately powered to assess the second part i.e. chemotherapy versus chemoRT in those with non-progressive disease, and if there really is any role for chemoRT so far down the line.

5 Evidence for Neoadjuvant Therapy

5.1 Published Studies

The attractiveness of neoadjuvant therapy lies in the fact that nearly 20–30 % of resected patients fail to receive adjuvant therapy on the grounds of delayed recovery from major surgery, co-morbidities, patient choice and early recurrence. The advantages with neoadjuvant treatment are a relatively fitter patient, earlier treatment of systemic micrometastases, the ability to in vivo assess tumour response, avoidance of unnecessary surgery in those with occult metastases, reducing risk of tumour spillage at surgery and potential for down staging disease from unresectable/borderline resectable to resectable. The disadvantages are difficulty in differentiating between pancreatic head and periampullary tumours, risk of exposure to chemotherapy in the absence of malignancy, the necessity for histology with the potential for attendant delays, loss of window of opportunity to pursue curative resection and risk of increased postoperative complications.

Drawing from the experience of neoadjuvant therapy in the advanced disease, Palmer et al. randomised 50 patients with resectable disease in a randomised phase 2 study to either receive neoadjuvant gemcitabine or gemcitabine plus cisplatin (Palmer et al. 2007). During the course of the trial, the gemcitabine cisplatin administration schedule was altered to reduce toxicity. The primary end point of resection rate was significantly higher in the combination arm (70% versus 38 %), without increased postoperative morbidity. Twelve month survival rate was also higher in the combination arm (62 % versus 42 %), suggesting further study of the combination arm in a phase 3 trial. An American phase 2 prospective study using the same combination obtained similar results (Heinrich et al. 2008a; Heinrich et al. 2008b).

Gemcitabine-based chemoRT (Evans et al. 2008), gemcitabine cisplatin-based chemoRT (Le Scodan et al. 2009) and docetaxel-based chemoRT (Turrini et al. 2010) were promising in phase 2 trials, though upfront gemcitabine plus cisplatin (4 cycles) followed by gemcitabine chemoRT did not confer any added advantage (Varadhachary et al. 2008). Comparison of gemcitabine chemoRT to gemcitabine, cisplatin, 5FU chemo followed by 5FU chemoRT in a randomised phase 2 trial revealed significantly greater toxicity in the combination arm (Landry et al. 2010). Moreover, this trial closed prematurely due to poor accrual.

5.2 Ongoing Studies

Despite the multitude of phase I/II trials, and observational studies in this area, there is only one phase 3 randomised study comparing resection followed by adjuvant chemotherapy to neoadjuvant chemoRT (gemcitabine + cisplatinum; 3 dimensional conformal RT at dose of 55.8 Gy to tumour and 50.4 to regional lymph nodes), followed by resection and adjuvant chemotherapy (Brunner et al. 2007). Disappointingly this trial has recruited less than a third of its planned 254 patients over 7 years, and will be closed before target accrual is reached (Gillen et al. 2010).

An Italian Co-operative group (Reni 2010) have launched a phase 2 randomised study, with one arm allocated to adjuvant therapy with gemcitabine for 6 months, a second arm to receive adjuvant treatment with cisplatin, epirubicin, capecitabine and gemcitabine (PEXG) for 6 months and a third arm assigned to 3 months PEXG neoadjuvant therapy followed by surgery and adjuvant 3 months of PEXG.

6 Evidence from Meta-Analyses

6.1 Adjuvant Therapy

An IPD meta-analyses (Stocken et al. 2005) evaluated the roles of adjuvant chemotherapy, and chemoradiation in patients with pancreatic ductal adenocarcinoma. Of the 5 eligible RCTs (939 patients), IPD were available in 4 studies (875 patients). Adjuvant chemotherapy resulted in 25 % reduction in the risk of death (hazard ratio = 0.75, 95 % CI: 0.64, 0.90, P_{strat} = 0.001) compared to no chemotherapy. In contrast, there was no significant difference between chemoradiation versus no chemoradiation (hazard ratio = 1.09, 95 % CI: 0.89, 1.32, P_{strat} = 0.43). Subgroup analyses based on age, tumour size, differentiation, resection margin status and nodal status revealed that chemotherapy was less effective (χ^2 = 7.3; p = 0.007) in the subgroup with positive resection margin, in comparison to chemoradiation which was more effective here ($\chi^2 = 4.2; p = 0.04$).

The influence of resection margin on survival was explored further by the Pancreatic Meta-analyses Group (Butturini et al. 2008) using the same IPD (Stocken et al. 2005). Resection margin status did not impact on overall survival (HR 1.10; 95 % CI 0.94–1.29), though there was a trend towards reduced survival in the R1 group (median survival 14.1 months; 95 % CI 11.9–16.4 months) compared to the R0 group (median survival 15.9 months; 95 % CI 14.6–17.4 months). Adjuvant chemotherapy resulted in a significant (35 %) reduction in risk of death (HR 0.65; 95 % CI 0.53–0.80) in the R0 group, with a 7 months survival advantage compared to the no chemotherapy arm. On the other hand, chemoradiation did not significantly reduce the risk of death in the R1 group (HR 0.72; 95 % CI 0.47–1.10).

A subsequent aggregate data meta-analyses (Boeck et al. 2007) of 5 RCTs (951 patients) of adjuvant treatment concluded that chemotherapy improved median survival by 3 months (95 % CI 0.3–5.7 months; $p = 0.03$), but did not impact on 5 years survival rates, possibly due to the low numbers at risk at this time point. It included two further RCTs on chemotherapy versus best supportive care (Kosuge et al. 2006; Oettle et al. 2007), compared to the previously published IPD meta-analyses, but did not include the 5 years results from the CONKO-001 trial. Chemotherapy with either 5FU and folinic acid, or gemcitabine was advocated, though significant inter-trial heterogeneity was noted. A criticism of this study was that the methodology of the meta-analyses, utilising median survival and rates at different time points. These have been shown to not be the ideal surrogate measures for meta-analyses of survival data (Michiels et al. 2005).

6.2 Neoadjuvant Therapy

In the absence of published randomised phase 3 trials of neoadjuvant therapy to date, a comprehensive systematic review by Gillen et al. of 111 prospective ($n = 78$), including phase I/II studies and retrospective ($n = 33$) studies has been carried out (Gillen et al. 2010). There was significant inter-trial heterogeneity, and potential for bias owing to the non-randomised nature of the studies. The majority (>90 %) of neoadjuvant treatment was in the form of chemoRT. In hospital mortality (5.3 %; 95 % CI 4.1–6.8 %) in resectable patients who received upfront treatment was at the upper limits of figures quoted for high volume centres.

The median survival for resectable patients who received neoadjuvant chemotherapy and went on to have a resection was 23.3 months (95 % CI 12–54 months), comparable with survival following resection and adjuvant treatment in the ESPAC-3v2 trial. Paradoxically in resectable patients who progressed on neoadjuvant therapy and did not undergo resection, the median survival was an abysmal 8.4 months (95 % CI 6–14 months). It appears likely that these patients lost their window of opportunity to undergo curative resection.

Two other meta-analyses on neoadjuvant therapy, one looking at 14 phase 2 clinical trials (536 patients) (Assifi et al. 2011) and another evaluating 20 prospective studies of preoperative/neoadjuvant gemcitabine (707 patients) (Andriulli et al. 2011) echoed the results of Gillen et al's exhaustive meta-analyses. The conclusion from all 3 meta-analyses was that currently neoadjuvant therapy appears to only benefit patients with borderline resectable/locally advanced disease.

7 Conclusions

Currently, there is strong level 1a evidence to support the continued use of adjuvant systemic chemotherapy with either 5FU/folinic acid or gemcitabine following curative resection. There is level 1b evidence to support adjuvant gemcitabine over 5FU/folinic acid on the grounds of reduced toxicity.

Despite advances in radiotherapy delivery techniques and quality assurance, there is still neither level 1a nor level 1b evidence to support the use of adjuvant chemoRT alone or with a follow on chemotherapy, over adjuvant chemotherapy. Based on available literature, there is insufficient evidence to support neoadjuvant therapy, intraoperative radiotherapy and regional chemotherapy.

8 Future Directions

Personalised chemotherapy using predictive biomarkers may enable us to utilise existing resources more effectively. Higher levels of hENT1 and human concentrative nucleoside transporter (h CNT) 1 and 3 expression may be associated with improved overall and disease-free survival in patients who received gemcitabine, but this notion has yet to be properly evaluated (Farrell et al. 2009; Marechal et al. 2009). Expanding this to assess the roles of other enzymes involved in gemcitabine metabolism such as cytidine deaminase, cytidine deoxy kinase and ribonucleoside reductase subunits 1 and 2, may predict sensitivity to gemcitabine (Tempero et al. 2003). Likewise in colorectal cancer, thymidylate synthase can predict sensitivity for fluorinated pyrimidines and this could be extended to the pancreatic cancer setting.

In addition to evaluating combinations of chemotherapy, translational research into prognostic and predictive biomarkers and new biological agents merit attention. Assessing neoadjuvant therapy in patients with borderline resectable disease, with clear cut definition of what constitutes this, would also be an area for future studies.

References

Abrams R, Lillemoe K, Piantadosi S (2001) Continuing controversy over adjuvant therapy of pancreatic cancer. Lancet 358:1565
Abrams RA, Winter KA, Regine WF, Safran H, Hoffman JP, Lustig R, Konski AA, Benson AB, Macdonald JS, Rich TA, Willett CG (2012) Failure to adhere to protocol specified radiation

therapy guidelines was associated with decreased survival in RTOG 9704-A phase III trial of adjuvant chemotherapy and chemoradiotherapy for patients with resected adenocarcinoma of the pancreas. Int J Radiat Oncol Biol Phys 82(2):809–816. doi:10.1016/j.ijrobp.2010.11.039

Andriulli A, Festa V, Botteri E, Valvano MR, Koch M, Bassi C, Maisonneuve P, Sebastiano PD (2011) Neoadjuvant/preoperative gemcitabine for patients with localized pancreatic cancer: a meta-analysis of prospective studies. Ann Surg Oncol. doi:10.1245/s10434-011-2110-8

Assifi MM, Lu X, Eibl G, Reber HA, Li G, Hines OJ (2011) Neoadjuvant therapy in pancreatic adenocarcinoma: a meta-analysis of phase II trials. Surgery 150(3):466–473. doi: 10.1016/j.surg.2011.07.006

Bakkevold K, Arnesjo B, Dahl O, Kambestad B (1993) Adjuvant combination chemotherapy (AMF) following radical resection of carcinoma of the pancreas and papilla of vater-results of a controlled, prospective, randomised multicentre study. Eur J Can 29A(5):698–703

Bao PQ, Ramanathan RK, Krasinkas A, Bahary N, Lembersky BC, Bartlett DL, Hughes SJ, Lee KK, Moser AJ, Zeh HJ 3rd (2011) Phase II study of gemcitabine and erlotinib as adjuvant therapy for patients with resected pancreatic cancer. Ann Surg Oncol 18(4):1122–1129. doi: 10.1245/s10434-010-1401-9

Bassi C, Stocken DD, Olah A, et al. (2005) The influence of surgical resection and post-operative complications on survival following adjuvant treatment for pancreatic cancer in the ESPAC-1 randomized controlled trial. Digestive Surgery in press

Berger AC, Garcia M Jr, Hoffman JP, Regine WF, Abrams RA, Safran H, Konski A, Benson AB 3rd, MacDonald J, Willett CG (2008) Postresection CA 19–9 predicts overall survival in patients with pancreatic cancer treated with adjuvant chemoradiation: a prospective validation by RTOG 9704. J Clin Oncol 26(36):5918–5922. doi:10.1200/JCO.2008.18.6288

Berlin J, Catalano PJ, Feng Y, Lowy AM, Blackstock AW, Philip PA, McWilliams RR, Abbruzzese JL, Benson AB (2010) ECOG 2204: an intergroup randomized phase II study of cetuximab (Ce) or bevacizumab (B) in combination with gemcitabine (G) and in combination with capecitabine (Ca) and radiation (XRT) as adjuvant therapy (Adj Tx) for patients (pts) with completely resected pancreatic adenocarcinoma (PC). J Clin Oncol 28[15 (May supplement)]:abstract 4034

Boeck S, Ankerst DP, Heinemann V (2007) The role of adjuvant chemotherapy for patients with resected pancreatic cancer: systematic review of randomized controlled trials and meta-analysis. Oncology 72(5–6):314–321. doi:10.1159/000113054

Brunner TB, Grabenbauer GG, Meyer T, Golcher H, Sauer R, Hohenberger W (2007) Primary resection versus neoadjuvant chemoradiation followed by resection for locally resectable or potentially resectable pancreatic carcinoma without distant metastasis. A multi-centre prospectively randomised phase II-study of the interdisciplinary working group gastrointestinal tumours (AIO, ARO, and CAO). BMC Cancer 7:41. doi:10.1186/1471-2407-7-41

Butturini G, Stocken DD, Wente MN, Jeekel H, Klinkenbijl JH, Bakkevold KE, Takada T, Amano H, Dervenis C, Bassi C, Buchler MW, Neoptolemos JP, Pancreatic Cancer Meta-Analysis G (2008) Influence of resection margins and treatment on survival in patients with pancreatic cancer: meta-analysis of randomized controlled trials. Arch Surg 143(1):75–83, discussion 83. doi 10.1001/archsurg.2007.17

Chua YJ, Cunningham D (2005) Adjuvant treatment for resectable pancreatic cancer. J Clin Oncol 23(20):4532–4537

Coquard R, Ayzac L, Gilly F et al (1997) Intraoperative radiotherapy in resected pancreatic cancer: feasibility and results. Radiother Oncol 44:271–275

Costello E, Neoptolemos JP (2011) Pancreatic cancer in 2010: new insights for early intervention and detection. Nat Rev Gastroenterol Hepatol 8(2):71–73. doi:10.1038/nrgastro.2010.214

Cunningham D, Chau I, Stocken D et al (2009) Phase III randomised comparison of gemcitabine versus gemcitabine plus capecitabine in patients with advanced pancreatic cancer. J Clin Oncol 27(33):5513–5518

Diener MK, Fitzmaurice C, Schwarzer G, Seiler CM, Antes G, Knaebel H, Büchler MW (2011) Pylorus-preserving pancreaticoduodenectomy (ppWhipple) versus pancreaticoduodenectomy (classicWhipple) for surgical treatment of periampullary and pancreatic carcinoma. In: Cochrane database of systematic reviewsed

Doughlass H (1987) Further evidence of effective adjuvant combined radiation and chemotherapy following curative resection of pancreatic cancer. Cancer 59:2006–2010

Evans DB, Varadhachary GR, Crane CH, Sun CC, Lee JE, Pisters PW, Vauthey JN, Wang H, Cleary KR, Staerkel GA, Charnsangavej C, Lano EA, Ho L, Lenzi R, Abbruzzese JL, Wolff RA (2008) Preoperative gemcitabine-based chemoradiation for patients with resectable adenocarcinoma of the pancreatic head. J Clin Oncol 26(21):3496–3502. doi:10.1200/JCO.2007.15.8634

Farrell JJ, Elsaleh H, Garcia M, Lai R, Ammar A, Regine WF, Abrams R, Benson AB, Macdonald J, Cass CE, Dicker AP, Mackey JR (2009) Human equilibrative nucleoside transporter 1 levels predict response to gemcitabine in patients with pancreatic cancer. Gastroenterology 136(1):187–195. doi:10.1053/j.gastro.2008.09.067

Fossati V, Cattaneo G, Zerbi A et al (1995) The role of intraoperative therapy by electron beam and combination of adjuvant chemotherapy and external radiotherapy in carcinoma of the pancreas. Tumori 81(1):23–31

Garofalo M, Flannery T, Regine W (2006) The case for adjuvant chemoradiation for pancreatic cancer. Best Pract Res Clin Gastroenterol 20(2):403–416

Gillen S, Schuster T, Meyer Zum Buschenfelde C, Friess H, Kleeff J (2010) Preoperative/ neoadjuvant therapy in pancreatic cancer: a systematic review and meta-analysis of response and resection percentages. PLoS medicine 7(4):e1000267. doi:10.1371/journal.pmed.1000267

Hardacre JM, Mulcahy MF, Small Jr. W, Talamonti M, Obel JC, Rocha Lima CS, Safran H, Lenz H, Chiorean EG, Link CJ (2011) Effect of the addition of algenpantucel-L immunotherapy to standard adjuvant therapy on survival in patients with resected pancreas cancer. J Clin Oncol 29(supplement 4):abstract 236

Hayashibe A, Kameyama M, Shinbo M, Makimoto S (2007) Clinical results on intra-arterial adjuvant chemotherapy for prevention of liver metastasis following curative resection of pancreatic cancer. Ann Surg Oncol 14(1):190–194. doi:10.1245/s10434-006-9110-0

Heinrich S, Schafer M, Weber A, Hany TF, Bhure U, Pestalozzi BC, Clavien PA (2008a) Neoadjuvant chemotherapy generates a significant tumor response in resectable pancreatic cancer without increasing morbidity: results of a prospective phase II trial. Ann Surg 248(6):1014–1022. doi:10.1097/SLA.0b013e318190a6da

Heinrich S, Pestalozzi BC, Schafer M, Weber A, Bauerfeind P, Knuth A, Clavien PA (2008b) Prospective phase II trial of neoadjuvant chemotherapy with gemcitabine and cisplatin for resectable adenocarcinoma of the pancreatic head. J Clin Oncol 26(15):2526–2531. doi: 10.1200/JCO.2007.15.5556

Hiraoka T, Uchino R, Kanemitsu K et al (1990) Combination of intraoperative radiation with resection of cancer of the pancreas. Int J Pancreatol 7(1–3):201–207

Hishinuma S, Ogata Y, Tomikawa M, Ozawa I, Hirabayashi K, Igarashi S (2006) Patterns of recurrence after curative resection of pancreatic cancer, based on autopsy findings. J Gastrointest Surg 10(4):511–518. doi:10.1016/j.gassur.2005.09.016

Jamieson NB, Carter CR, McKay CJ, Oien KA (2011) Tissue biomarkers for prognosis in pancreatic ductal adenocarcinoma: a systematic review and meta-analysis. Clin Cancer Res 17(10):3316–3331. doi:10.1158/1078-0432.CCR-10-3284

Jemal A, Siegel R, Xu J, Ward E (2010) Cancer statistics. CA Cancer J Clin 60(5):277–300. doi: 10.3322/caac.20073

Kalser M, Ellenberg S (1985) Pancreatic cancer: adjuvant combined radiation and chemotherapy following curative resection. Arch Surg 120:899–903

Klinkenbijl J, Jeekel J, Sahmoud T et al (1999) Adjuvant radiotherapy and 5-fluorouracil after curative resection of cancer of the pancreas and periampullary region. Phase III trial of the EORTC gastrointestinal tract cancer cooperative group. Ann Surg 230(6):776–784

Knaebel HP, Marten A, Schmidt J, Hoffmann K, Seiler C, Lindel K, Schmitz-Winnenthal H, Fritz S, Herrmann T, Goldschmidt H, Mansmann U, Debus J, Diehl V, Buchler MW (2005) Phase III trial of postoperative cisplatin, interferon alpha-2b, and 5-FU combined with external radiation treatment versus 5-FU alone for patients with resected pancreatic adenocarcinoma—CapRI: study protocol [ISRCTN62866759]. BMC Cancer 5(1):37

Koshy M, Landry J, Cavanaugh S et al (2005) A challenge to the therapeutic nihilism of ESPAC-1. Int J Radiat Oncol Biol Phys 61(4):965–966

Kosuge T, Kiuchi T, Mukai K, Kakizoe T (2006) A multicenter randomised controlled trial to evaluate the effect of adjuvant cisplatin and 5-Fluorouracil therapy after curative resection in cases of pancreatic cancer. Jpn J Clin Oncol 36(3):159–165

Landry J, Catalano PJ, Staley C, Harris W, Hoffman J, Talamonti M, Xu N, Cooper H, Benson AB 3rd (2010) Randomized phase II study of gemcitabine plus radiotherapy versus gemcitabine, 5-fluorouracil, and cisplatin followed by radiotherapy and 5-fluorouracil for patients with locally advanced, potentially resectable pancreatic adenocarcinoma. J Surg Oncol 101(7):587–592. doi: 10.1002/jso.21527

Le Scodan R, Mornex F, Girard N, Mercier C, Valette PJ, Ychou M, Bibeau F, Roy P, Scoazec JY, Partensky C (2009) Preoperative chemoradiation in potentially resectable pancreatic adenocarcinoma: feasibility, treatment effect evaluation and prognostic factors, analysis of the SFRO-FFCD 9704 trial and literature review. Ann Oncol 20(8):1387–1396. doi:10.1093/annonc/mdp015

Li D, Moughan J, Crane CH, Hoffman JP, Regine W, Abrams RA, Safran H, Freedman GM, Guha C, Abbruzzese JL (2011) Association of RecQ1 A159C polymorphism with overall survival of patients with resected pancreatic cancer: a replication study in RTOG 9704. J Clin Oncol 29(supplement 4):abstract 156

Linehan DC, Tan MC, Strasberg SM, Drebin JA, Hawkins WG, Picus J, Myerson RJ, Malyapa RS, Hull M, Trinkaus K, Tan BR Jr (2008) Adjuvant interferon-based chemoradiation followed by gemcitabine for resected pancreatic adenocarcinoma: a single-institution phase II study. Ann Surg 248(2):145–151. doi:10.1097/SLA.0b013e318181e4e9

Maeda A, Boku N, Fukutomi A, Kondo S, Kinoshita T, Nagino M, Uesaka K (2008) Randomized phase III trial of adjuvant chemotherapy with gemcitabine versus S-1 in patients with resected pancreatic cancer: Japan adjuvant study group of pancreatic cancer (JASPAC-01). Jpn J Clin Oncol 38(3):227–229. doi:10.1093/jjco/hym178

Marechal R, Mackey JR, Lai R, Demetter P, Peeters M, Polus M, Cass CE, Young J, Salmon I, Deviere J, Van Laethem JL (2009) Human equilibrative nucleoside transporter 1 and human concentrative nucleoside transporter 3 predict survival after adjuvant gemcitabine therapy in resected pancreatic adenocarcinoma. Clin Cancer Res 15(8):2913–2919. doi:10.1158/1078-0432.CCR-08-2080

Marten A, Schmidt J, Ose J, Harig S, Abel U, Munter MW, Jager D, Friess H, Mayerle J, Adler G, Seufferlein T, Gress T, Schmid R, Buchler MW (2009) A randomized multicentre phase II trial comparing adjuvant therapy in patients with interferon alpha-2b and 5-FU alone or in combination with either external radiation treatment and cisplatin (CapRI) or radiation alone regarding event-free survival—CapRI-2. BMC Cancer 9:160. doi:10.1186/1471-2407-9-160

Marten A, Schmidt J, Debus J, Harig S, Lindel K, Klein J, Bartsch D, Capussotti L, Zülke C, Buchler M (2010) CapRI: final results of the open-label, multicenter, randomized phase III trial of adjuvant chemoradiation plus interferon- 2b (CRI) versus 5-FU alone for patients with resected pancreatic adenocarcinoma (PAC). J Clin Oncol 28[18 (June 20 Supplement)]:LBA4012

Michalski CW, Kleeff J, Wente MN, Diener MK, Buchler MW, Friess H (2007) Systematic review and meta-analysis of standard and extended lymphadenectomy in pancreaticoduodenectomy for pancreatic cancer. Br J Surg 94(3):265–273. doi:10.1002/bjs.5716

Michiels S, Piedbois P, Burdett S et al (2005) Meta-analysis when only the median survival times are known: a comparison with individual patient data results. Int J Technol Assess Health Care 21(1):119–125

Morak MJ, van der Gaast A, Incrocci L, van Dekken H, Hermans JJ, Jeekel J, Hop WC, Kazemier G, van Eijck CH (2008) Adjuvant intra-arterial chemotherapy and radiotherapy versus surgery alone in resectable pancreatic and periampullary cancer: a prospective randomized controlled trial. Ann Surg 248(6):1031–1041. doi:10.1097/SLA.0b013e318190c53e

Morak MJ, Pek CJ, Kompanje EJ, Hop WC, Kazemier G, van Eijck CH (2010) Quality of life after adjuvant intra-arterial chemotherapy and radiotherapy versus surgery alone in resectable pancreatic and periampullary cancer: a prospective randomized controlled study. Cancer 116(4):830–836. doi:10.1002/cncr.24809

Neoptolemos J, Dunn J, Stocken D et al (2001) Adjuvant chemoradiotherapy and chemotherapy in resectable pancreatic cancer: a randomised controlled trial. Lancet 358(9293):1576–1585

Neoptolemos J, Stocken D, Freiss H et al (2004) A randomised trial of chemoradiotherapy and chemotherapy after resection of pancreatic cancer. N Engl J Med 350:1200–1210

Neoptolemos JP, Stocken DD, Bassi C, Ghaneh P, Cunningham D, Goldstein D, Padbury R, Moore MJ, Gallinger S, Mariette C, Wente MN, Izbicki JR, Friess H, Lerch MM, Dervenis C, Olah A, Butturini G, Doi R, Lind PA, Smith D, Valle JW, Palmer DH, Buckels JA, Thompson J, McKay CJ, Rawcliffe CL, Buchler MW (2010) European study group for Pancreatic C. Adjuvant chemotherapy with fluorouracil plus folinic acid vs gemcitabine following pancreatic cancer resection: a randomized controlled trial. JAMA 304 (10):1073–1081. doi 10.1001/jama.2010.1275

Neuhaus P, Riess H, Post S, Gellert K, Ridwelski K, Schramm H, Zuelke C, Fahlke J, Langrehr J, Oettle H (2008) CONKO-001: final results of the randomized, prospective, multicenter phase III trial of adjuvant chemotherapy with gemcitabine versus observation in patients with resected pancreatic cancer. J Clin Oncol 26 (15S):LBA4504, (May 20 Supplement)

Oettle H, Post S, Neuhaus P et al (2007) Adjuvant chemotherapy with gemcitabine versus observation in patients undergoing curative-intent resection of pancreatic cancer. A randomised controlled trial. JAMA 297(3):267–277

Office for National Statistics (2010) Cancer statistics registration: registration of cancers diagnosed in 2008, England

Office for National Statistics (2010) Mortality statistics: deaths registered in England and wales 2008

Palmer DH, Stocken DD, Hewitt H, Markham CE, Hassan AB, Johnson PJ, Buckels JA, Bramhall SR (2007) A randomized phase 2 trial of neoadjuvant chemotherapy in resectable pancreatic cancer: gemcitabine alone versus gemcitabine combined with cisplatin. Ann Surg Oncol 14(7):2088–2096. doi:10.1245/s10434-007-9384-x

Pérez-Mancera PA, Guerra C, Barbacid M, Tuveson DA (2012) What the mouse has told us about human pancreatic cancer. Gastroenterology in press

Picozzi V, Kozarek R, Traverso L (2003) Interferon-based adjuvant chemoradiation therapy after pancreaticoduodenectomy for pancreatic adenocarcinoma. Am J Surg 185:476–480

Picozzi VJ, Abrams RA, Decker PA, Traverso W, O'Reilly EM, Greeno E, Martin RC, Wilfong LS, Rothenberg ML, Posner MC, Pisters PW (2011) American college of surgeons oncology gmulticenter phase II trial of adjuvant therapy for resected pancreatic cancer using cisplatin, 5-fluorouracil, and interferon-alfa-2b-based chemoradiation: ACOSOG Trial Z05031. Ann Oncol 22(2):348–354. doi:10.1093/annonc/mdq384

Regine WF, Winter KA, Abrams RA, Safran H, Hoffman JP, Konski A, Benson AB, Macdonald JS, Kudrimoti MR, Fromm ML, Haddock MG, Schaefer P, Willett CG, Rich TA (2008) Fluorouracil vs gemcitabine chemotherapy before and after fluorouracil-based chemoradiation following resection of pancreatic adenocarcinoma: a randomized controlled trial. JAMA 299(9):1019–1026. doi:10.1001/jama.299.9.1019

Regine WF, Winter KA, Abrams R, Safran H, Hoffman JP, Konski A, Benson AB, Macdonald JS, Rich TA, Willett CG (2011) Fluorouracil-based chemoradiation with either gemcitabine or fluorouracil chemotherapy after resection of pancreatic adenocarcinoma: 5-year analysis of the U.S. Intergroup/RTOG 9704 phase III trial. Ann Surg Oncol 18(5):1319–1326. doi:10.1245/s10434-011-1630-6

Reni M (2010) Neoadjuvant treatment for resectable pancreatic cancer: time for phase III testing? World J Gastroenterol 16(39):4883–4887

Reni M, Panucci M, Ferreri A et al (2001) Effect of local control and survival of electron beam intraoperative irradiation for resectable pancreatic adenocarcinoma. Int J Radiat Oncol Biol Phys 50(3):651–658

Rizzato C, Campa D, Giese N, Werner J, Rachakonda PS, Kumar R, Schanne M, Greenhalf W, Costello E, Khaw KT, Key TJ, Siddiq A, Lorenzo-Bermejo J, Burwinkel B, Neoptolemos JP, Buchler MW, Hoheisel JD, Bauer A, Canzian F (2011) Pancreatic cancer susceptibility loci and their role in survival. PLoS ONE 6(11):e27921. doi:10.1371/journal.pone.0027921

Shore S, Raraty M, Ghaneh P, Neoptolemos J (2003) Chemotherapy for pancreatic cancer. Aliment Pharmacol Ther 18(11–12):1049–1069

Showalter TN, Winter KA, Berger AC, Regine WF, Abrams RA, Safran H, Hoffman JP, Benson AB, MacDonald JS, Willett CG (2011) The influence of total nodes examined, number of positive nodes, and lymph node ratio on survival after surgical resection and adjuvant chemoradiation for pancreatic cancer: a secondary analysis of RTOG 9704. Int J Radiat Oncol Biol Phys 81(5):1328–1335. doi:10.1016j.ijrobp.2010.07.1993

Sindelar W, Kinsella T (1986) Randomised trial of intraoperative radiotherapy in resected carcinoma of the pancreas. Int J Radiat Oncol Biol Phys 12(suppl. 1):148

Smeenk HG, van Eijck CH, Hop WC, Erdmann J, Tran KC, Debois M, van Cutsem E, van Dekken H, Klinkenbijl JH, Jeekel J (2007) Long-term survival and metastatic pattern of pancreatic and periampullary cancer after adjuvant chemoradiation or observation: long-term results of EORTC trial 40891. Ann Surg 246(5):734–740. doi:10.1097/SLA.0b013e318156eef3

Smith RA, Tang J, Tudur-Smith C, Neoptolemos JP, Ghaneh P (2011) Meta-analysis of immunohistochemical prognostic markers in resected pancreatic cancer. Br J Cancer 104(9):1440–1451. doi:10.1038/bjc.2011.110

Sperti C, Pasquali C, Piccoli A et al (1997) Recurrence after resection for ductal adenocarcinoma of the pancreas. World J Surg 21:195–200

Stathis A, Moore M (2010) Advanced pancreatic carcinoma: current treatment and future challenges. Nat Rev Clin Oncol 7:163–172

Stocken D, Buchler M, Dervenis C, et al. (2005) Meta-analysis of randomised adjuvant therapy trials for pancreatic cancer. Br J Cancer, pp 1–10

Sultana A, Tudur Smith C, Cunningham D, Starling N, Neoptolemos J, Ghaneh P (2007) Meta-analyses of chemotherapy for locally advanced and metastatic pancreatic cancer. J Clin Oncol 25(18):2607–2615

Takada T, Amano H, Yasuda H et al (2002) Is postoperative adjuvant chemotherapy useful for gall bladder carcinoma? A phase III multicentre prospective randomised controlled trial in patients with resected pancreaticobiliary carcinoma. Cancer 95(8):1685–1695

Tempero M, Plunkett W, Ruiz Van Haperen V et al (2003) Randomised phase II comparison of dose-intense gemcitabine: thirty-minute infusion and fixed-dose rate infusion in patients with pancreatic adenocarcinoma. J Clin Oncol 21(18):3383–3384

Turrini O, Ychou M, Moureau-Zabotto L, Rouanet P, Giovannini M, Moutardier V, Azria D, Delpero JR, Viret F (2010) Neoadjuvant docetaxel-based chemoradiation for resectable adenocarcinoma of the pancreas: new neoadjuvant regimen was safe and provided an interesting pathologic response. Eur J Surg Oncol 36(10):987–992. doi:10.1016/j.ejso.2010.07.003

Tuveson D, Hanahan D (2011) Translational medicine: cancer lessons from mice to humans. Nature 471(7338):316–317. doi:10.1038/471316a

Tuveson DA, Neoptolemos JP (2012) Understanding metastasis in pancreatic cancer: a call for new clinical approaches. Cell 148:1–4. doi:10.1016/j.cell.2011.12.021

Ueno H, Kosuge T, Matsuyama Y, Yamamoto J, Nakao A, Egawa S, Doi R, Monden M, Hatori T, Tanaka M, Shimada M, Kanemitsu K (2009) A randomised phase III trial comparing gemcitabine with surgery-only in patients with resected pancreatic cancer: Japanese study group of adjuvant therapy for pancreatic cancer. Br J Cancer 101(6):908–915. doi 10.1038/sj.bjc.6605256

Van Laethem JL, Hammel P, Mornex F, Azria D, Van Tienhoven G, Vergauwe P, Peeters M, Polus M, Praet M, Mauer M, Collette L, Budach V, Lutz M, Van Cutsem E, Haustermans K (2010) Adjuvant gemcitabine alone versus gemcitabine-based chemoradiotherapy after curative resection for pancreatic cancer: a randomized EORTC-40013-22012/FFCD-9203/GERCOR phase II study. J Clin Oncol 28(29):4450–4456. doi:10.1200/JCO.2010.30.3446

Van Laethem JL, Verslype C, Iovanna JL, Michl P, Conroy T, Louvet C, Hammel P, Mitry E, Ducreux M, Maraculla T, Uhl W, Van Tienhoven G, Bachet JB, Marechal R, Hendlisz A, Bali M, Demetter P, Ulrich F, Aust D, Luttges J, Peeters M, Mauer M, Roth A, Neoptolemos JP, Lutz M (2011) New strategies and designs in pancreatic cancer research: consensus guidelines report from a European expert panel. Ann Oncol. doi:10.1093/annonc/mdr351

Varadhachary GR, Wolff RA, Crane CH, Sun CC, Lee JE, Pisters PW, Vauthey JN, Abdalla E, Wang H, Staerkel GA, Lee JH, Ross WA, Tamm EP, Bhosale PR, Krishnan S, Das P, Ho L, Xiong H, Abbruzzese JL, Evans DB (2008) Preoperative gemcitabine and cisplatin followed by gemcitabine-based chemoradiation for resectable adenocarcinoma of the pancreatic head. J Clin Oncol 26(21):3487–3495. doi:10.1200/JCO.2007.15.8642

Yoshitomi H, Togawa A, Kimura F, Ito H, Shimizu H, Yoshidome H, Otsuka M, Kato A, Nozawa S, Furukawa K, Miyazaki M, Pancreatic Cancer Chemotherapy Program of the Chiba University Department of General Surgery Affiliated Hospital G (2008) A randomized phase II trial of adjuvant chemotherapy with uracil/tegafur and gemcitabine versus gemcitabine alone in patients with resected pancreatic cancer. Cancer 113(9):2448–2456. doi 10.1002/cncr.23863

Zerbi A, Fossati V, Parolini D (1994) Intraoperative radiation therapy adjuvant to resection in the treatment of pancreatic cancer. Cancer 73:2930–2935

Radiotherapy of the Pancreas: State of the Art in 2012

F. Mornex, M. Hatime, S. Touch, B. Elmorabit, G. Pigne, C. Enachescu, O. Diaz and Y. Elkhoti

Contents

1 The Role of Radiotherapy in the Therapeutic Management of Pancreatic Cancer........... 90
   1.1 Adjuvant Approach 90
   1.2 Neoadjuvant Approach... 92
   1.3 Approach of Unresectable Pancreatic Tumors... 93
2 Techniques of Radiation Therapy Planning and Delivery... 94
   2.1 Radiation Dose Escalation 95
   2.2 Intensity-Modulated Radiation Therapy 95
   2.3 Image-Guided Radiation Therapy and Stereotactic Body Radiation Therapy........... 97
3 Conclusions.. 99
References... 99

Pancreatic adenocarcinoma (PA) is a rare tumor; it represents 2–3 % of all new cancer cases in Europe and USA, and 95 % of malignant pancreatic tumors (Parkin et al. 2001). PA is an aggressive disease with a poor prognosis, one-year survival rate of 25 % and a five-year survival rate of less than 5 % (Evans et al. 2001). PA is among the top five causes of cancer-related death in adults in most industrialized countries, with over 70,000 deaths per year in Europe and the USA (Fernandez et al. 1994; Bramhall et al. 1995; Bramhall et al. 1998; Parkin et al. 2001; Jemal et al. 2002).

Surgery is mainly the only hope for cure of PA. However, only 5–25 % of patients with PA are amenable to resection, due to the presence of borderline resectable, locally advanced, or metastatic disease in the majority of patients. After radical resection of a localized PA, the median survival rate is about 12–18 months and 5-year survival rate is approximately 10–15 % (Edis et al. 1980; Manabe et al. 1989; Baumel et al. 1994;

F. Mornex (✉) · M. Hatime · S. Touch · B. Elmorabit ·
G. Pigne · C. Enachescu · O. Diaz · Y. Elkhoti
Radiation Oncology Department, Centre Hospitalier Lyon Sud,

F. Otto and M. P. Lutz (eds.), *Early Gastrointestinal Cancers*,
Recent Results in Cancer Research 196, DOI: 10.1007/978-3-642-31629-6_6,
© Springer-Verlag Berlin Heidelberg 2012

Table 1 Clinical classification of pancreatic cancer

Staging	Characteristics
Resectable	– No radiographic evidence of superior mesenteric vein and portal vein abutment; distortion, tumor thrombus, or venous encasement
	– Clear fat planes around the celiac axis; hepatic artery; and superior mesenteric artery
	– No distant metastases
Borderline resectable	– SMV or PV encased, neighboring arteries not encased
	– SMV or PV occluded with patent vessel proximal and distal
	– Tumor encases less than half the circumference of SMA
	– GD encased up to HA; but not extending to CA
	– No distant metastases
Locally advanced or unresectable	– Involvement of nodes outside resection field
	– Tumor abuts or encases more than half circumference of CA suitable vessel for reconstruction
	– Aorta invaded or encased
	– No distant metastases
Metastatic	– Distant metastases

Abbreviation: *CA* celiac axis; *GD* Gastroduodenal artery; *HA* hepatic artery; *PV* portal vein; *SMA* superior mesenteric artery; *SMV* superior mesenteric vein

Janes et al. 1996). A local recurrence will be observed in 50–80 % of cases (Griffin et al. 1990; Westerdahl et al. 1993). In case of locally advanced or metastatic PA, median overall survival is 6–12 months and 3–6 months, respectively (Haller 2003). The tumor will recur in the peritoneum or liver in more than 75 % of cases (Griffin et al. 1990; Westerdahl et al. 1993). Table 1 describes these clinical situations.

In this context of a very poor prognosis, there is a major need of a better understanding regarding the complex biology of this tumor, as well as of new therapeutic strategies, including especially the field of modern radiotherapy development. This review will describe (1) the role of radiotherapy, alone or combined to chemotherapy, in different settings, corresponding to the clinical situations observed with this disease, (2) the new techniques of radiation, which make currently the conventional radiotherapy totally obsolete.

1 The Role of Radiotherapy in the Therapeutic Management of Pancreatic Cancer

1.1 Adjuvant Approach

The goal of radiation is to eradicate tumor in the upper abdomen. Even if the tumor is fully resected, the outcome in patients with early pancreatic cancer is disappointing. Local recurrences are observed after radical surgery, expressing the fact that cancerous cells have been left locally, which must be eradicated. In this context of the need for adjuvant therapy, radiation, chemotherapy, and combined chemoradiation have been tested in several trials. A standard radiation field includes the presurgery tumor volume and, often, prophylactic treatment of the celiac and portal lymph nodes. Chemotherapeutic agents have been shown to make cancer cells more susceptible to death by radiation than the surrounding healthy cells. The mechanism that produces cytotoxicity is often not the same mechanism that increases the sensitivity to radiation.

Combination of adjuvant radiation and chemotherapy has been assessed in several phase I and phase II studies (Alfieri 2001; Johnstone and Sindelar 1993; Willett et al. 1993; Klinkenbijl et al. 1999; Lee et al. 2000; Mehta et al. 2000). Four randomized trials have been reported (Table 2); they evaluate the impact of postoperative adjuvant therapy in patients with resected pancreatic cancer. All these trials have been largely criticized, regarding the quality of radiation, the split course scheme, the use of Cobalt 60 and 2D radiotherapy, often without any central review or quality control, especially in the ESPAC 1 trial; Bolus of 5FU was also described as a suboptimal chemotherapy (Neoptolemos et al. 2004).

Because of these concerns, despite the results unfavorable to radiation, there has not been universal abandonment of postoperative chemoradiation as shown below.

The RTOG adjuvant phase III study 97-04, which compared two regimens of chemotherapy, did not help to evaluate the role of CRT because all the patients received this treatment (Regine et al. 2008). These results are similar to those of large institutions series incorporating also radiation therapy (Hidalgo 2010).

The only published randomized trial of adjuvant CRT and maintenance chemotherapy randomly allocated 43 patients with R0 resected PA to either observation alone or the same regimen as that developed by the Gastrointestinal Tumor Group for patients with locally advanced PA (Moertel et al. 1969, 1981).

On the other hand, the feasibility of postoperative administration of gemcitabine alone, followed by concurrent gemcitabine and irradiation after curative resection for PA has been evaluated. Twenty-two patients with stage II and III curatively resected tumors were included with a good tolerance, showing that this treatment was feasible (Van Laethem et al. 2003). The EORTC 40013 randomized phase II trial was designed to compare adjuvant gemcitabine-based CRT followed by gemcitabine with chemotherapy with gemcitabine alone, and demonstrated that combined chemotherapy and modern radiation was not deleterious and feasible, with encouraging results without excessive toxicity (Van Laethem et al. 2010).

As a result, reasonable options for adjuvant treatment following curative resection include chemoradiation, alone or followed by chemotherapy, or chemotherapy alone (Ducreux et al. 2007).

Finally, it can be concluded that postoperative approach combining CT and RT has shown conflicting results and the true impact of postoperative RT-CT remains questionable. Far away from the old fashioned 2D radiotherapy used in EORTC and ESPAC trials, modern radiotherapy and gemcitabine in expert centers is

Table 2 Randomized studies in adjuvant therapy for pancreatic cancer

Trials	No. patients	Method	Median survival
ESPAC-1 (Neoptolemos et al. 2004)	144	No chemoradiation	17.9 vs 15.9 months (p = NS)
	145	Chemoradiation	
GITSG (Moertel et al. 1981)	25	Surgery + radiation alone (60 Gy)	5 months vs 10,1 - 10,6 months (p < 0.001)
	169	Surgery + chemoradiation (40–60 Gy)	
RTOG 9704 (Regine WF et al. 2008)	230 221	Surgery + chemoradiation + chemotherapy (5-FU) Surgery + chemoradiation + chemotherapy (Gemcitabine)	16,9 vs 20,5 months vs 22 vs 31 % for a 3 year survival (p = .09, 95 % confidence interval, .65-1.03)
EORTC-40013-22012 (Van Laethem et al. 2010)	45	Surgery + chemotherapy (gemcitabine)	24 months for both arms
	45	Surgery + chemoradiation (gemcitabine + RT)	First local recurrent 24 vs 11 %

EORTC European Organization of Research and Treatment of Cancer; *ESPAC* European Study Group for Pancreatic Cancer; *GITSG*, Gastrointestinal Tumor Study Group; *RTOG* Radiation Therapy Oncology Group

feasible. Well-conducted chemoradiation phase II trials are not deleterious, as shown for example in the EORTC 40013 trial (Van Laethem et al. 2010). A SEER analysis reported that modern chemoradiation was suggested to be better than observation (Stessin et al. 2008; Hsu et al. 2010).

Postoperative adjuvant therapy improves survival in patients with resected adenocarcinoma of the pancreas. Unfortunately, the current results urge to clarify the role of chemotherapy, radiation, and newer therapies. New trials including modern radiation should be designed to assess the real impact of modern chemoradiation.

1.2 Neoadjuvant Approach

Neoadjuvant therapy can be proposed to downstage a locally advanced tumor and to decrease the rate of local failures and positive margins. (Ducreux et al. 2007; Hidalgo 2010; Mornex et al. 2006; Le Scodan et al. 2009). It has also been proposed after observing that many patients (more than 30 %), following pancreatic tumor resection, will not be able to receive an adjuvant treatment due to complications. (Wey et al. 2005). Preoperative (chemo)radiotherapy provides better survival than both postoperative (chemo)radiotherapy and surgery alone (Hsu et al. 2010; Evans et al. 2008).

Some phase II trials have been conducted, showing that it was possible to perform surgery of pancreatic neoplasms after completion of a CRT schedule, (Hoffman et al. 1995, 1998), the most recent including gemcitabine. These non-randomized chemoradiation phase II trials suggest this approach is at least as effective as postoperative treatment and may decrease the rate of local failures and positive resection margins after surgery (Hidalgo 2010).

Neoadjuvant chemoradiation appears to have a potential benefit in resectable, and also borderline resectable pancreatic cancer. The definition of locally advanced PA depends largely on the expertise of the local PA team (Talamonti et al. 2000). Provided that this expertise is available, patients with locally advanced PA (and without metastases) are eligible for radiotherapy, chemotherapy, or both. Studies are frequently hampered by the inclusion of ampullary or biliary cancers, and variations in the definition of 'unresectable locally advanced PA', as up to two-thirds of cases of so-called 'unresectable PA' could eventually be resected by specialized surgical teams (Sohn et al. 1999). About 20–34 % of initially unresectable tumors can be converted to resectable disease, at the price of increased but manageable toxicities (Laurence et al. 2011). An extensive meta-analysis investigated 111 studies of neoadjuvant treatment, 56 of which were in patients with tumors considered unresectable. In these studies of patients with initially unresectable tumors, 33.2 % of patients underwent a successful resection. Remarkably, the R0 resection rate (79.2 %) and the median survival (20.5 months) in this group were similar to those seen in the studies of primarily resected patients (Gillen et al. 2010; Ceha et al. 2000).

Future studies should overcome selection biases, uniform standard for reporting pathology, and study endpoints must be developed; modern radiotherapy, especially including modulated intensity radiotherapy, must be used to avoid toxicity in the surrounding radiosensitive organs. All these efforts should continue in order to define an active optimal neoadjuvant treatment that can be evaluated against surgery or in order to make borderline resectable tumors amenable to curative surgery, with equivalent prognosis to those obtained with resectable tumors (Van Tienhoven et al. 2011).

1.3   Approach of Unresectable Pancreatic Tumors

Approximately 30 % of patients with pancreatic cancer receive a diagnosis of advanced locoregional disease, and an additional 30 % of patients will have local recurrence of tumors after treatment for early disease. The optimal management of these patients is still controversial, management options range from systemic chemotherapy alone to combined forms of treatment with chemoradiation therapy and chemotherapy. Furthermore, adding to the debate, several trials have been published comparing the different treatment modalities with conflicting results (Chauffert et al. 2008).

Since local tumor growth is often a factor of importance causing severe pain, it is logical to consider radiotherapy or chemoradiotherapy as a treatment option, with median duration of pain relief of 6 months (Ceha et al. 2000). Generally, it is believed that radiation alone is a suboptimal treatment for locally advanced pancreatic cancer as most of the patients will die of systemic disease, even if new radiotherapy techniques are found to give better results.

A series of randomized trials conducted over the last two decades established that chemoradiation was superior to radiation alone and superior to best supportive care (Sultana et al. 2007; Van Tienhoven et 2011; Bichenbach et al. 2011).

Several drugs have been combined to radiation, 5FU, capecitabine, taxanes have also been studied, and, more recently, gemcitabine has been introduced in this setting of combined chemoradiation, especially for its radiosensitization properties. When radiation used fields confined to the tumor alone, high doses of gemcitabine were able to be administered weekly, doses two to three times higher than studies that used regional, larger fields (Huang et al. 2011).

If the common treatment is often chemoradiation, an alternative strategy is the use of induction chemotherapy followed by chemoradiation. This approach has the advantage of excluding patients with rapidly progressive and occult metastatic disease who may not benefit from primary local treatment (Gillmore 2010).

Targeted therapies have been tested in the treatment of metastatic pancreatic carcinoma with various results. The addition of bevacizumab (an anti-angiogenic antibody) to gemcitabine was not active (Kindler et al. 2007). Similarly, the addition of cetuximab, an epidermal growth factor receptor (EGFR) inhibitor, to gemcitabine does not show any benefit (Philip et al. 2007). However, the addition of erlotinib, another EGFR inhibitor, to gemcitabine has given positive results with a statistically significant improvement in overall survival (Moore et al. 2007). This drug has obtained approval in the USA and Europe.

In locally advanced pancreatic cancer, molecular therapies may play a role as radiosensitizer. The mechanisms of potential radiosensitization produced by bevacizumab are not clear but could include enhanced lethality of endothelial cells and/or tumor cells (Gorski et al. 1999; Wey et al. 2005). However, real sensitization of radiotherapy with bevacizumab has been demonstrated in the treatment of rectal cancer (Willett et al. 2006). The induction of EGFR targeting with cetuximab in radiation-based therapy of solid tumors has yielded promising results. Thus, trimodal therapy with gemcitabine-based CRT and cetuximab was evaluated in locally advanced inoperable pancreatic cancer (Krempien et al. 2007). These results seem to be very promising but they need to be confirmed.

Overall, there is no doubt that radiation therapy is useful in this setting, especially when combined to chemotherapy. Modern radiation should be tested, especially with limited fields, as allowed by IMRT, in order to improve the results without increasing the toxicity. Definitive results are warranted to clarify the situation and close the debate.

2 Techniques of Radiation Therapy Planning and Delivery

The poor results observed for pancreatic cancer justify the search for a therapeutic improvement. Radiation dose escalation has shown disease control benefits for various cancer sites, such as prostate or lung cancer. For pancreatic cancer, although systemic relapse is a predominant feature, dose escalation may provide better long-term disease control for selected patients. It is noteworthy that the longest median survival rates were achieved in series in which a higher dose was given by using either brachytherapy or intraoperative radiotherapy (IORT), suggesting a dose–response relation in terms of local disease control (Bouchard et al. 2009).

However, pancreas is a deep organ surrounded by radiosensitive organs, which can be damaged by radiation; this situation being a real challenge, the proximity of organs at risk (OAR) can hamper external beam dose escalation because the appropriate tumoricidal dose level needed to eradicate the bulk of the tumor can exceed the maximally tolerated radiation dose.

Three-dimensional reconstruction of the target area, beam conformation, and three-dimensional treatment planning allow minimization of the radiation dose delivered to the stomach, duodenum, kidneys, liver, and spinal cord. Consequently, tumor doses can be increased, with normal tissue doses kept below chosen limits.

2.1 Radiation Dose Escalation

In a phase II study, the primary objective was to investigate the feasibility of delivering doses above 70 Gy by external beam therapy using multiple small, conformal fields. Elective lymph node areas were not treated. From the results, it can be concluded that a total dose of 72 Gy over 7 weeks is feasible using conformal radiotherapy, with a satisfying sparing of normal surrounding tissues, low toxicity, but disappointing results.

2.2 Intensity-Modulated Radiation Therapy

With recent advances in radiotherapy planning and delivery, it is now possible to benefit from improvements in radiation treatment techniques, especially with intensity-modulated photon-radiation therapy: IMRT (Bouchard et al. 2009). This technique allows dose escalation with minimal normal tissue damage. For pancreatic cancer, dosimetric studies have shown the benefits of IMRT over three-dimensional photon-radiation therapy (3DCRT) in achieving dose escalation (Bouchard et al. 2009).

An early phase I trial of concurrent gemcitabine and IMRT was closed early due to excessive toxicity (Crane et al. 2001). However, additional studies have demonstrated favorable toxicity profiles with IMRT and chemotherapy. Ben-Josef reported a phase I study using IMRT and concurrent gemcitabine with doses ranging from 50 to 60 Gy that attempted to intensify local therapy for patients presenting with locally advanced pancreatic cancer. Treatment volumes included a 1 cm margin around the primary tumor, with additional measures taken to account for tumor movement. This study was well tolerated and demonstrated a very promising median survival of 23.1 months, with local progression in only one patient (Ben-Josef et al. 2009).

Table 3 IMRT in pancreatic cancer

Author	Years	Methods	Treatment technique	Median survival	Toxicity
Milano et al.	2003 Retrospective study	– 17 unresectable tumors 25 unresectable pancreatic cancers : – 8 resected tumors,	50.4–59.4 Gy CT + IMRT : 45–50.4 Gy	- 14.3 months - 17.3 months	– chronic small bowel obstruction (Grade 2) in 1 patient – Grade 4 late liver toxicity in 1 patient
Ben-Josef et al.	2004 Retrospective study	15 unresectable pancreatic cancers : – 7 as adjuvant therapy after curative resection – 8 unresectable disease	CT + IMRT : 45–54 Gy 54–55 Gy	8.5 months	– Grade 3 gastric ulceration toxicity in 1 patient – Weight loss in nine patients
Ben-Josef et al.	2009 Phase I	27 unresectable pancreatic cancers	IMRT with active breathing control: 50, 52.5, 55, 57.5 and 60 Gy	23.1 months -	– G3 anorexia, nausea vomiting, and/or dehydration in 5 patients – duodenal bleed in 1 patient.

Abreviation: *CT* chemotherapy

Milano et al. treated 25 patients having pancreatic and bile duct cancer, with IMRT and concurrent 5-FU. This study found that IMRT was well tolerated and reduced the mean dose to the small bowel, stomach, liver, and kidneys, with 80 % of patients experiencing grade 2 toxicity only (Milano et al. 2004; Willett et al. 2003). In an other study, the IMRT, with concomitant capecetabine used to a dose 54 Gy to the GTV and 45 Gy to the draining lymph nodes in a simultaneous boost method, is likely to be safely delivered (Ben Josef et al. 2004; Roy and Maraveyas 2010). Even with IMRT, the proximity of tail tumors to the stomach and the proximity of pancreatic head tumors to the duodenum make sparing of the surrounding normal tissues challenging. Motion of the primary tumor due to respiration presents a problem in the design of highly conformal radiation fields (Johung et al. 2012). The recent introduction of respiratory-gated four-dimensional computed tomography (4D-CT) acquisition technique has shown the potential to improve radiotherapy target definition by the inclusion of personalized information based on the lesion movement due to breathing (Mori et al. 2009; Pan et al. 2004; Rietzel et al. 2005).

In the Cattaneo study, the center of mass motion was estimated during quiet breathing in the CE-4D-CT (contrast-enhanced 4D-CT) images to define ITV for RT plan comparing 4D and population-based approach, and to evaluate intraobserver variability in ITV definition.

By synchronizing the CT acquisition to the respiratory curve, the 4D technique describes breathing motion and defines the volume within which the lesion moves. Thereby GTV margins can be reduced with a better sparing of normal tissues surrounding the tumor lesion, even more in IMRT planning in which dose gradients between target and OAR are higher (Rietzel et al. 2005; Xi et al. 2007).

Overall, results of these preliminary studies indicate that the use of IMRT provides a promising means of intensifying treatment without adding excessive toxicity. The position of IMRT and other concurrent irradiation techniques for local control needs randomized clinical trials with conventional comparators Table 3.

2.3 Image-Guided Radiation Therapy and Stereotactic Body Radiation Therapy

The emergence of image-guided radiation therapy (IGRT) combined with sophisticated linear accelerators and micromultileaf collimators gives now access to stereotactic body radiation therapy (SBRT), a technique able to deliver very high radiation doses, regarded as ablative. The SBRT is a minimally invasive treatment usually indicated to treat small and hard-to-target lesions. In order to deliver such high doses to selected cases, some specific devices (usually implanted gold-fiducial seeds) or bony structures are used as reference points to track the tumor motion and surrounding organs during the treatment. Visualized by four-dimensional CT scan (4-D CT), a gross tumor volume (GTV) movement is adjusted due to the respiration. A 2–3 mm margin is added to define planning target volume (PTV) for assuring the setup error. To decrease the normal tissue exposure and provide rapid fall-off of the radiation dose, multiple non-coplanar fixed-beams or arc fields are applied (Chang and Saif 2008; Chang et al. 2008). The improved ability to shape the radiation beam and spare surrounding tissues has led to a greater interest of SBRT be time saving, as it is typically delivered in 1–5 fractions with very high dose per fraction (vary from 8 to 25 Gy) which radio-biologically achieves ablative doses (Chang and Saif 2008; Chang et al. 2008; Mahadevan et al. 2010; Schelleberg et al. 2011).

With rigorous quality assurance, the SBRT would be an optimal choice to treat small tumors (<5 cm) which recur locally with ability to sterilize them and to decrease the systemic toxicity. Positive margins patients after surgery might benefit from ablative dose of SBRT to complete objective of R0 resection. Recently, several trials have demonstrated the feasibility and efficacy of SBRT for pancreatic cancer (Chang and Saif 2008; Chang et al. 2008).

In 2009, a study reported by Chang aims to show the efficacy of local control and toxicity in unresectable pancreatic cancer by using SBRT at dose of 25 Gy in one fraction. Seventy-five patients were eligible to be recruited, 45 patients had locally advanced disease, 11 patients had medically inoperable disease, 15 patients had metastatic disease, and 6 patients had locally recurrent disease. Excellent local control of 91 % and 84 % of freedom from local progression (FFLP) were observed at 6 and 12 months respectively. Regarding high grade toxicity (Grade $\geq$ 3), the authors recommend paying much attention on the treatment planning and delivery (Chang et al. 2008).

A group in Boston has published a retrospective analysis of 36 patients (non-metastatic, locally advanced, or unresectable PA). The patients were treated with hypofractionated SBRT by using three categories of doses (8, 10 or 12 Gy per fraction) with total doses of 24–36 Gy in three fractions followed by gemcitabine. With an overall median follow-up of 24 months (range, 12–33), a high rank of local control was obtained in 78 % and the median survival time was 14.3 months. Factors determining progression-free survival (PFS) were carbohydrate antigen 19-9 and computed tomography, which were 7.9 and 9.6 months, respectively. The acute and late toxicity was also concluded to be safely acceptable (Mahadevan et al. 2010).

A phase II trial was performed by Schellenberg to evaluate the toxicity, local control, and overall survival in 20 patients treated with single-fraction SBRT (25 Gy) with sequential gemcitabine. In result, no acute grade $\geq$3 gastrointestinal toxicity was reported; whereas one patient (5 %) experienced late grade 4 gastrointestinal toxicity, which needed surgery for duodenal perforation. Median survival was 11.8 months; the survival rate of 50 and 20 % was applied in the first and second year, respectively. Serial computed tomography was used to define the FFLP which was very high (94 %) at 1 year (Schelleberg et al. 2011). These studies are summarized in Table 4.

Once again, improvements are facing technical problems and difficulties, such as organ motion, definition of the extent of the disease, and surrounding organs: the proximity of the duodenum poses a particular challenge, as hypofractionated radiation to the bowel can cause late stenosis, ulceration, hemorrhage or perforation, as observed in clinical trials.

Table 4 SBRT results in pancreatic cancer

Author	No. patients	Method of treatment	Median survival (months)
Chang et al. (2008)	77	25 Gy × 1	6.7
Mahadevan et al. (2010)	36	8–12 Gy × 3 => Gem × 6 months	14.3
Shellenberg et al. (2011)	20	Gem at days 1, 8, 15 follow by 25 Gy × 1 SBRT day 29	11.8

Further prospective studies are required to determine the optimal dose fractionation scheme to maximize therapeutic ratio, and to examine whether improved local control with SBRT can ultimately be translated into a survival benefit.

3 Conclusions

There is no doubt that the role of radiotherapy in pancreatic carcinoma is important, most of the time in combination with chemotherapy, using several schemes, in different settings. The advent of modern radiation techniques, such as IMRT for normal tissues sparing, or SBRT, sustained by IGRT, by increasing the radiation dose for an optimized tumoricidal effect, may deeply modify the landscape of this disease, by producing new positive results. The previous and current indications of radiation and chemoradiation should be revisited at the light of the modern techniques to redefine the precise role of this powerful tool in oncology, whose role has been jeopardized in pancreatic cancer by obsolete studies.

References

Alfieri S, Morganti AG, Di Giorgio A et al (2001) Improved survival and local control after intraoperative radiation therapy and postoperative radiotherapy: a multivariate analysis of 46 patients undergoing surgery for pancreatic head cancer. Arch Surg 136:343–347

Baumel H, Huguier M, Manderscheid JC et al (1994) Results of resection for cancer of the exocrine pancreas: a study from the French association of surgery. Br J Surg 81:102–110

Ben-Josef E, Griffith K, Francis IR et al (2009) Phase I radiation dose –escalation trial of intensity-modulated radiotherapy (IMRT) with concurrent fixed dose-rate gemcitabine (FDRG) for unresecatable pancreatic cancer. J Clin Oncol 27:a4602

Ben-Josef E, Shields AF, Vaishampayan U et al (2004) Intensity-modulated radiotherapy (IMRT) and concurrent capecitabine for pancreatic cancer. Int J Radiat Oncol Biol Phys 59:454–459

Bichenbach KA, Gonen M,Tang LH et al. (2011) Down staging in pancreatic cancer: a matched analysis of patients resected following systemic treatment of initially locally unresectable disease. Annal surgical oncol. doi: 10.124/s10434-011-2156-7

Bouchard M, Amos RA, Briere TM et al (2009) Dose escalation with proton or photon radiation treatment for pancreatic cancer. Radiother Oncol 92:238–243

Bramhall SR, Allum WH, Jones AG et al (1995) Treatment and survival in 13,560 patients with pancreatic cancer, and incidence of the disease, in the West Midlands: an epidemiological study. Br J Surg 82:111–115

Bramhall SR, Dunn J, Neoptolemos JP et al. (1998) Epidemiology of pancreatic cancer. In: Carr-Locke (ed); the pancreas, Blackwell Scientific, Boston pp 889–906

Chang BW, Saif MW (2008) Stereotactic body radiation therapy (SBRT) in Pancreatic Cancer: is it ready for prime time. JOP. J Pancreas (Online) 9(6):676–682

Ceha HM, Van Tienhoven G, Gouma DJ et al (2000) Feasibility and efficacy of high dose conformal radiotherapy for patients with locally advanced pancreatic carcinoma. Cancer 89:2222–2229

Chauffert B, Mornex F, Bonnetain F et al (2008) Phase III trial comparing initial chemoradiotherapy (intermittent cisplatine and infusional 5-FU) followed by gemcitabine vs. gemcitabine alone in patients with locally advanced non metastatic pancreatic cancer: a FFCD-SFRO study. Ann Oncol 19:1592–1599

Crane CH, Antolak JA, Rosen II et al (2001) Phase I study of concomitant gemcitabine and IMRT for patient with unresecable adenocarcinoma of the pancreatic head. Int J Gastrointest cancer 30:123–132

Chang DT, Schellenberg D, Shen J et al. (2008) Stereotactic radiotherapy for unresectable adenocarcinoma of the pancreas. Cancer 2009. doi: 10.1002/cncr.24059

Ducreux M, Boige V, Goéré D et al (2007) Pancreatic cancer: from pathogenesis to cure. Best Pract Res Clin Gastroenterol 21(6):997–1014

Edis AJ, Kiernan PD, Taylor WF (1980) Attempted curative resection of ductal carcinoma of the pancreas. Review of Mayo clinic experience, 1951–1975. Mayo Clin Proc 55:531–536

Evans DB, Abbruzzese JL, Willett CG et al. (2001) Cancer of the pancreas. Principles and practice of oncology. In: Hellman S, Rosenberg SA (eds), Lippincott Williams and Wilkins, Philadelphia 1126–1161

Evans DB, Varadhachary GR, Crane CH et al (2008) Preoperative gemcitabine-based chemoradiation for patients with resectable adenocarcinoma of the pancreatic head. J Clin Oncol 26:3496–3502

Fernandez E, La Vecchia C, Porta M et al (1994) Trends in pancreatic cancer mortality in Europe, 1955–1989. Int J Cancer 57:786–792

Gillen S, Schuster T, Meyer Zum Büschenfelde C et al (2010) Preoperative/neoadjuvant therapy in pancreatic cancer: a systematic review and meta-analysis of response and resection percentages. PLoS Med 7(4): e1000267

Gillmore R, Laurence V, Raouf S et al (2010) Chemoradiotherapy with or without induction chemotherapy for locally advanced pancreatic cancer: a UK multi-institutional experience. Clin Oncol (R Coll Radiol) 22(7): 564–569

Gorski DH, Beckett MA, Jaskowiak NT et al (1999) Blockage of the vascular endothelial growth factor stress response increases the antitumor effects of ionizing radiation. Cancer Res 59:3374–3378

Griffin JF, Smalley SR, Jewell W et al (1990) Patterns of failure after curative resection of pancreatic carcinoma. Cancer 66:56–61

Haller DG (2003) Chemotherapy for advanced pancreatic cancer. Int J Radiat Oncol Biol Phys 56:16–23

Hidalgo M (2010) Pancreatic cancer. N E J Med 362:1605–1617

Hoffman JP, Lipsitz S, Pisansky T et al (1998) Phase II trial of preoperative radiation therapy and chemotherapy for patients with localized, resectable adenocarcinoma of the pancreas: an eastern cooperative oncology group study. J Clin Oncol 16:317–323

Hoffman JP, Weese JL, Solin LJ et al (1995) A pilot study of preoperative chemoradiation for patients with localized adenocarcinoma of the pancreas. Am J Surg 169:71–77

Hsu CC, Herman JM, Corsini MM et al (2010) Adjuvant chemoradiation for pancreatic adenocarcinoma: the Johns Hopkins hospital-mayo clinic collaborative study. Ann Surg Oncol 17:981–990

Huang J, M.robertson J, Margolis J and al (2011) Long-term results of full-dose gemcitabine with radiation therapy compared TO 5-FLUOROURACIL radiation therapy for locally advanced pancreas cancer. doi:10.1016/j.radonc.2011.05.038

Janes RH, Niederhuber JE, Chmiel JS et al (1996) National patterns of care for pancreatic cancer. Results of a survey by the commission on cancer. Ann Surg 223:261–272

Jemal A, Thomas A, Murray T et al (2002) Cancer statistics. CA Cancer J Clin 52:23–47

Johnstone PA, Sindelar WF (1993) Patterns of disease recurrence following definitive therapy of adenocarcinoma of the pancreas using surgery and adjuvant radiotherapy: correlations of a clinical trial. Int J Radiat Oncol Biol Phys 27:831–834

Johung K, Saif MW, Chang BW (2012) Treatment of locallyadvanced pancreatic cancer: the role of radiation therapy. Int J Radiat Oncol Biol Phys 82(2):508–518

Kindler HL, Niedzwiecki D, Hollis D, et al (2007) A double-blind, placebo-controlled, randomized phase III trial of gemcitabine (G) plus bevacizumab (B) versus gemcitabine plus placebo (P) in patients (pts) with advanced pancreatic cancer (PC): a preliminary analysis of cancer and leukemia group B (CALGB) 80303. In Proceedings of the GI ASCO symposium, abstract no 108. http://www.asco.org/ASCOv2/Meetings/Abstracts?vmview=abst_detail_view&abstractID=10557&confID=45

Klinkenbijl HL, Jeekel J, Sahmoud T et al (1999) Adjuvant radiotherapy and 5-fluorouracil after curative resection of cancer of the pancreas and periampullary region: phase III trial of the EORTC gastrointestinal tract cancer cooperative group. Ann Surg 230:776–782

Krempien R, Munter MW, Timke C et al. (2007) Cetuximab in combination with intensity modulated radiotherapy (IMRT) and gemcitabine for patients with locally advanced pancreatic cancer: a prospective phase II trial [PARC-Study ISRCTN56652283]. Proc Am Soc Clin Oncol, 25:4573

Laurence JM, Tran PD, Morarji K, Eslick GD, Lam VW, Sandroussi C (2011) A systematic review and meta-analysis of survival and surgical outcomes following neoadjuvant chemoradiotherapy for pancreatic cancer. J Gastrointest Surg 15(11):2059–2069. doi:10.1007/s11605-011-1659

Le Scodan R, Mornex F, Girard N et al (2009) Preoperative chemoradiation in potentially resectable pancreatic adenocarcinoma: feasibility, treatment effect evaluation and prognostic factors, analysis of the SFRO-FFCD 9704 trial and literature review. Ann Oncol 20(8): 1387–1396

Lee JH, Whittington R, Williams NN et al (2000) Outcome of pancreaticoduodenectomy and impact of adjuvant therapy for ampullary carcinomas. Int J Radiat Oncol Biol Phys 47:945–953

Mahadevan A, Jain S, Goldstein M et al (2010) Stereotactic body radiotherapy and gemcitabine for locally advanced pancreatic cancer. Int J Radiation Oncology Biol Phys 78(3):735–742

Manabe T, Ohshio G, Baba N et al (1989) Radical pancreatectomy for ductal cell carcinoma of the head of the pancreas. Cancer 64:1132–1137

Mehta VK, Fisher GA, Ford JM et al (2000) Adjuvant radiotherapy and concomitant 5-fluorouracil by protracted venous infusion for resected pancreatic cancer. Int J Radiat Oncol Biol Phys 48:1483–1487

Milano MT, Chmura SJ, Garofalo MC et al (2004) Intensity-modulated radiotherapy in treatment of pancreatic and bile duct malignancies: toxicity and clinical outcome. Int J Radiat Oncol Biol Phys 59:445–453

Moertel CG, Childs DS, Reitemeier RJ et al (1969) Combined 5-fluorouracil and supervoltage radiation therapy of locally unresectable gastrointestinal cancer. Lancet 2:865–867

Moertel CG, Frytak S, Hahn RG et al (1981) Therapy of locally unresectable pancreatic carcinoma: a randomized comparison of high dose (6000 Rads) radiation alone, moderate dose radiation (4000 Rads + 5-fluorouracil), and high dose radiation + 5-fluorouracil. Gastrointest Tumor Study Group Cancer 48:1705–1710

Moore MJ, Goldstein D, Hamm J et al (2007) Erlotinib plus gemcitabine compared with gemcitabine alone in patients with advanced pancreatic cancer: a phase III trial of the national cancer institute of canada clinical trials group. J Clin Oncol 25:1960–1966

Mori S, Hara R, Yanagi T et al (2009) Four-dimensional measurement of intrafractional respiratory motion of pancreatic tumours using a 256 multi-slice CT scanner. Radiother Oncol 92:231–237

Mornex F, Girard N, Scoazec JY et al (2006) Feasibility of preoperative combined radiation therapy and chemotherapy with 5-fluorouracil and cisplatin in potentially resectable pancreatic adenocarcinoma: the French SFRO-FFCD 97-04 phase II trial. Int J Radiat Oncol Biol Phys 65(5): 1471–1478

Neoptolemos JP, Stocken DD, Friess H (2004) A randomized trial of chemoradiotherapy and chemotherapy after resection of pancreatic cancer. N Engl J Med 350:1200–1210

Pan T, Lee TY, Rietzel E et al (2004) 4D-CT imaging of a volume influenced by Respiratory motion on multi-slice CT. Med Phys 31:333–340

Parkin DM, Bray FI, Devesa SS (2001) Cancer burden in the year 2000. The global picture. Eur J Cancer 37(Suppl. 8):S4–S66

Philip PA, Benedetti C, Fenoglio-Preiser Cet al (2007). Phase III study of gemcitabine (G) plus cetuximab (C) versus gemcitabine in patients (pts) with locally advanced or metastatic pancreatic adenocarcinoma (PC): SWOG S025 study. Proc Am Soc Clin Oncol, 25:[LBA4509]

Rietzel E, Chen GT, Choi NC et al (2005) Four-dimensional image-based treatment planning target volume segmentation and dose calculation in the presence of respiratory motion. Int J Radiat Oncol Biol Phys 61:535–555

Regine WF, Winter KA, Abrams RA, Safran H, Hoffman JP, Konski A, et al. (2008) Fluorouracil vs gemcitabine chemotherapy before and after fluorouracil-based chemoradiation following resection of pancreatic adenocarcinoma: a randomized controlled trial. JAMA 299:1019–1026. [PMID18319412]

Roy R, Maraveyas A (2010) Chemoradiation in pancreatic adenocarcinoma: a literature review. Oncologist 15:259–269

Schellenberg D, Kim J, Christman-Skieller C et al (2011) Single-fraction stereotactic body radiation therapy and sequential gemcitabine for the treatment of locally advanced pancreatic cancer. Int J Radiat Oncol Biol Phys 81(1):181–188

Sohn TA, Lillemoe KD, Cameron JL et al (1999) Reexploration for periampullary carcinoma: resectability, perioperative results, pathology, and long-term outcome. Ann Surg 229:393–400

Stessin AM, Meyer JE, Sherr DL (2008) Neoadjuvant radiation is associated with improved survival in patients with resectable pancreatic cancer: an analysis of data from the surveillance, epidemiology, and end results (SEER) registry. Int J Radiat Oncol Biol Phys 72(4): 1128–1133

Sultana A, Tudur Smith C, Cunningham D et al (2007) Systematic review, including meta-analyses, on the management of locally advanced pancreaticcancer using radiation/combined modality therapy. Br J Cancer 96(8):1183–1190

Talamonti MS, Catalano PJ, Vaughn DJ et al (2000) Eastern Cooperative Oncology Group phase I trial of protracted venous infusion fluorouracil plus weekly gemcitabine with concurrent radiation therapy in patients with locally advanced pancreas cancer: a regimen with unexpected early toxicity. J Clin Oncol 18:3384–3389

Van Laethem JL, Demols A, Gay F et al (2003) Postoperative adjuvant gemcitabine and concurrent radiation after curative resection of pancreatic head carcinoma: a phase II study. Int J Radiat Oncol Biol Phys 56:974–980

Van Laethem JL, Hammel P, Mornex F, Azria D, et al. (2010) Adjuvant gemcitabine alone versus gemcitabine-based chemoradiotherapy after curative resection for pancreatic cancer: a randomized EORTC-40013-22012/FFCD-9203/GERCOR Phase II Study. J Clin Oncol 2010. doi: 10.1200/JCO.2010.30.3446

Van Tienhoven JL, Gouma J, Richel D (2011) Neoadjuvant chemoradiotherapy has a potential role in pancreatic carcinoma. Ther Adv Med Oncol 3(1) 27_33

Westerdahl J, Andren-Sandberg A, Ihse I (1993) Recurrence of exocrine pancreatic cancer—local or hepatic. Hepatogastroenterology 40:384–387

Wey JS, Fan F, Gray MJ et al (2005) Vascular endothelial growth factor receptor-1 promotes migration and invasion in pancreatic carcinoma cell lines. Cancer 104:427–438

Willett CG, Kozin SV, Duda DG et al (2006) Combined vascular endothelial growth factor-targeted therapy and radiotherapy for rectal cancer: theory and clinical practice. Semin Oncol 33:S35–S40

Willett CG, Lewandrowski K, Warshaw AL et al (1993) Resection margins in carcinoma of the head of the pancreas. Implications for radiation therapy. Ann Surg 217:144–148

Willett CG, Safran H, Abrams RA et al (2003) Clinical research in pancreatic cancer: the radiation therapy oncology group trials. Int J Radiat Oncol Biol Phys 56:31–37

Xi M, Liu MZ, Deng XW, Zhang L, Huang XY, Liu H et al (2007) Defining internal target volume (ITV) for hepatocellular carcinoma using four-dimensional CT. Radiother Oncol 8:272–278

Part III
Different Cancer Types in the Oesophagus and Stomach

Adenocarcinoma of the GEJ: Gastric or Oesophageal Cancer?

J. Rüschoff

Abstract

According to WHO (2010) adenocarcinomas of the esophagogastric junction (GEJ) are defined as tumors that cross the most proximal extent of the gastric folds regardless of where the bulk of the tumor lies. In addition, these neoplasms are now classified as esophageal cancers by UICC (2010). Recent studies, however, revealed two types of carcinogenesis in the distal oesophagus and at the GEJ, one of intestinal type (about 80 %) and the other of gastric type (about 20 %). These are characterized by marked differences in morphology, tumor stage at diagnosis, and prognosis. Furthermore, both cancer types show different targetable biomarker expression profiles such as Her2 in the intestinal and EGFR in the non-intestinal pathway indicating new therapy options. Due to the fact that carcinomas of the intestinal pathway were typically associated with Barrett's mucosa which was not the case in the non-intestinal-type tumors, this challenges the paradigm "no goblets no Barrett's". Moreover, even the cancer risk of intestinal-type metaplasia has seriously been questioned by a Danish population-based study where Barrett's mucosa turned out to be only a weak indicator of esophageal and GEJ cancer (1 case in 860 patients years). Thus, two biologically different types of cancer arise at the GEJ—esophageal and gastric type that open distinctive targeted treatment options and also question our current concept about the diagnostics of potential precursor lesions as well as the associated screening and surveillance strategy.

J. Rüschoff (✉)
Institut für Pathologie Nordhessen, Germaniastraße 7, 34119 Kassel, Germany
e-mail: rueschoff@patho-nordhessen.de

F. Otto and M. P. Lutz (eds.), *Early Gastrointestinal Cancers*,
Recent Results in Cancer Research 196, DOI: 10.1007/978-3-642-31629-6_7,
© Springer-Verlag Berlin Heidelberg 2012

Contents

1	Introduction	108
2	Challenges of the Current Barrett's Concept	108
	2.1 Evidence of Two Pathways	108
	2.2 Evidence of Different Targets for Therapy	110
	2.3 Evidence for Surveillance Recommendations	111
References		112

1 Introduction

Adenocarcinomas of the esophagus and stomach are two different types of tumors that showed marked changes of incidence with constant rise of esophageal and decrease of gastric cancers during the last three decades in the Western World (Pohl and Welch 2005). Both types arise by two different etiological mechanisms—reflux and Barrett metaplasia in esophageal and H. pylori infection in gastric cancers (Wijetunge et al. 2010). However, much confusion exists about the tumors at the distal third of esophagus and gastric cardia. Adenocarcinomas at the gastroesophageal junction (GEJ) have recently been defined as a third tumor type (GEJ cancer) by WHO Classification of Tumours of the Digestive System (Bosman et al. 2010). This classification is replacing the anatomic system of Siewert suggesting that type I (distal esophegeal) is different from type II (cardiac) and type III (subcardiac) adenocarcinomas (Siewert et al. 2006). Due to common epidemiology with increasing incidence of all three types at the GEJ these tumors have now been grouped within the esophageal category by UICC Cancer Staging Manual (Wittekind and Meyer 2010) (Fig. 1).

Besides this new classification, a multistep model of carcinogenesis in GEJ cancer is widely accepted where intestinal metaplasia is the initial lesion (Barrett's mucosa). This then proceeds to dysplasia (low grade and high grade) and finally shows invasion, i.e., adeno- (Barrett's) carcinoma develops. In addition, these steps are accompanied by accumulation of chromosomal and distinct genetic changes (Baretton and Aust 2012).

2 Challenges of the Current Barrett's Concept

Although the definition and classification of GEJ cancer including the molecular model of multi-step carcinogenesis have only quite recently been developed, there are already new data available that raise questions about this concept.

2.1 Evidence of Two Pathways

Demicco et al. (2011) from Harvard Medical School investigated a series of 157 consecutively resected carcinomas of distal esophagus and GEJ (type I/II acc. to Siewert's classification). When they divided the tumors in those accompanied

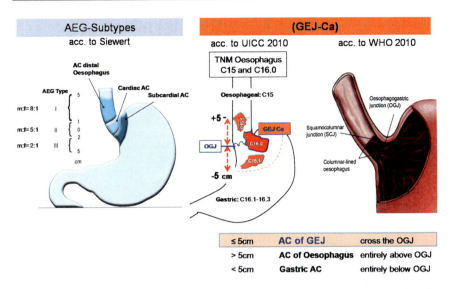

Fig. 1 Classification of adenocarcinomas of lower esophagus and gastroesophageal junction (GEJ). AEG-subtypes according to Siewert (2006) are replaced by WHO (2010) as GEJ cancer and included into UICC's TNM classification of the esophagus (2010)

by intestinal Barrett's metaplasia (n = 108) and those without goblet cell metaplasia (cardiac type mucosa) they observed a number of highly significant differences suggestive of a dichotomy in the carcinogenesis of the distal esophagus and esophagogastric junction. Accordingly, Barrett-associated carcinomas were much more often ($p < 0.0001$) associated with a history of reflux (67 vs. 28 %) and showed a well to moderate grade of differentiation (67 vs 39 %). They were less often in an advanced stage (pT3: 33 vs 88 %) and lymphovascular invasion was less frequent (LV1: 46 vs 88 %). Interestingly, there were also significant differences in the expression of biomarkers. Intestinal-type mucins were typically expressed in Barrett mucosa-associated carcinomas (53 vs 36 %, $p = .0015$). The same holds true when CDX2 (59 vs 16 %, $p = 00.2$) and beta catenin (46 vs 22 % $p = 0.008$) were investigated. They could also show that cardiac-type mucosa-associated carcinomas had a significant higher prevalence of EGFR gene amplification and overexpression (19 % vs 4 %, $p = 0.005$). These associations could even be confirmed if only the larger tumors (>3 cm) were considered demonstrating that overgrowth of adjacent Barrett's mucosa did not play a significant role.

This concept of a two pathway carcinogenesis at the GEJ is supported by other recent studies giving evidence of different types of precursor lesions. In fact, it has been shown that two types of dysplasia could be histologically delineated. One, so-called adenomatous type, is very similar to tubular adenomas in other parts of the gastrointestinum. These lesions may express intestinal-type mucins such as MUC2 and also CDX2 and villin. In contrast, there is another type of precursor lesion that shows a villous architecture with more eosinophilic polarized

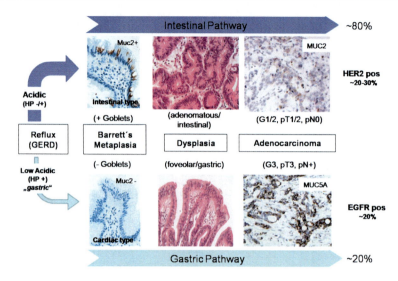

Fig. 2 Proposal of a two pathway concept of carcinogenesis at the GEJ

cells. Immunohistochemically, expression of foveolar-type mucin MUC5A has been shown corresponding to a so-called foveolar-type dysplasia. Again these observations are in favor of two different pathways of carcinogenesis at the GEJ (Brown et al. 2010; Khor et al. 2012).

Even from the clinical point of view there are data supporting this concept of a two pathway carcinogenesis. Horii et al. (2011) performed a gastric acid secretion study in a series of 46 consecutive patients with mainly early type of GEJ cancer (Siewert II, mostly pT1b). They divided the patients into those with Barrett's and those without such metaplasia (23 pts each). *H pylori* (HP) was present in 35 % of the former and 47 % of the latter group. They measured gastric acid secretion [H + mEq/10 min] using an adapted endoscopic pentagastrin test. Interestingly, high level of gastric acid secretion (3.4–5.1 mEq/10 min) was preserved in Barrett-associated carcinomas irrespective of HP status. However, in the non-Barrett's group HP + patients had significantly lower acid secretion values than those without HP (1.8 vs 4.7 mEq/10 min, $p < 0.05$). This gives evidence that there might be a low acid secretion "pathway" in non-Barrett-associated carcinomas at the GEJ resembling distal gastric cancer. In sum these data fit to a novel concept of a two pathway concept of carcinogenesis at the GEJ (Fig. 2).

2.2 Evidence of Different Targets for Therapy

The question raises as to whether such a two-sided pathway concept may also translate into different options of (targeted) tumor therapy. In fact, we could show that GEJ cancer often shows Her2 positivity. In the ToGA trial, this was the case in up to 33 % of the carcinoma specimen taken from the GEJ which could only be observed in about

16 % of the distal gastric tumors. Thereby, these tumors had a gland-forming growth pattern corresponding to intestinal-type tumors of G1 and G2 grade. For the first time, the ToGA trial showed that trastuzumab (Herceptin) is a new efficient targeted therapy option for these Her2-positive intestinal-type adenocarcinomas at GEJ (Bang et al. 2010). Thereby, a new scoring system specifically adapted to gastric and GEJ cancer was developed by our group (Hofmann et al. 2008; Rüschoff et al. 2012) and proved to be predictive in the ToGA trial. Quite recently these observations could be confirmed by a group from Mayo Clinic, Rochester (Yoon et al. 2012). In a large series of n = 713 resected adenocarcinomas at GEJ (Siewert type I and II) Her2 testing was done according to the new scoring roles following the EMA algorithm for Her2 positivity (IHC3 + or IHC2 + and amplification). Overall, 17 % of GEJ carcinomas were Her2 positive, which was correlated to lower tumor grade, less invasiveness, fewer metastatic nodes, and the presence of adjacent Barrett's mucosa strongly confirming the association between Her2 and the intestinal-type pathway of carcinogenesis at GEJ. Demonstration of Barrett's mucosa adjacent to the GEJ cancers and good histological differentiation could independently predict the Her2 positivity. In GEJ adenocarcinomas with adjacent Barrett's mucosa Her2 positivity was a strong prognostic marker toward higher disease-specific survival ($p = 0.0047$).

In contrast, EGFR amplification and overexpression seems to be associated with the gastric/foveolar type pathway of GEJ cancer. Demicco et al. (2012) observed EGFR positivity in 19 % of these tumors and Marx et al. (2010) could clearly show that this is associated with poor prognosis. However, up to now we do not really know whether these tumors show improved response to anti-EGFR-directed therapy, e.g., of cetuximab (Han et al. 2009). Only phase II studies have been performed so far and the biomarker analysis lacked standardization, i.e., we do not know the optimal predictive cut-off in immunohistochemical analyses and how to read in situ hybridization analyses properly (Varella-Garcia 2009).

2.3 Evidence for Surveillance Recommendations

Finally, the question raises as to whether the new data may also have an impact on the screening recommendations for Barrett's metaplasia as a risk indicator of GEJ cancer. According to AGA recommendations endoscopic surveillance is restricted to patients with proven intestinal-type metaplasia following the principle: no goblets no Barrett's. In fact, the new two pathway concept gives evidence that also cardiac-type metaplasia may dispose to cancer at the GEJ. But due to the lack of clear data about the cancer risk associated with non-intestinal columnar-type epithelium in the esophagus (Chandrasoma et al. 2012) this lesion is still excluded from surveillance (http://www.gastro.org/mobiletools/mobile-guidelines/aga-medical-position-statement-on-the-management-of-barrett-s-esophagus). More remarkably even the risk of intestinal (goblet cell)-type metaplasia (Barrett's mucosa sensu strictu) has very recently been questioned by the largest population-based study about the incidence of adenocarcinoma among patients with Barrett's esophagus in Denmark (Hvid-Jensen et al. 2011). The database comprises the entire Danish population of 5.4 million persons and involved all patients with Barrett's esophagus (intestinal type) during the period from 1992 to 2009. The follow-up for median 5.2 years was analyzed for 11028 patients with Barrett's within this time period. The incidence rate for adenocarcinomas was 1.2 cases per 1,000 person years with an annual risk of esophageal adenocarcinoma of 0.12 %. According to previous risk estimates of about 5.3–7.0 cases per 1,000 person years this study indicates a significantly lower cancer risk associated with Barrett's esophagus. Only the demonstration of low grade dysplasia reached the value of 5.1 cases per 1,000 person years on which the current surveillance guidelines are based upon. Thus, these data challenge our present screening and surveillance concepts of patients with Barrett's esophagus, neither cost-effectiveness nor a reduction of mortality from esophageal adenocarcinoma has been shown (Kahrilas 2011).

References

Bang YJ, Van Cutsem E, Feyereislova A, Chung HC, Shen L, Sawaki A, Lordick F, Ohtsu A, Omuro Y, Satoh T, Aprile G, Kulikov E, Hill J, Lehle M, Rüschoff J, Kang YK (2010) ToGA Trial Investigators Trastuzumab in combination with chemotherapy versus chemotherapy alone for treatment of HER2-positive advanced gastric or gastro-oesophageal junction cancer (ToGA): a phase 3, open-label, randomised controlled trial. Lancet 376:687–697

Baretton GB, Aust DE (2012) Barrett-ösophagus. Aktueller Stand Pathologe 33:5–16

Bosman FT, Carneiro F, Hruban RH, Theise ND (2010) WHO classification of tumours of the digestive system. IARC, Lyon

Brown IS, Whiteman DC, Lauwers GY (2010) Foveolar type dysplasia in Barrett esophagus. Mod Pathol 23:834–843

Chandrasoma P, Wijetunge S, DeMeester S, Ma Y, Hagen J, Zamis L, DeMeester T (2012) Columnar-lined esophagus without intestinal metaplasia has no proven risk of adenocarcinoma. Am J Surg Pathol 36:1–7

Demicco EG, Farris AB 3rd, Baba Y, Agbor-Etang B, Bergethon K, Mandal R, Daives D, Fukuoka J, Shimizu M, Dias-Santagata D, Ogino S, Iafrate AJ, Gaissert HA, Mino-Kenudson M (2011) The dichotomy in carcinogenesis of the distal esophagus and esophagogastric junction: intestinal-type vs cardiac-type mucosa-associated adenocarcinoma. Mod Pathol 24(9):1177–1190

Han SW, Oh DY, Im SA, Park SR, Lee KW, Song HS, Lee NS, Lee KH, Choi IS, Lee MH, Kim MA, Kim WH, Bang YJ, Kim TY (2009) Phase II study and biomarker analysis of cetuximab combined with modified FOLFOX6 in advanced gastric cancer. Br J Cancer 100:298–304

Hvid-Jensen F, Pedersen L, Drewes AM, Sørensen HT, Funch-Jensen P (2011) Incidence of adenocarcinoma among patients with Barrett's esophagus. N Engl J Med 365:1375–1383

Hofmann M, Stoss O, Shi D, Büttner R, van de Vijver M, Kim W, Ochiai A, Rüschoff J, Henkel T (2008) Assessment of a HER2 scoring system for gastric cancer: results from a validation study. Histopathology 52:797–805

Horii T, Koike T, Abe Y, Kikuchi R, Unakami H, Iijima K, Imatani A, Ohara S, Shimosegawa T (2011) Two distinct types of cancer of different origin may be mixed in gastroesophageal junction adenocarcinomas in Japan: evidence from direct evaluation of gastric acid secretion. Scand J Gastroenterol 46:710–719

Kahrilas PJ (2011) The problems with surveillance with Barretts esophagus. N Engl J Med 365:1437–1438

Khor TS, Alfaro EE, Ooi EM, Li Y, Srivastava A, Fujita H, Park Y, Kumarasinghe MP, Lauwers GY (2012) Divergent expression of MUC5AC, MUC6, MUC2, CD10, and CDX-2 in dysplasia and intramucosal adenocarcinomas with intestinal and foveolar morphology: is this evidence of distinct gastric and intestinal pathways to carcinogenesis in Barrett Esophagus? Am J Surg Pathol 36:331–342

Marx AH, Zielinski M, Kowitz CM, Dancau AM, Thieltges S, Simon R, Choschzick M, Yekebas E, Kaifi JT, Mirlacher M, Atanackovic D, Brümmendorf TH, Fiedler W, Bokemeyer C, Izbicki JR, Sauter G (2010) Homogeneous EGFR amplification defines a subset of aggressive Barrett's adenocarcinomas with poor prognosis. Histopathology 57:418–426

Pohl H, Welch G (2005) The role of over diagnosis and reclassification in the marked increase of esophageal adenocarcinoma incidence. J Natl Cancer Inst 97:142–146

Rüschoff J, Hanna W, Bilous M, Hofmann M, Osamura RY, Penault-Llorca F, van de Vijver M, Viale G (2012) HER2 testing in gastric cancer: a practical approach. Mod Pathol 25:637–650

Siewert JR, Stein HJ, Lordick F (2006) Ösophaguskarzinom. In Siewert JR, Rothmund M, Schumpelick V (eds) Praxis der viszeralchirurgie. Springer, Heidelberg

Varella-Garcia M, Diebold J, Eberhard DA, Geenen K, Hirschmann A, Kockx M, Nagelmeier I, Rüschoff J, Schmitt M, Arbogast S, Cappuzzo F (2009) EGFR fluorescence in situ hybridisation assay: guidelines for application to non-small-cell lung cancer. J Clin Pathol 62:970–977

Wijetunge S, Ma Y, DeMeester S, Hagen J, DeMeester T, Chandrasoma P (2010) Association of adenocarcinomas of the distal esophagus, "gastroesophageal junction," and "gastric cardia" with gastric pathology. Am J Surg Pathol 34:1521–1527

Wittekind C, Meyer H-J (2010) TNM Klassifikation maligner Tumoren 7. Auflage. Wiley-VHC, Weinheim

Yoon HH, Shi Q, Sukov WR, Wiktor AE, Khan M, Sattler CA, Grothey A, Wu TT, Diasio RB, Jenkins RB, Sinicrope FA (2012) Association of HER2/ErbB2 expression and gene amplification with pathologic features and prognosis in esophageal adenocarcinomas. Clin Cancer Res 18:546–554

Why is There a Change in Patterns of GE Cancer?

Prarthana Thiagarajan and Janusz A. Jankowski

Abstract

Recent decades have seen a worrying trend in incidence rates of distal oesophageal and proximal gastric cancers. Fuelled by radical changes in lifestyle, diet, physical activity and environmental exposures, as well as an ageing population and host genetic predisposition, the incidence of oesophageal adenocarcinoma (OAC) is on the rise in Western populations. While overall incidence of gastric cancers is declining, the ageing of society means that an increase in absolute numbers is expected over coming years. Both cancers tend to present at an advanced stage, hence prognosis remains poor despite increasingly effective screening and treatment strategies. The development of gastric and oesophageal malignancies is influenced by myriad factors, not least geographical, racial and socioeconomic differences in addition to lifestyle choices. The multidimensional nature of these risk factors requires a holistic

P. Thiagarajan
Department of Emergency Medicine, Balmoral Building,
Leicester Royal Infirmary, Leicester, LE1 5WW United Kingdom

J. A. Jankowski
Digestive Disease Centre, Level 4, Windsor Building,
Royal Infirmary, Leicester, LE1 5WW United Kingdom

J. A. Jankowski (✉)
Department of Oncology, University of Oxford, Oxford, OX3 7DQ
United Kingdom
e-mail: j.a.jankowski@qmul.ac.uk

J. A. Jankowski
Centre for Digestive Diseases, Queen Mary University of London,
London, E1 7AT United Kingdom

F. Otto and M. P. Lutz (eds.), *Early Gastrointestinal Cancers*,
Recent Results in Cancer Research 196, DOI: 10.1007/978-3-642-31629-6_8,
© Springer-Verlag Berlin Heidelberg 2012

understanding of their net influence in the development of malignancy. This review explores the evidence base for established and putative risk factors in the development of gastric and oesophageal cancers. It is hoped that with a clear understanding of important risk factors, a multidisciplinary approach including effective primary prevention, regular screening of high-risk groups and continued research into the molecular biology of gastrointestinal carcinogenesis may facilitate a reduction in incidence rates, as well as early detection and optimal management of upper gastrointestinal malignancies.

Contents

1	Introduction	117
2	An Ageing Population	118
	2.1 Factors Leading to Improved Life Expectancy	118
	2.2 Implications of an Ageing Population on Management of Upper GI Cancers	118
3	Colonisation with Helicobacter Pylori	119
	3.1 Mechanisms of Oncogenesis	119
	3.2 H. pylori Eradication and Decline in Prevalence	119
	3.3 Association Between H. pylori and Oesophageal Cancers	120
4	The Role of Obesity	120
5	Bile Acids and Dietary Fat	122
6	Tobacco and Alcohol	123
	6.1 Smoking and Gastric Cancer	123
	6.2 Alcohol, GORD and Oesophageal Cancers	123
7	Gastric Polyps	124
	7.1 Epidemiology of Gastric polyps	124
	7.2 Adenomatous Polyps and Risk of Malignancy	124
	7.3 Hereditary Polyposis Syndromes	125
8	Other Medical Conditions	125
	8.1 Pernicious Anaemia	125
	8.2 Partial Gastrectomy	126
	8.3 Plummer-Vinson Syndrome	126
	8.4 Coeliac Disease	127
	8.5 Oeosphageal Achalasia	127
	8.6 Hereditary Tylosis (Familial Palmoplantar Keratosis)	128
9	Anti-Inflammatory Drugs	128
10	Family History	129
	10.1 Sporadic Gastric cancer	129
	10.2 Inherited Cancer Syndromes	130
11	Having Other Cancers	130
12	Radiation Exposure	131
13	Reduced Immunity	131
14	Work Chemicals	132
15	Hormone Replacement Therapy	132
16	Physical Activity	133
17	Conclusion	133
References		135

1   Introduction

Gastric and oesophageal malignancies continue to present a significant health threat to diverse populations worldwide. Despite modern advances in multimodal investigative and therapeutic strategies, these cancers remain associated with high patient morbidity and mortality, as the majority are diagnosed at advanced stages when curative management options are limited. While a decline in the incidence rate of distal gastric carcinomas and oesophageal squamous cell carcinomas has been observed in recent years, the rate of proximal gastric cancers and oesophageal adenocarcinomas (OACs) continues to rise rapidly, particularly in Western nations and among Caucasian males (Ahmed et al. 2006). This is likely to reflect changes in diet and lifestyle, leading to an increased incidence of obesity, gastro-oesophageal reflux and ultimately, the premalignant condition Barrett's oesophagus (Crew and Neugut 2004). In addition, cultural, environmental and nutritional factors are influencing the gradual shift in anatomical location, histological subtype and patient demographic of gastro-oesophageal cancers seen in recent years.

Stomach cancer currently ranks as the 4th most common malignancy worldwide, and remains the 2nd-leading cause of cancer-related deaths (Vial et al. 2010; Polk and Peek 2010). Despite a reduction in overall incidence rate, the mean population age is increasing, resulting in an absolute increase in gastric cancers. Incidence and anatomical location vary widely between continents, implying a substantial role for environmental factors in the development of stomach cancers. For example, gastric cancers are relatively common in Northeast Asian countries, where incidence may reach up to 69 cases per 100,000 people per year (Parkin 2004). Conversely, North America, Southern Asia and Africa are considered low-risk regions, with an incidence of 4–10 per 100,000 per year. Furthermore, distal (antro-pyloric) cancers are seen more commonly in Japan and Korea, whereas proximal tumours of the gastric cardia, fundus and oesophagus are becoming increasingly common in the west (Yamaoka et al. 2008). This may reflect the relative prevalence of *Helicobacter Pylori,* which is a well established risk factor for distal gastric cancer, as well as lifestyle factors and the obesity epidemic faced by Western countries.

Oesophageal malignancy is the 8th most common cancer worldwide, accounting for 5.4 % of cancer-related deaths in 2008 (Sasako et al. 2010). Its incidence is rising rapidly in western nations, with the United Kingdom estimated to have the highest reported incidence of OAC worldwide (Ferlay et al. 2010). That the prognosis of oesophageal cancer remains bleak despite breakthroughs in evidence-based therapies is worrying: 5-year survival is less than 10 % (Bollschweiler et al. 2001), leading physicians to consider a shift in focus from treatment towards prevention. Epidemiological studies indicate that among Caucasian males, the incidence of OAC has risen by >350 % from the mid-1970s to the mid-1990s. This was paralleled by a lesser increase in the incidence of gastric cardia tumours, and both upward trends were noted to be more significant in elderly male populations (Enzinger and Mayer 2003).

This review focuses on the multifactorial reasons governing the change in patterns of gastric and oesophageal cancers observed in recent decades. Established and putative risk factors are discussed, as well as the role of lifestyle, nutrition, socioeconomic and environmental factors and the key influence of *H. pylori*. With a clear evidence base for risk factors and the relative roles of lifestyle and environmental exposures, physicians may begin to focus on interventions aiming to prevent these aggressive malignancies, as well as developing more effective therapeutic strategies for the future.

2 An Ageing Population

While incidence rates for gastric cancer have declined worldwide, the absolute number of newly diagnosed patients is rising yearly, due to the ageing of society (Devesa et al. 1998). Similarly, longer life expectancy has resulted in increasing numbers of elderly patients developing oesophageal malignancies and being referred for surgical treatment (Munoz 2002).

2.1 Factors Leading to Improved Life Expectancy

In the United Kingdom, average male life expectancy is 78.2 years as of 2011, representing an increase of 8 years since 1970 (Ruol et al. 2007). This upward trend is paralleled in several other Western European nations, as well as Japan and the United States. Several reasons have been postulated as to the improved life expectancy observed in current times, including healthier diet, better sanitation and recent breakthroughs in medical interventions. Morbidity and mortality from ischaemic heart disease have fallen dramatically in recent years with the advent of novel therapeutic approaches, including thrombolysis, percutaneous coronary angioplasty and stenting, as well as aggressive risk factor management with angiotensin converting enzyme (ACE) inhibitors and statins and a reduction in prevalence of cardiovascular risk factors such as smoking (Leon 2011).

2.2 Implications of an Ageing Population on Management of Upper GI Cancers

A recent Japanese review emphasised the increasing importance of early endoscopic diagnosis and treatment of oesophageal malignancies in a society in which the mean population age is rapidly increasing (Ford et al. 2007). The group called for age-specific research into optimal management of elderly patients with oesophageal malignancies, as current studies are based mainly on populations less than 75 years of age, and results may not be applicable to an elderly cohort. This concern is echoed by, Kato and Nakajima (2011) who discuss the increasing burden of oesophageal cancer with the ageing of society, while highlighting the lack of conclusive evidence as to the safety and efficacy of standard surgical interventions and chemoradiotherapy (Nakui et al. 2010).

The elderly represent a high-risk population for treatment of upper gastrointestinal cancer, due to the greater prevalence of comorbid conditions and reduced physiological reserve, thereby potentially decreasing ability to withstand the stress of complex surgical or pharmacological intervention. However, a recent study indicated that complication rates and mortality following oesophagectomy for cancer were not significantly different between elderly (>70 years) and non-elderly (<70 years) populations ($p > 0.05$), and had similar success rates between the two groups (Kato and Nakajima 2011).

3   Colonisation with Helicobacter Pylori

3.1   Mechanisms of Oncogenesis

Epidemiological data have demonstrated that colonisation with *Helicobacter Pylori* is the strongest known single risk factor for the development of gastric adenocarcinoma (Vial et al. 2010; Alibakhshi et al. 2009). Through inducing a chronic superficial gastritis, this bacterium promotes inflammation of the gastric mucosa, ultimately leading to cellular transformation and neoplasia. In recent years, there has been much research into the mechanisms of *H. pylori*-induced oncogenesis and the influence of genetically diverse virulence strains. A 2001 meta-analysis demonstrated the propensity for *H. pylori* to increase the risk of distal (non-cardia) gastric carcinomas (Odds ratio 2.97), while no association was shown between *H. pylori* and cancers of the gastric cardia (Bornschein and Malfertheiner 2011). Furthermore, infection with the more virulent *cagA* strain of *H. pylori* has been shown to result in a 1.64-fold increase in the risk of developing non-cardia cancers (Helicobacter and Cancer Collaborative Group 2001).

3.2   H. pylori Eradication and Decline in Prevalence

Eradication of *H. pylori* has been shown to result in regression of precancerous lesions and gastric lymphomas. Recent work by (Kodama et al. 2012) followed 118 patients for 8.6 years after successful *H. pylori* eradication, taking endoscopic biopsies from the gastric antrum and corpus. The group demonstrated a significant decline in gastric atrophy ($p < 0.001$) and intestinal metaplasia ($p < 0.05$) in patients who had undergone successful *H. pylori* eradication, suggesting that this may decrease the risk of gastric carcinomas (Fuccio et al. 2007).

In recent years, the decline in prevalence of *H. pylori* among Western populations (reported to be due to better sanitation, less crowding and increased use of antimicrobial therapy) has been reflected by a fall in incidence of distal gastric

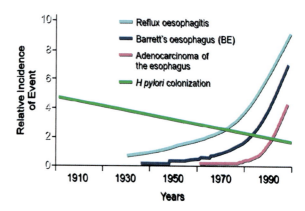

Fig. 1 Changing incidence of GI diseases and H. pylori infection

cancers. However, we are simultaneously observing a rise in number of patients with proximal gastric cancers and oesophageal malignancies, which are thought to be secondary to lifestyle changes, including obesity, acid reflux and ultimately, Barrett's Metaplasia (Fig. 1) (Kodama et al. 2012).

3.3 Association Between H. pylori and Oesophageal Cancers

It has been postulated that carriage of *H. pylori* confers a protective effect against oesophagitis and oesophageal malignancies (Peek and Blaser 2002). Indeed, successful antimicrobial *H. pylori* eradication is associated with an increased risk of symptomatic gastro-oesophageal reflux disease (GORD). Whiteman and colleagues (2010) conducted a population-based case-control study to determine the effect of *H. pylori* seropositivity on development of OACs, concluding that infection with *H. pylori* was inversely associated with OACs and gastro-oesophageal junctional carcinomas (OR 0.45 and 0.41, respectively) but had no effect on the development of squamous cell carcinomas of the oesophagus (Islami and Karmangar 2008). Therefore, the decline in *H. pylori* prevalence may be an independent contributing factor to the rising burden of oesophageal malignancy in the West.

4 The Role of Obesity

The alarmingly rapid rise in incidence of OAC seen in Western countries has been paralleled by an increase in symptomatic GORD, itself a function of high rates of obesity (Fig. 2) (Whiteman et al. 2010). Results from several population-based studies provide evidence for a causal association between obesity and GORD and its complications, Barrett's metaplasia, erosive oesophagitis and OAC. A 2005 meta-analysis demonstrated that obesity (defined as BMI > 25 kg/m^2) resulted in a statistically significant rise in the risk of developing GORD, erosive oesophagitis and OAC (Odds Ratio 2.78 for OAC) (Hongo et al. 2009). The group additionally demonstrated a 'dose–response' relationship, with increasing BMI resulting in a

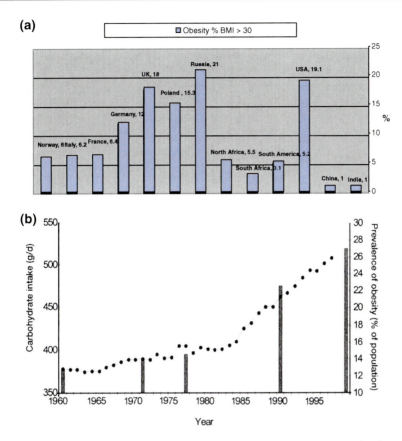

Fig. 2 Increasing prevalence of Obesity, **a** by % BMI > 30 in different countries, **b** overall prevalence of obesity and carbohydrate intake (% of population)

higher prevalence of GORD symptoms and OAC. Avazi and colleagues (2009) analysed data from 1659 patients with GORD symptoms undergoing oesophageal pH monitoring, and concluded that raised BMI was positively correlated with increased acid exposure (Hampel et al. 2005). Interestingly, patients defined as obese (BMI > 30 kg/m^2) were also found to be twice as likely to have defective lower oesophageal sphincter function, which may contribute further to the development of GORD and ultimately Barrett's oesophagus in these populations.

However, while this relationship has been well established in literature studying Western populations, a 2008 cross-sectional study of over 5000 Iranian adults demonstrated no association between BMI and symptomatic GORD (OR 0.88), implying that in this population, reflux symptoms may occur independently of BMI (Ayazi et al. 2009).

In recent decades, OAC has overtaken oesophageal squamous cell carcinoma (OSCC) as the dominant histological subtype in Caucasian males, with a ratio of 1:0.43 in the late 1990s (Whiteman et al. 2010; Solhpour et al. 2008). Reasons for this are thought to be multifactorial, and include the decline in prevalence of *H. pylori* in Western nations, as well as an increase in acid reflux and obesity. However, in Eastern Asian countries, OSCC remains the dominant subtype.

While it is well established that an elevated BMI is associated with greater risk of GORD and OAC, the mechanisms underlying this are not clear. Factors such as increased rates of hiatus hernia, increased intra-abdominal pressure gradients and decreased lower oesophageal sphincter tone have all been postulated to have a role in increasing lower oesophageal exposure to gastric acid (Kubo and Corley 2004). Additionally, a role has been proposed for endogenous peptides such as the adipocytokines adiponectin and lectin, which are produced by adipose tissue and influence cell growth, thereby potentially orchestrating neoplastic change (Kubo and Corley 2004).

Pooled results from several observational studies indicate that an elevated BMI is also independently associated with an increased risk of gastric cardia malignancies, possibly through similar mechanisms of reflux and gastric acid exposure (Quigley et al. 2011; Kubo and Corley 2006). The strength of association also increases with rising BMI, in a similar manner to that of OAC.

5 Bile Acids and Dietary Fat

Bile acids have been implicated as endogenous carcinogens in cancers of the GI tract, through inducing oxidative stress and reactive oxygen species (ROS), DNA damage, cellular mutation and apoptosis (Yang et al. 2009). Individuals with high levels of dietary fat intake are most at risk of bile acid exposure; hence modern dietary patterns among Western populations, which include high levels of saturated fat, are conducive to increased bile reflux and its deleterious effects.

Bernstein et al. (2009) discuss the fact that increased prevalence of acid reflux exposes the oesophagus further to bile acids from the duodenum, as well as gastric acidity, thereby inducing oxidative stress and leading to the development of Barrett's oesophagus and OAC (Yang et al. 2009). Indeed, patients with GORD and Barrett's oesophagus have been shown to have increased levels of bile acid in the refluxate, implying a causal association between bile acid exposure and development of Barrett's metaplasia Bernstein et al. (2009). Nakos and colleagues (2009) histologically evaluated gastric mucosa to look for evidence of bile acid-induced damage following endoscopic biopsies in subjects with and without symptomatic GORD. The group demonstrated that in patients with GORD, 47 % had evidence of bile reflux gastropathy, compared with just 13 % of control subjects. Furthermore, the degree of bile reflux was shown to be associated with disease severity: in subjects with severe oesophagitis or Barrett's metaplasia, 72 % had evidence of bile acid-induced mucosal damage, whereas in subjects with mild or no lesions, this number was only 34 %.

The aetiology of adenocarcinomas of the gastric cardia is thought to be similar to that of OAC, meaning that reflux is again implicated as a significant contributing factor. Dixon et al. (2002) studied the effect of bile reflux on histology of the gastric cardia in 267 dyspeptic patients, concluding that a high level of bile reflux was an independent risk factor for intestinal metaplasia of the cardia. However, there was no significant association between bile reflux and intestinal metaplasia of the gastric antrum, thus lending further support to differing aetiologies of cardia and antral malignancies (Menges and Müller 2001).

6 Tobacco and Alcohol

Smoking and alcohol are well established risk factors for the development of oesophageal and gastric malignancies. Numerous studies have implicated smoking as a causal factor in the development of OSCC, largely thought to be driven by exposure to tobacco constituents such as nitrosamines and aromatic hydrocarbons (Dixon et al. 2002; International Agency for Research on Cancer 1986; Wang et al. 2007). Similarly, high alcohol intake has been shown to increase the risk of developing OSCC, but its role in the aetiology of adenocarcinomas of the oesophagus is less clear (Stoner and Gupta 2001).

6.1 Smoking and Gastric Cancer

Smoking is an important environmental risk factor for the development of gastric cancer (Pandeya et al. 2009). The EPIC study, a large multicentre prospective cohort study including data from over 500,000 individuals, estimated that 17.6 % of gastric cancer cases may be attributable to smoking alone (Ladeiras-Lopes et al. 2008). A 2006 systematic review evaluated the association between tobacco smoking and gastric cancer among the Japanese population, concluding that tobacco moderately increases the risk of cancer (relative risk 1.79 among Japanese men) (Nishino et al. 2006; González et al. 2003). In a large population-based cohort study of 669,570 Korean men, a moderate association was found between smoking and upper-third gastric cancers, as well as tumours of the gastric cardia (adjusted relative risk, 2.2) (Sung et al. 2007). The group also found that combined tobacco and alcohol consumption further increased risk for upper-third and cardia cancers of the stomach.

6.2 Alcohol, GORD and Oesophageal Cancers

The role of alcohol in the development of OAC and gastric cardia cancers is contentious, with various studies reporting positive associations between alcohol intake and Barrett's oesophagus, whereas others have shown no effect or indeed inverse associations (Lindblad et al. 2005; Gammon et al. 1997). However, there have been reports of a positive association between alcohol consumption and GORD symptoms (Nocon et al. 2006). It is thought that alcohol may increase GORD through relaxation of lower oesophageal sphincter tone, thereby predisposing to erosive oesophagitis, Barrett's metaplasia and OAC.

A 2009 report used data collected from the Irish case–control Factors INfluencing the Barrett's Adenocarcinoma Relationship (FINBAR) study, to evaluate the effect of alcohol intake at various ages on development of reflux oesophagitis, Barrett's oesophagus and OAC. The group demonstrated that alcohol consumption in early adulthood (age 21) was associated with an increased risk of reflux oesophagitis but not Barrett's oesophagus or OAC. However, there was no relationship observed between more recent alcohol intake (5 years prior to interview date) and development of these lesions. In fact, wine consumption appeared to be inversely associated with risk of reflux oesophagitis and Barrett's oesophagus (OR 0.45) (Anderson et al. 2009).

7 Gastric Polyps

Gastric polyps are generally asymptomatic and are found incidentally on endoscopic investigation. They may represent precancerous lesions in that some polyps have the potential to undergo malignant transformation, resulting in adenocarcinomas. Therefore, any polyp found at endoscopy must be biopsied for histological examination before dysplasia can be excluded, despite the frequent presence of characteristic appearances at endoscopy.

7.1 Epidemiology of Gastric polyps

Epithelial polyps arise commonly in the stomach and may be classified as hyperplastic, fundic-gland and adenomatous. Factors influencing the epidemiology of each lesion include the local prevalence of *H. pylori*, use of proton pump inhibitor (PPI) therapy and age and gender of the study population. For example, fundic-gland polyps are associated with PPI use and occur more commonly than hyperplastic polyps in the west, due to the increasing prevalence of GORD and PPI consumption, together with decreasing prevalence of *H. pylori* infection. By the same token, hyperplastic polyps, which are commonly associated with atrophic gastritis, are declining in Western populations, in parallel with the reduction in prevalence of *H. pylori*.

7.2 Adenomatous Polyps and Risk of Malignancy

Adenomatous polyps are neoplastic, and may be divided into 3 histological subtypes; tubular, villous and tubulovillous. Malignant potential increases with increasing size: it has been reported that >50 % of adenomatous polyps >2 cm contain a focus of adenocarcinoma, the risk being greatest in villous adenomas (Rubin and Strayer 2008; Carmack et al. 2009). The presence of adenomatous polyps at endoscopy should prompt a search for mucosal abnormalities throughout the stomach, as well as regular endoscopic follow-up (Goddard et al. 2010). As the association between adenomatous polyps and malignancy increases with age, it becomes increasingly important to recognise and resect these neoplasms in an increasingly elderly population.

7.3 Hereditary Polyposis Syndromes

Although the majority occur sporadically, polyps may also constitute part of hereditary polyposis syndromes, such as familial adenomatous polyposis (FAP) and hamartomatous polyps, such as in juvenile polyposis, Cowden disease and Peutz-Jehger's syndrome. In these contexts, regular endoscopic surveillance is recommended, with a view to detecting and treating early malignant transformation. Most authorities recommend surveillance every 2–3 years for individuals with FAP and Peutz-Jehger's syndrome, in whom the presence of gastroduodenal polyposis is well-recognised and the risk of gastric cancer may be as high as 30 % (Carmack et al. 2009).

8 Other Medical Conditions

8.1 Pernicious Anaemia

Pernicious anaemia is a macrocytic anaemia secondary to cobalamin deficiency, itself a consequence of chronic atrophic gastritis and lack of intrinsic factor. The association between long-standing pernicious anaemia and development of gastric carcinoid tumours and gastric adenocarcinoma is well established, and is likely to reflect hypochlorhydria and hypergastrinaemia occurring as a result of atrophic gastritis (Hagarty et al. 2000; Annibale et al. 2011). It has been proposed that hypergastrinaemia, occurring secondary to hypochlorhydria in patients with pernicious anaemia, promotes hyperplasia of enterochromaffin cell lines, ultimately leading to gastric carcinoid tumours (Massironi et al. 2009). Another mechanism which has been proposed is that hypochlorhydria leads to a high intragastric pH, providing a milieu in which nitrosamine producing bacteria may flourish and generate *N-nitroso* compounds which act as endogenous carcinogens (Correa 1992).

A recent Italian study reported an annual incidence rate for gastric cancer of 0.1 % among individuals with atrophic gastritis. The authors report that annual incidence rate in the general Italian population is approximately 0.01 %, thereby confirming that individuals with atrophic gastritis are at increased risk for the development of gastric neoplasms (Vannella et al. 2010).

In terms of endoscopic surveillance in patients with pernicious anaemia, consensus is divided as to cost-effectiveness and clinical need. Kokkola and colleagues (1998) suggest that routine gastroscopic follow-up is not required in view of the relatively benign nature of gastric carcinoid tumours, and that only patients with premalignant lesions (e.g. ECL hyperplasia) and those with gastrointestinal symptoms should undergo regular endoscopic surveillance at 5-year intervals (Kokkola et al. 1998). Vannella et al. (2010) suggest that endoscopic-histological surveillance may be worthwhile in a subset of patients with atrophic gastritis, who are either over 50 years of age or have evidence of atrophic pangastritis or intestinal metaplasia on initial endoscopy, as these patients are at higher risk of gastric malignancy (Vannella et al. 2010).

8.2 Partial Gastrectomy

Now an almost obsolete surgical procedure, partial gastrectomy was historically a popular management option for patients with peptic ulcer disease. A number of studies have suggested that the procedure confers increased long-term risk of subsequent gastric cancers, purportedly through increased enterogastric reflux and therefore exposure of remaining gastric tissue to endogenous carcinogens (La Vecchia et al. 1992; Fisher et al. 1993). However, an Australian retrospective case-control study including 569 patients reported no significant increase in the risk of gastric cancer following partial gastrectomy (Bassily et al. 2000).

The utility of endoscopic screening in this patient population is disputed, with the weight of current opinion against regular endoscopic surveillance as there is no evidence that it improves survival (Tersmette et al. 1995). Furthermore, with diminishing popularity of partial gastrectomy, the patient cohort in question are currently elderly and therefore unlikely to be suitable candidates for radical surgery if a focus of malignancy were to be found at endoscopy.

8.3 Plummer-Vinson Syndrome

The Plummer Vinson syndrome (PVS) comprises a triad of iron deficiency anaemia, oesophageal webs and post-cricoid dysphagia (Novacek 2006). There have been various case reports in the literature of an association between this condition and subsequent development of squamous cell malignancies of the oesophagus and hypopharynx (Jain 2009; Messmann 2001; Hoffman and Jaffe 1995). This complication is estimated to affect approximately 10 % of patients with PVS (Larsson et al. 1975). Rarely, PVS is associated with gastric cancer: a 2005 case report describes the development of gastric cardia cancer in a 43-year old woman with PVS, who recovered following radical total gastrectomy with D2 nodal dissection (Kim et al. 2005).

Treatment includes dilatation of any existing oesophageal webs, as well as iron supplementation and regular endoscopic surveillance. For patients without any evidence of malignancy, the prognosis of this condition is excellent. However, progression to oesophageal dysplasia results in dramatic worsening of prognosis. The prevalence of PVS and its complications have declined dramatically over the past 30 years, presumably due to improved nutritional status and reduced rates of severe iron deficiency anaemia (Chen and Chen 1994).

8.4 Coeliac Disease

Coeliac disease is a genetically-determined autoimmune disorder, resulting from impaired immune responses to gliadin fractions of gluten in wheat. It is relatively common with a reported prevalence of approximately 1 % in Western populations (Dubé et al. 2005). There is a well established association between coeliac disease and oesophageal squamous cell cancers, as well as small bowel adenocarcinomas and non-Hodgkin's lymphomas (Green et al. 2003; Lohi et al. 2009). It has been suggested that the majority of this risk occurs prior to the diagnosis of coeliac disease, and that risk may be substantially reduced by strict adherence to a gluten-free diet. With improved methods and widespread availability of diagnostic testing, in particular sensitive and specific serological assays, earlier detection of coeliac disease is possible. This will enable prompt intervention and improved education of coeliac patients, in turn leading to an anticipated decline in complications of this disease in the future (Green and Cellier 2007).

8.5 Oeosphageal Achalasia

Patients with long-standing achalasia have a 140-fold increased risk of developing oesophageal malignancies compared with the general population (Brücher et al. 2001). Diagnosis is frequently delayed, due to adaptation of many patients to a degree of dysphagia associated with achalasia itself, and therefore failure to recognise further dysphagia due to stenosis from an encroaching oesophageal cancer. A recent prospective cohort study of 448 patients with achalasia with a mean follow-up period of 9.6 years demonstrated an annual incidence rate of 0.34 and relative hazard rate of 28 for development of oesophageal cancer, compared with age and gender matched control populations (Leeuwenburgh et al. 2010). Prognosis of oesophageal cancer in patients with achalasia is generally poor, due to diagnostic delay until the malignancy reaches an advanced stage; hence regular endoscopic surveillance of high-risk populations has been suggested.

8.6 Hereditary Tylosis (Familial Palmoplantar Keratosis)

Tylosis is an autosomal dominant disorder characterised by palmoplantar hyperkeratosis, oral hairy leukoplakia and a high lifetime risk for the development of oesophageal squamous cell carcinomas (von Brevern et al. 1998). The genetic locus has been found on the long arm of chromosome 17 (17q25) (Thiers et al. 2009), and there have been reports that this locus is frequently deleted in patients with sporadic oesophageal squamous cell carcinoma, implying that a tumour suppressor gene may map to this region (Iwaya et al. 1998). A recent study identified a missense mutation the tylosis oesophageal carcinoma (TOC)-associated gene RHBDF2 as the underlying cause for hereditary oesophageal cancer in tylosis (Blaydon et al. 2012). The authors report altered distribution of the protease encoded for by this gene in tylotic skin compared to normal skin, and suggest that immortalised tylotic keratinocytes may have impaired epidermal growth factor signalling. The authors also suggest that dysregulation of RHBDF2 may also occur in sporadic oesophageal cell carcinomas, and hence targeting of RHBDF2 pathways may represent a novel therapeutic focus for reducing the hyperproliferative nature of both sporadic and inherited oesophageal squamous cell cancers.

Regular endoscopic follow-up is recommended for patients with hereditary tylosis from the age of 30 years (Hirota et al. 2006).

9 Anti-Inflammatory Drugs

A growing body of evidence suggests that aspirin and other non-steroidal anti-inflammatory drugs (NSAIDs) have chemoprotective effects on gastrointestinal mucosa, reducing the development of cancers by up to 30 % (Jankowska et al. 2010). Population-based cohort and case-control studies have assessed the effect of NSAID use in patients with Barrett's oesophagus, reporting statistically significant reductions in risk of developing OAC in patients taking regular NSAIDs (Nguyen et al. 2010; Kastelein et al. 2011).

Aspirin is currently the most widely consumed drug worldwide (Fuster and Sweeny 2011). With an increasing awareness of its cardioprotective effects, the number of high-risk individuals taking aspirin is likely to increase: it is anticipated that this will result in the added benefit of reducing malignant transformation in the population with Barrett's oesophagus, many of whom also carry significant cardiovascular comorbidities (Moayyedi et al. 2008).

To date, high-quality data from randomised controlled trials (RCTs) researching the effect of aspirin on gastrointestinal malignancies is lacking. It is hoped that the Aspirin Esomeprazole Chemoprevention Trial (AspECT) -a large, multicentre, phase III RCT—will shed light on uncertainties regarding the use of aspirin as a chemoprotective agent in Barrett's oesophagus and will help to guide clinical practice by providing much needed quantitative data to clarify the role of aspirin and PPIs in GI chemoprevention.

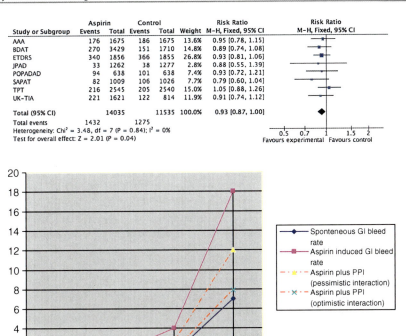

Fig. 3 a The role of aspirin in GI cancer prevention. **b** Risk of aspirin-induced GI bleeding by age, compared to spontaneous GI bleeding and bleeding risk with aspirin plus a proton pump inhibitor (*PPI*)

Recent meta-analyses have also supported a role for aspirin in reducing the risk of non-cardia gastric cancers in a dose-dependent manner (Wang et al. 2003; Yang et al. 2010). The risk of gastrointestinal toxicity, including peptic ulceration and haemorrhage, must be weighed against the putative benefits of aspirin when assessing its potential for chemoprevention on a large scale (Fig. 3).

10 Family History

10.1 Sporadic Gastric cancer

Both genetic and environmental factors influence the development of gastric cancer. A positive family history of gastric cancer has been reported to affect patient survival both favourably and negatively in different studies. A recent retrospective review of 1273 patients undergoing curative-intent surgery for stage III or IV gastric cancer concluded that having a first degree relative with gastric cancer was associated with improved disease-free survival, recurrence free survival and overall survival (P = 0.012, 0.066 and 0.005, respectively) (Han et al. 2012). This has important implications for screening of first degree relatives of patients with gastric cancer, and may be due to genetic characteristics which predispose to improved survival, as well as differences in health behaviour, for example higher rates of smoking cessation among first degree relatives (Nadauld and Ford 2012).

10.2 Inherited Cancer Syndromes

Inherited cancer syndromes which may feature gastric adenocarcinoma include hereditary diffuse gastric cancer (HDGC), FAP, Peutz-Jehger's syndrome and the Li Fraumeni syndrome. HDGC is inherited in an autosomal dominant manner, and results from a germline mutation in the E-cadherin gene CDH1 in 40–50 % of cases (Lynch et al. 2008). This mutation confers an approximately 75 % lifetime risk of developing gastric cancer (Ford 2002). Women with this mutation are also at increased risk of lobular breast carcinoma. Patients with HDGC characteristically demonstrate signet ring cells on histological examination of biopsied specimens (Han and Lauwers 2010). The only known preventative treatment is prophylactic gastrectomy.

Early onset gastric cancer has been reported as a component of the Li Fraumeni syndrome, an inherited cancer syndrome associated with germline mutations in the p53 gene (Masciari et al. 2011). This supports the need for early and regular endoscopic surveillance in this high-risk population, especially among individuals with a family history of gastric cancer.

Gastric polyposis has been reported to occur with a frequency of up to 50 % in individuals with FAP (Lynch et al. 2011). While the majority of polyps are of the fundic-gland type, adenomatous polyps do occur and regular endoscopic surveillance is advised. Peutz-Jegher's syndrome confers an increased risk of gastric malignancy in the order of 5–10 %. Current recommendations for early detection of malignant transformation of hamartomatous polyps include 3-yearly endoscopy from 25 years of age in individuals diagnosed with this condition (Dunlop 2002).

11   Having Other Cancers

The presence of other malignancies can predispose to subsequent primary cancers of the stomach in certain cases. A 2006 study used data collected over a 26-year period (1975–2001) from the United States Surveillance Epidemiology and End Results (SEER) program to demonstrate that sporadic colorectal carcinoma increases the risk of subsequent gastric cancer in male subjects (Ahmed et al. 2006). Likewise, survivors of thyroid cancer have been shown to be at increased risk of second primary malignancies, including gastric cancer (Subramanian et al. 2007). A large multicentre, multinational population-based study demonstrated that primary oesophageal cancer can increase the risk of subsequent gastric cancer diagnoses, although this may in part be due to surveillance bias, given the proximity of the two sites (Chuang et al. 2008). Other primary malignancies which have been linked with subsequent development of stomach cancer include breast cancer in men, as well as testicular cancer (Satram-Hoang et al. 2007; Travis et al. 2005).

It has also been established that individuals with hereditary non-polyposis colon cancer (HNPCC) carry a substantially higher risk of developing gastric cancer than the general population. The relative risk in HNPCC patients and first degree relatives has been reported to be 4-fold. However, Park et al. (2000) demonstrated that younger generations carry a much greater risk: 11.3-fold in the 30 s and 5.5-fold in the 40 s (Park et al. 2000). As a result, the authors recommend an age-specific cancer surveillance programme in areas where gastric cancer is endemic, to facilitate its early detection and treatment, thereby leading to improved patient outcome.

12   Radiation Exposure

Radiotherapy plays an integral role in the successful treatment of many cancers; however, it also risks incidental exposure of surrounding tissue to irradiation, thereby increasing the risk of developing a second primary malignancy. This is an important consideration in the context of improved long-term survival associated with radiotherapy use. Using data from the SEER program, Maddams et al. (2011) estimated that oesophageal cancer is one of the most common radiation-related malignancies (13.3 % of the total) (Maddams et al. 2011). The group estimated that second cancers occurred most frequently among female survivors of breast cancer, who had been treated with radiotherapy. In this group, 7.5 % of subsequent gastric cancers were attributable to radiotherapy for initial breast cancer.

The view that radiotherapy is responsible to a high degree for development of a second malignancy in cancer survivors is contested in recent research by Berrington et al. (2011), who also used data from the SEER program to conduct a systematic analysis of cancer sites routinely tested with radiotherapy. The group argue that a relatively small proportion of second cancers (8 %) are attributable to ionising radiotherapy for initial cancers, and propose that lifestyle, genetic and environmental factors play a more important role in influencing the development of second cancers.

13   Reduced Immunity

The concept of cancers associated with immune deficiency has gained credence in recent years, as data has become available regarding long-term morbidities for patients with HIV infection (as survival has improved dramatically following the introduction of highly active antiretroviral therapy), and also in solid organ transplant recipients, for whom pharmacological and surgical advances have resulted in more successful long-term outcomes.

Research by Grulich et al. (2007) demonstrated that these populations have an approximately 2-fold increased risk of developing gastric cancer (relative risk 1.90 in HIV patients and 2.04 in transplant recipients), and highlight that the similar pattern of increased cancer risk provides compelling evidence that immune deficiency is the key cause (Grulich et al. 2007). Furthermore, the authors suggest that the mechanism for increased risk in these populations is through increased likelihood of colonisation with culpable organisms in cancers which are well-known to be infection-related: for example, individuals who are immunosuppressed are at greater risk *of H. pylori* infection, which may ultimately become manifest as stomach cancer.

14 Work Chemicals

Exposure to industrial carcinogens has been linked with development of gastric cancer, particularly in individuals working with metal dusts present in quarries, mines and construction sites (Aragonés et al. 2002). Sjödhal and colleagues (2007) conducted a prospective cohort study among Swedish men to demonstrate that in working environments such as construction sites, the risk of non-cardia gastric cancer was increased with airborne exposure to harmful chemicals, particularly in workers exposed to cement dust, quartz dust and diesel exhaust (Incidence rate ratios 1.5, 1.4 and 1.3, respectively) Sjödahl et al. (2007). Furthermore, a dose-response relationship was observed for such exposures, supporting the aetiological role of airborne exposures in the development of non-cardia cancers. The authors suggest that these findings might in part explain the large male preponderance of gastric cancers, as most of these industries are male-dominated.

Rushton et al. (2010) estimated that the occupational-attributable fraction of stomach cancers in the UK is approximately 2 %, highlighting the impact of passive exposure to carcinogens in the workplace, and calling for focussed efforts to reduce exposure in high-risk working environments as part of a long-term risk reduction strategy.

15 Hormone Replacement Therapy

The largely unexplained male predominance of gastric and oesophageal cancers has led to the hypothesis that endogenous oestrogens may confer a protective effect to females. Indeed, an inverse association between the age of menopause and the risk of OSCC was noted by Gallus et al. (2001), thereby supporting the theory that female hormones may act as protective agents against oesophageal carcinogenesis (Gallus et al. 2001).

Lindblad et al. (2006) conducted a case-control study to determine the effect of oestrogens in the development of gastric and oesophageal cancers. The group demonstrated that women using hormone replacement therapy (HRT) had a 50 %

reduced risk of gastric adenocarcinoma (OR 0.48). Interestingly, this inverse association was strongest for non-cardia cancers of the stomach, and there was no association proven between use of HRT and oesophageal cancers (OR 1.17) (Lindblad et al. 2006). One mechanism suggested to account for this observation is that oestrogens reduce bile acid concentration, which may serve to decrease exposure of the gastric mucosa to this potentially carcinogenic source.

16 Physical Activity

There is a good evidence that regular physical activity may reduce the risk of several cancer types, including breast cancer and colorectal cancer (Thune and Furberg 2001; Kruk 2007). However, the relationship between physical activity and upper gastrointestinal cancers is less well established.

Data gained from the EPIC study have supported the benefits of physical activity in risk reduction for upper GI malignancies. Results demonstrated that non-cardia tumours of the stomach were reduced in populations who undertook regular physical activity, including cycling (hazard ratio 0.69) (Huerta et al. 2010). However, no association was observed between physical activity and tumours of the gastric cardia, or OACs.

This is in contrast to a case-control study by Vigen et al. (2006), who reported an inverse association between lifetime occupational physical activity (Total Activity Index, TAI) and OAC (OR 0.61), but no association between TAI and tumours of the gastric cardia or distal stomach (Vigen et al. 2006).

Such discrepancies may be explained by differing types of physical activity evaluated, and differing methods of evaluating physical activity (e.g. the EPIC study focused on all physical activity, whereas Vigen et al. (2006) looked only at occupational physical activity) as well as several confounding factors including the local prevalence of *H. pylori*, tobacco smoking, age and socioeconomic status (the latter were adjusted for in the study by Vigen et al. (2006) but not in the EPIC study).

Further investigation is needed to explain the mechanisms whereby physical activity can lead to a reduction in overall or site-specific cancer risk, although current hypotheses include a beneficial effect of physical activity on endogenous antioxidant properties, immunological defences and the favourable consequences of maintained weight loss.

17 Conclusion

The public health implications for rising rates of proximal gastric and distal oesophageal carcinomas are considerable. Although incidence of gastric cancer is declining, the absolute number of patients with gastric malignancies is expected to rise over the next decade and beyond. In addition, the rapidly increasing prevalence of OAC in Western populations is worrying as it is associated with an extremely poor prognosis (Griffin and Wahed 2011). It is therefore imperative to identify modifiable risk factors to enable early intervention and promote preventative strategies.

Much of the increasing burden of upper GI malignancies is expected to affect the growing proportion of elderly individuals in society. With their comorbidities, increased risk of frailty and decreased physiological reserve, the capacity of these patients to withstand radical surgical treatment options is brought into question. This further supports the urgent need to focus on preventative strategies in order to reduce the incidence of upper GI malignancies in the future. There is a promising role for aspirin as a chemopreventive agent, although objective evidence for its benefits in reducing oesophageal malignancies is lacking, and results from RCT-sare awaited.

The rising pattern of distal oesophageal and proximal gastric malignancies in Western populations suggests a common aetiology. In particular, the influence of lifestyle and environmental circumstances has been questioned in recent decades. Most notably, the prevalence of obesity is rising, with industrialised nations facing an obesity epidemic: in the United Kingdom, it is estimated that 23 % of men and 25 % of women have a BMI > 30 kg/m^2, according to 2002 data (Rennie and Jebb 2005). The role of increased BMI in the development of gastric and oesophageal cancers has been explored in this review, with current evidence suggesting a positive association through increased acid reflux, erosive oesophagitis and Barrett's oesophagus, which are harbingers of malignancy .

The impact of other lifestyle factors, including tobacco smoking, alcohol consumption, medications and physical activity have all been discussed, but further research is required to accurately assess the individual contributions of these factors towards development of upper GI cancers. While some individuals possess an inherited predisposition towards developing gastrointestinal cancers, it is their interaction with the local environment which influences manifestation of the phenotype. For example, individuals with genetic risk who eat healthily, partake in regular physical activity and do not smoke or drink alcohol may never develop gastric or oesophageal cancers despite perhaps inheriting a predisposition towards them. By contrast, persons without genetic risk factors may develop these malignancies through environmental exposures alone.

Effective prevention strategies for the future may be modelled on individual risk profiles, including host genetic factors as well as environmental exposures and lifestyle modification (Hartgrink et al. 2009). A clear and evidence-based understanding of factors predisposing to the development of gastric and oesophageal malignancies will pave the way for effective primary prevention based on education of the general population regarding specific risks. Combined with screening of high-risk groups to detect early cancer, further research into the molecular characterisation of gastric and oesophageal tumours will enhance our understanding of carcinogenic pathways, thereby guiding the development of novel therapeutic targets for the future.

References

Ahmed F, Goodman MT, Kosary C, Ruiz B, Wu XC, Chen VW, Correa CN (2006) Excess risk of subsequent primary cancers among colorectal carcinoma survivors, 1975–2001. Cancer 107(5 Suppl):1162–1171

Alibakhshi A, Aminian A, Mirsharifi R, Jahangiri Y, Dashti H, Karimian F (2009) The effect of age on the outcome of esophageal cancer surgery. Ann Thorac Med 4(2):71–74

Anderson LA, Cantwell MM, Watson RG, Johnston BT, Murphy SJ, Ferguson HR, McGuigan J, Comber H, Reynolds JV, Murray LJ (2009) The association between alcohol and reflux esophagitis, barrett's esophagus, and esophageal adenocarcinoma. Gastroenterology 136(3):799–805

Annibale B, Lahner E, Fave GD (2011) Diagnosis and management of pernicious anemia. Curr Gastroenterol Rep 13(6):518–524

Aragonés N, Pollán M, Gustavsson P (2002) Stomach cancer and occupation in Sweden: 1971–89. Occup Environ Med 59(5):329–337

Ayazi S, Hagen JA, Chan LS, DeMeester SR, Lin MW, Ayazi A, Leers JM, Oezcelik A, Banki F, Lipham JC, DeMeester TR, Crookes PF (2009) Obesity and gastroesophageal reflux: quantifying the association between body mass index, esophageal acid exposure, and lower esophageal sphincter status in a large series of patients with reflux symptoms. J Gastrointest Surg 13(8):1440–1447

Bassily R, Smallwood RA, Crotty B (2000) Risk of gastric cancer is not increased after partial gastrectomy. J Gastroenterol Hepatol 15(7):762–765

Bernstein H, Bernstein C, Payne CM, Dvorak K (2009) Bile acids as endogenous etiologic agents in gastrointestinal cancer. World J Gastroenterol 15(27):3329–40

Berrington de Gonzalez A, Curtis RE, Kry SF, Gilbert E, Lamart S, Berg CD, Stovall M, Ron E (2011) Proportion of second cancers attributable to radiotherapy treatment in adults: a cohort study in the US SEER cancer registries. Lancet Oncol 12(4):353–360

Blaydon DC, Etheridge SL, Risk JM, Hennies HC, Gay LJ, Carroll R, Plagnol V, McRonald FE, Stevens HP, Spurr NK, Bishop DT, Ellis A, Jankowski J, Field JK, Leigh IM, South AP, Kelsell DP (2012) RHBDF2 mutations are associated with tylosis, a familial esophageal cancer syndrome. Am J Hum Genet 10;90(2):340–346

Bollschweiler E, Wolfgarten E, Gutschow C, Hölscher AH (2001) Demographic variations in the rising incidence of esophageal adenocarcinoma in white males. Cancer 92(3):549–555

Bornschein J, Malfertheiner P (2011) Gastric carcinogenesis. Langenbecks Arch Surg 396(6):729–742

Brücher BL, Stein HJ, Bartels H, Feussner H, Siewert JR (2001) Achalasia and esophageal cancer: incidence, prevalence, and prognosis. World J Surg 25(6):745–749

Carmack SW, Genta RM, Graham DY, Lauwers GY (2009) Management of gastric polyps: a pathology-based guide for gastroenterologists. Nat Rev Gastroenterol Hepatol 6(6):331–341

Chen TS, Chen PS (1994) Rise and fall of the plummer-vinson syndrome. J Gastroenterol Hepatol 9(6):654–658

Chuang SC, Hashibe M, Scelo G, Brewster DH, Pukkala E, Friis S, Tracey E, Weiderpass E, Hemminki K, Tamaro S, Chia KS, Pompe-Kirn V, Kliewer EV, Tonita JM, Martos C, Jonasson JG, Dresler CM, Boffetta P, Brennan P (2008) Risk of second primary cancer among esophageal cancer patients: a pooled analysis of 13 cancer registries. Cancer Epidemiol Biomark Prev 17(6):1543–1549

Correa P (1992) Human gastric carcinogenesis: a multistep and multifactorial process—first American cancer society award lecture on cancer epidemiology and prevention. Cancer Res 52:6735–6740

Crew KD, Neugut AI (2004) Epidemiology of upper gastrointestinal malignancies. Semin Oncol 31:450–446

Devesa SS, Blot WJ, Fraumeni JF Jr (1998) Changing patterns in the incidence of esophageal and gastric carcinoma in the United States. Cancer 83:2049–2053

Dixon MF, Mapstone NP, Neville PM, Moayyedi P, Axon AT (2002) Bile reflux gastritis and intestinal metaplasia at the cardia. Gut 51(3):351–355

Dubé C, Rostom A, Sy R, Cranney A, Saloojee N, Garritty C, Sampson M, Zhang L, Yazdi F, Mamaladze V, Pan I, Macneil J, Mack D, Patel D, Moher D (2005) The prevalence of celiac disease in average-risk and at-risk western European populations: a systematic review. Gastroenterology 128(4 Suppl 1):S57–S67

Dunlop MG (2002) British society for gastroenterology; association of coloproctology for great Britain and Ireland. Guidance on gastrointestinal surveillance for hereditary non polyposis colorectal cancer, familial adenomatous polypolis, juvenile polyposis, and peutz-jeghers syndrome. Gut 51 Suppl 5:V21–7

Enzinger PC, Mayer RM (2003) Esophageal cancer. N Engl J Med 349:206–221

Ferlay J, Shin HR, Bray F, Forman D, Mathers C, Parkin DM (2010) Estimates of worldwide burden of cancer in 2008: GLOBOCAN 2008. Int J Cancer 127:2893–2917

Fisher SG, Davis F, Nelson R, Weber L, Goldberg J, Haenszel W (1993) A cohort study of stomach cancer risk in men after gastric surgery for benign disease. J Natl Cancer Inst 85(16):1303–1310

Ford JM (2002) Inherited susceptibility to gastric cancer: advances in genetics and guidelines for clinical management. ASCO Educational Book pp 116–125

Ford ES, Ajani UA, Croft JB, Critchley JA, Labarthe DR, Kottke TE, Giles WH, Capewell S (2007) Explaining the decrease in U.S. deaths from coronary disease, 1980–2000. N Engl J Med 356:2388–2398

Fuccio L, Zagari RM, Minardi ME, Bazzoli F (2007) Systematic review: helicobacter pylori eradication for the prevention of gastric cancer. Aliment Pharmacol Ther 25(2):133–141

Fuster V, Sweeny J (2011) Contemporary reviews in cardiovascular medicine. Circulation 123(7):768–778

Gallus S, Bosetti C, Franceschi S, Levi F, Simonato L, Negri E, La Vecchia C (2001) Oesophageal cancer in women: tobacco, alcohol, nutritional and hormonal factors. Br J Cancer 85(3):341–345

Gammon MD, Schoenberg JB, Ahsan H, Risch HA, Vaughan TL, Chow WH, Rotterdam H, West AB, Dubrow R, Stanford JL, Mayne ST, Farrow DC, Niwa S, Blot WJ, Fraumeni JF Jr (1997) Tobacco, alcohol, and socioeconomic status and adenocarcinomas of the esophagus and gastric cardia. J Natl Cancer Inst 89(17):1277–1284

Goddard AF, Badreldin R, Pritchard DM, Walker MM (2010) Warren B; British Society of Gastroenterology. The management of gastric polyps. Gut 59(9):1270–1276

González CA, Pera G, Agudo A, Palli D, Krogh V, Vineis P, Tumino R, Panico S, Berglund G, Simán H, Nyrén O et al (2003) Smoking and the risk of gastric cancer in the European prospective investigation into cancer and nutrition (EPIC). Int J Cancer 107:629–634

Green PH, Cellier C (2007) Celiac disease. N Engl J Med 357:1731–1743

Green PH, Fleischauer AT, Bhagat G, Goyal R, Jabri B, Neugut AI (2003) Risk of malignancy in patients with celiac disease. Am J Med 115:191–195

Griffin SM, Wahed S (2011) Oesophageal Cancer. Surgery 29(11):557–562

Grulich AE, van Leeuwen MT, Falster MO, Vajdic CM (2007) Incidence of cancers in people with HIV/AIDS compared with immunosuppressed transplant recipients: a meta-analysis. Lancet 370(9581):59–67

Hagarty S, Hüttner I, Shibata H, Katz S (2000) Gastric carcinoid tumours and pernicious anemia: case report and review of the literature. Can J Gastroenterol 14(3):241–245

Hampel H, Abraham NS, El-Serag HB (2005) Meta-analysis: obesity and the risk for gastroesophageal reflux disease and its complications. Ann Intern Med 2(143):199–211

Han HS, Lauwers GY (2010) Gastric Carcinoma. D Connection 15:20–25

Han MA, Oh MG, Choi IJ, Park SR, Ryu KW, Nam BH, Cho SJ, Kim CG, Lee JH, Kim YW (2012) Association of family history with cancer recurrence and survival in patients with gastric cancer. J Clin Oncol 30(7):701–708

Hartgrink HH, Jansen EP, van Grieken NC, van de Velde CJ (2009) Gastric cancer. Lancet 374(9688):477–490

Helicobacter and Cancer Collaborative Group (2001) Gastric cancer and helicobacter pylori: a combined analysis of 12 case control studies nested within prospective cohorts. Gut 49:347–353

Hirota WK, Zuckerman MJ, Adler DG, Davila RE, Egan J, Leighton JA, Qureshi WA, Rajan E, Fanelli R, Wheeler-Harbaugh J, Baron TH (2006) Standards of practice committee, American society for gastrointestinal endoscopy. ASGE guideline: the role of endoscopy in the surveillance of premalignant conditions of the upper GI tract. Gastrointest Endosc 63(4):570–580

Hoffman RM, Jaffe PE (1995) Plummer-vinson syndrome. A case report and literature review. Arch Intern Med 9(155):2008–2011

Hongo M, Nagasaki Y, Shoji T (2009) Epidemiology of esophageal cancer: orient to occident. Effects of chronology, geography and ethnicity. J Gastroenterol Hepatol 24(5):729–735

Huerta JM, Navarro C, Chirlaque MD, Tormo MJ, Steindorf K, Buckland G, Carneiro F, Johnsen NF, Overvad K, Stegger J, Tjønneland A et al (2010) Prospective study of physical activity and risk of primary adenocarcinomas of the oesophagus and stomach in the EPIC (European Prospective Investigation into Cancer and nutrition) cohort. Cancer Causes Control 21(5):657–669

International Agency for Research on Cancer (1986) Tobacco smoking. IARC Monogr Eval Carcinog Risk Chem Hum 38:35–394

Islami F, Karmangar F (2008) Helicobacter pylori and esophageal cancer risk: a meta-analysis. Cancer Prev Res 1:329–338

Iwaya T, Maesawa C, Ogasawara S, Tamura G (1998) Tylosis esophageal cancer locus on chromosome 17q25.1 is commonly deleted in sporadic human esophageal cancer. Gastroenterology 114(6):1206–1210

Jain P (2009) Plummer-Vinson Syndrome Associated with Celiac Disease. Clin Exp Med J 2009(3):509–512

Jankowska H, Hooper P, Jankowski JA (2010) Aspirin chemoprevention of gastrointestinal cancer in the next decade. A review of the evidence. Pol Arch Med Wewn 120(10):407–412

Kastelein F, Spaander MC, Biermann K, Steyerberg EW, Kuipers EJ, Bruno MJ (2011) Probar-study group. Nonsteroidal anti-inflammatory drugs and statins have chemopreventative effects in patients with Barrett's esophagus. Gastroenterology 141(6):2000–2008 quiz e13-4

Kato H, Nakajima M (2011) Multimodal treatment for esophageal cancer in elderly patients. Esophagus 8:71–77

Kim KH, Kim MC, Jung GJ (2005) Gastric cancer occurring in a patient with plummer-vinson syndrome: a case report. World J Gastroenterol 28;11(44):7048–7050

Kodama M, Murakami K, Okimoto T, Abe T, Nakagawa Y, Mizukami K, Uchida M, Inoue K, Fujioka T (2012) Helicobacter pylori eradication improves gastric atrophy and intestinal metaplasia in long-term observation. Digestion 85(2):126–130

Kokkola A, Sjöblom S-M, Haapiainen R et al (1998) The risk of gastric carcinoma and carcinoid tumours in patients with pernicious anaemia. Scand J Gastroenterol 33:88–92

Kruk J (2007) Lifetime physical activity and the risk of breast cancer: a case-control study. Cancer Detect Prev 31(1):18–28

Kubo A, Corley DA (2004) Marked multi-ethnic variation of esophageal and gastric cardia carcinomas within the United States. Am J Gastroenterol 99:582–588

Kubo A, Corley DA (2006) Body mass index and adenocarcinomas of the esophagus or gastric cardia: a systematic review and meta-analysis. Cancer Epidemiol Biomarkers Prev 15(5):872–878

La Vecchia C, Negri E, D'Avanzo B, Moller H, Franceschi S (1992) Partial gastrectomy and subsequent gastric cancer risk. J Epidemiol Community Health 46(1):12–14

Ladeiras-Lopes R, Pereira AK, Nogueira A et al (2008) Smoking and gastric cancer: systematic review and meta-analysis of cohort studies. Cancer Causes Control 19:689–701

Larsson LG, Sandström A, Westling P (1975) Relationship of plummer-vinson disease to cancer of the upper alimentary tract in Sweden. Cancer Res 35 (11 pt2):3308–3316

Leeuwenburgh I, Scholten P, Alderliesten J, Tilanus HW, Looman CW, Steijerberg EW, Kuipers EJ (2010) Long-term esophageal cancer risk in patients with primary achalasia: a prospective study. Am J Gastroenterol 105(10):2144–2149

Leon DA (2011) Trends in European life expectancy: a salutary view. Int J Epidemiol 40(2):271–277

Lindblad M, Rodríguez LA, Lagergren J (2005) Body mass, tobacco and alcohol and risk of esophageal, gastric cardia, and gastric non-cardia adenocarcinoma among men and women in a nested case-control study. Cancer Causes Control 16(3):285–294

Lindblad M, García Rodríguez LA, Chandanos E, Lagergren J (2006) Hormone replacement therapy and risks of oesophageal and gastric adenocarcinomas. Br J Cancer 94:136–141

Lohi S, Maki M, Rissanen H et al (2009) Prognosis of unrecognized coeliac disease as regards mortality: a population-based cohort study. Ann Med 41:508–515

Lynch HT, Kaurah P, Wirtzfeld D, Rubinstein WS, Weissman S, Lynch JF, Grady W, Wiyrick S, Senz J, Huntsman DG (2008) Hereditary diffuse gastric cancer: diagnosis, genetic counseling, and prophylactic total gastrectomy. Cancer 112:2655–2663

Lynch HT, Lynch JF, Shaw TG (2011) Hereditary gastrointestinal cancer syndromes. Gastrointest Cancer Res 4(4 Suppl 1):S9–S17

Maddams J, Parkin DM, Darby SC (2011) The cancer burden in the United Kingdom in 2007 due to radiotherapy. Int J Cancer 129(12):2885–2893

Masciari S, Dewanwala A, Stoffel EM, Lauwers GY, Zheng H, Achatz MI, Riegert-Johnson D, Foretova L, Silva EM, Digianni L, Verselis SJ, Schneider K, Li FP, Fraumeni J, Garber JE, Syngal S (2011) Gastric cancer in individuals with li-fraumeni syndrome. Genet Med 13(7):651–657

Massironi S, Sciola V, Spampatti MP, Peracchi M, Conte D (2009) Gastric carcinoids: between underestimation and overtreatment. World J Gastroenterol 15:2177–2183

Menges M, Müller M (2001) Zeit z M. Increased acid and bile reflux in Barrett's esophagus compared to reflux esophagitis, and effect of proton pump inhibitor therapy. Am J Gastroenterol 96:331–333

Messmann H (2001) Squamous cell cancer of the oesophagus. Best Pract Res Clin Gastroenterol 15:249–265

Moayyedi P, Burch N, Akhtar-Danesh N et al (2008) Mortality rates in patients with Barrett's oesophagus. Aliment Pharmacol Ther 27:316–320

Munoz N (2002) Epidemiology of gastric cancer (Chapter 10). In: Posner MC, Vokes EE, Weichselbaum RR, Decker BC Cancer of the upper gastrointestinal tract, pp 206–217

Nadauld LD, Ford JM (2012) Family history as a positive prognostic factor in gastric cancer. J Clin Oncol 30(7):683–684

Nakos A, Zezos P, Liratzopoulos N, Efraimidou E, Manolas K, Moschos J, Molivas E, Kouklakis G (2009) The significance of histological evidence of bile reflux gastropathy in patients with gastroesophageal reflux disease. Med Sci Monit 15(6):313–318

Nakui M, Chino O, Ozawa S (2010) Treatment of esophageal cancer in elderly patients. Gan To Kagaku Ryoho 37(13):2813–2816. [Article in Japanese]

Nguyen DM, Richardson P, El-Serag HB (2010) Medications (NSAIDs, statins, proton pump inhibitors) and the risk of esophageal adenocarcinoma in patients with Barrett's esophagus. Gastroenterology 138(7):2260–2266

Nishino Y, Inoue M, Tsuji I, Wakai K, Nagata C, Mizoue T, Tanaka K (2006) Research group for the development and evaluation of cancer prevention strategies in Japan. Tobacco smoking and gastric cancer risk: an evaluation based on a systematic review of epidemiologic evidence among the Japanese population. Jpn J Clin Oncol 36(12):800–807

Nocon M, Labenz J, Willich SN (2006) Lifestyle factors and symptoms of gastro-oesophageal reflux—a population-based study. Aliment Pharmacol Ther 23:169–174

Novacek G (2006) Plummer-Vinson syndrome. Orphanet J Rare Dis 1:36

Pandeya N, Williams G, Green AC, Webb PM (2009) Australian cancer study. Alcohol consumption and the risks of adenocarcinoma and squamous cell carcinoma of the esophagus. Gastroenterology 136(4):1215–1224

Park YJ, Shin KH, Park JG (2000) Risk of gastric cancer in hereditary nonpolyposis colorectal cancer in Korea. Clin Cancer Res 6(8):2994–2998

Parkin DM (2004) International variation. Oncogene 23:6329–6340

Peek RM, Blaser MJ (2002) Helicobacter pylori and gastrointestinal tract adenocarcinomas. Nature Rev Cancer 2:28–37

Polk DB, Peek RM Jr (2010) Helicobacter pylori: gastric cancer and beyond. Nat Rev Cancer 10(6):403–414

Quigley EM, Jacobson BC, Lenglinger J, Rubenstein JH, El-Serag H, Cicala M, McCallum RW, Levine MS, Gore RM (2011) Barrett's esophagus: clinical features, obesity, and imaging. Ann N Y Acad Sci 1232:36–52

Rennie KL, Jebb SA (2005) Prevalence of obesity in Great Britain. Obes Rev 6(1):11–12

Rubin E, Strayer D (eds) (2008) Rubin's pathology: clinicopathologic foundations of medicine, 6th edn. Lippincott Williams & Wilkins, Maryland, Chapter 13, pp 611

Ruol A, Portale G, Zaninotto G, Cagol M, Cavallin F, Castoro C, Sileni VC, Alfieri R, Rampado S, Ancona E (2007) Results of esophagectomy for esophageal cancer in elderly patients: age has little influence on outcome and survival. J Thorac Cardiovasc Surg 133(5):1186–1192

Rushton L, Bagga S, Bevan R, Brown TP, Cherrie JW, Holmes P, Fortunato L, Slack R, Van Tongeren M, Young C, Hutchings SJ (2010) Occupation and cancer in Britain. Br J Cancer 102(9):1428–1437

Sasako M, Inoue M, Lin JT, Khor C, Yang HK, Ohtsu A (2010) Gastric cancer working group report. Jpn J Clin Oncol 40(Suppl 1):i28–i37

Satram-Hoang S, Ziogas A, Anton-Culver H (2007) Risk of second primary cancer in men with breast cancer. Breast Cancer Res 9(1):R10

Sjödahl K, Jansson C, Bergdahl IA, Adami J, Boffetta P, Lagergren J (2007) Airborne exposures and risk of gastric cancer: a prospective cohort study. Int J Cancer 120(9):2013–2018

Solhpour A, Pourhoseingholi MA, Soltani F, Zarghi A, Habibi M, Ghafarnejad F, Tajik Z, Rostaminejad M, Ramezankhani A, Zali MR (2008) Gastro-esophageal reflux symptoms and body mass index: no relation among the Iranian population. Indian J Gastroenterol 27(4):153–155

Stoner GD, Gupta A (2001) Etiology and chemoprevention of esophageal squamous cell carcinoma. Carcinogenesis 22:1737–1746

Subramanian S, Goldstein DP, Parlea L, Thabane L, Ezzat S, Ibrahim-Zada I, Straus S, Brierley JD, Tsang RW, Gafni A, Rotstein L, Sawka AM (2007) Second primary malignancy risk in thyroid cancer survivors: a systematic review and meta-analysis. Thyroid 17(12):1277–1288

Sung NY, Choi KS, Park EC, Park K, Lee SY, Lee AK, Choi IJ, Jung KW, Won YJ, Shin HR (2007) Smoking, alcohol and gastric cancer risk in Korean men: the national health insurance corporation study. Br J Cancer 97(5):700–704

Tersmette AC, Giardiello FM, Tytgat GN, Offerhaus GJ (1995) Carcinogenesis after remote peptic ulcer surgery: the long-term prognosis of partial gastrectomy. Scand J Gastroenterol Suppl 212:96–99

Thiers BH, Sahn RE, Callen JP (2009) Cutaneous manifestations of internal malignancy. CA Cancer J Clin 59(2):73–98

Thune I, Furberg AS (2001) Physical activity and cancer risk: dose-response and cancer, all sites and site-specific. Med Sci Sports Exerc 33(6 Suppl):S530–S550

Travis LB, Fosså SD, Schonfeld SJ, McMaster ML, Lynch CF, Storm H, Hall P, Holowaty E, Andersen A, Pukkala E, Andersson M, Kaijser M, Gospodarowicz M, Joensuu T, Cohen RJ, Boice JD Jr, Dores GM, Gilbert ES (2005) Second cancers among 40,576 testicular cancer patients: focus on long-term survivors. J Natl Cancer Inst 97(18):1354–1365

Vannella L, Lahner E, Osborn J, Bordi C, Miglione M, Delle Fave G, Annibale B (2010) Risk factors for progression to gastric neoplastic lesions in patients with atrophic gastritis. Aliment Pharmacol Ther 31(9):1042–1050

Vial M, Grande L, Pera M (2010) Epidemiology of adenocarcinoma of the esophagus, gastric cardia, and upper gastric third. Recent Results Cancer Res 182:1–17

Vigen C, Bernstein L, Wu AH (2006) Occupational physical activity and risk of adenocarcinomas of the esophagus and stomach. Int J Cancer 118(4):1004–1009

von Brevern M, Hollstein MC, Risk JM, Garde J, Bennett WP, Harris CC, Muehlbauer KR, Field JK (1998) Loss of heterozygosity in sporadic oesophageal tumors in the tylosis oesophageal cancer (TOC) gene region of chromosome 17q. Oncogene 22:2101–2105

Wang WH, Huang JQ, Zheng GF, Lam SK, Karlberg J, Wong BC (2003) Non-steroidal anti-inflammatory drug use and the risk of gastric cancer: a systematic review and meta-analysis. J Natl Cancer Inst 3;95(23):1784–1791

Wang JM, Xu B, Rao JY, Shen HB, Xue HC, Jiang QW (2007) Diet habits, alcohol drinking, tobacco smoking, green tea drinking, and the risk of esophageal squamous cell carcinoma in the Chinese population. Eur J Gastroenterol Hepatol 19(2):171–176

Whiteman DC, Parmar P, Fahey P, Moore SP, Stark M, Zhao ZZ, Montgomery GW, Green AC, Hayward NK, Webb PM (2010) Australian cancer study. Association of Helicobacter pylori infection with reduced risk for esophageal cancer is independent of environmental and genetic modifiers. Gastroenterology 139(1):73–83

Yamaoka Y, Kato M, Asaka M (2008) Geographic differences in gastric cancer incidence can be explained by differences between helicobacter pylori strains. Intern Med 47:1077–1083

Yang P, Zhou Y, Chen B, Wan HW, Jia GQ, Bai HL, Wu XT (2009) Overweight, obesity and gastric cancer risk: results from a meta-analysis of cohort studies. Eur J Cancer 45(16):2867–2873

Yang P, Zhou Y, Chen B, Wan HW, Jia GQ, Bai HL, Wu XT (2010) Aspirin use and the risk of gastric cancer: a meta-analysis. Dig Dis Sci 55(6):1533–1539

Part IV
Choosing the Best Treatment for Oesophageal Cancer

Endoscopic Treatment for Esophageal Squamous Cell Carcinoma

Tsuneo Oyama

Contents

1	Introduction	143
2	Indications of Endoscopic Resection for Esophageal SCC	144
	2.1 Absolute Indication	144
	2.2 Relative Indications	144
3	Endoscopic Mucosal Resection	145
	3.1 Procedures	145
	3.2 Advantage and Disadvantage of EMR	145
4	Endoscopic Submucosal Dissection (ESD)	145
	4.1 Procedure	145
	4.2 Marking and Submucosal Injection	146
	4.3 Mucosal incision	146
	4.4 Submucosal Dissection	148
	4.5 Hemostasis	150
	4.6 Prevention of Bleeding	150
5	Complications of Esophageal EMR/ESD	151
References		153

1 Introduction

Esophageal endoscopic mucosal resection (EMR) was developed in the late 1980s (Makuuchi 1996; Yoshida T 2004; Inoue et al. 1993; Pech et al. 2004). And EMR was widely accepted as the treatment for superficial esophageal squamous cell carcinoma (SCC). However, there was limitation in size, and precise resection was

---

T. Oyama (✉)
Department of Gastroenerology, Saku Central Hospital, Nagano, Japan
e-mail: oyama@coral.ocn.ne.jp

F. Otto and M. P. Lutz (eds.), *Early Gastrointestinal Cancers*,
Recent Results in Cancer Research 196, DOI: 10.1007/978-3-642-31629-6_9,
© Springer-Verlag Berlin Heidelberg 2012

impossible. Piecemeal resection was performed for big lesions, and local recurrence after piece meal EMR was high (Momma 2007). Therefore, a novel endoscopic treatment, endoscopic submucosal dissection (ESD) was developed to resolve such disadvantage of EMR (Oyama and Kikuchi 2002; Oyama et al. 2005; Fujishiro et al. 2006; Ishihara et al. 2008; Hiroaki et al. 2010).

The other endoscopic treatment is ablation method such as radio frequent ablation. However, pathological findings, such as invasion depth, histological type, and lymphatic or venous permeation, could not be learned by ablation therapy. Therefore, the first choice endoscopic treatment is EMR/ESD rather than ablation therapy.

2 Indications of Endoscopic Resection for Esophageal SCC

2.1 Absolute Indication

The indication of endoscopic resection is esophageal cancer without lymph node metastasis. According to Japanese criteria, the invasion depth of mucosal SCC (T1a) was divided into three groups, as follows:
T1a EP: SCC those remaining in the mucosal epithelium (EP).
T1a LPM: SCC those remaining in the lamina propria mucosae (LPM).
T1a MM: SCC those contact or invade muscularis mucosae (MM).
And, the invasion depth of submucosal SCC was divided into two groups, as follows:
T1b SM1: SCC those invaded submucosal layer 200 micrometer or less.
T1b SM2: SCC those invaded submucosal layer 201 micrometer or deep.

The incidence of lymph node metastasis of T1a EP and LPM is extremely rarely (Oyama Oyama 2011). Therefore, T1a EP or LPM SCC was defined as the indications for endoscopic resection by the guidelines of Japan Esophageal Society (Kuwano et al. 2008).

2.2 Relative Indications

The incidence of lymph node metastasis of T1a MM, T1b SM1, and T1b SM2 reported as 9.3, 19.30, and 40 %, respectively (Oyama et al. 2002). The standard treatment for T1a MM or T1b SM is esophagectomy with lymph node dissection. However, the quality of life (QOL) after esophagectomy is not good. Therefore, T1a MM or T1b SM1 with clinical N0 (no lymph node swelling by CT and EUS) was defined as relative indications of endoscopic resection.

In addition, lymphatic or venous involvement and infiltrative growth have been reported as the risk factors. However, precise pathological diagnosis is impossible by the piecemeal resected specimen. Therefore, an en bloc resection is necessary for the treatment of superficial esophageal SCC.

3 Endoscopic Mucosal Resection

3.1 Procedures

Many EMR methods have been reported. Especially, EMRC method has been widely accepted. At first, a transparent hood was attached at the tip of the scope and saline was injected into the submucosal layer to separate mucosal cancer from the proper muscular layer. After that, a snare was inserted from the working channel of the scope and opened on the cancer. The cancer was sucked into the transparent hood and snared. Finally, the cancer could be resected using a high frequency generator.

3.2 Advantage and Disadvantage of EMR

The skill of EMR is easy, and the procedure duration is short. However, the size of resected specimens was small, 10–20 mm or less, and piecemeal resection was performed for larger lesions. A precise pathological examination of piecemeal-resected specimens was impossible. And local recurrent rate has been reportedly high after piecemeal resection.

According to the report by Ishihara et al. (Fujishiro et al. 2006), since the results of EMR and ESD were comparable in achieving en bloc complete resection of lesions less than 15 mm diameter, they recommended the easier EMR method in this situation.

4 Endoscopic Submucosal Dissection (ESD)

The risk of perforation in esophageal ESD is higher than gastric ESD, because the esophageal proper mucosal layer is thinner than that of stomach. The maneuverability of scope is more difficult, because the space of esophagus is narrow, and bended by compression with heart, aorta, and vertebra. Therefore, ESD should be performed carefully.

4.1 Procedure

Many endo knives have been developed for ESD. Usually, the hook knife (KD-620LR, Olympus, Tokyo) has been selected for esophageal ESD, because it is the safest knife. The tip of the knife is bent at right angle. The length of hook part is 1.3 mm and that of the arm part is 4.5 mm (Fig. 1). The hook knife has a handle on the proximal side and the direction of hook can be controlled with the handle rotation. It is a useful device to cut mucosa, submucosal fibers, vessels, and to stop minor bleeding (Oyama et al. 2006). The direction of the hook knife should be controlled, and kept parallel with the muscular layer to prevent perforation during ESD. A therapeutic scope that has water jet system is useful for ESD. We usually use GIFQ260 J, Olympus, Tokyo, Japan, and a high-frequency generator (VIO 300D; ERBE Elektromedizin, Tübingen, Germany).

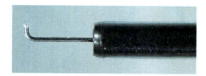

Fig. 1 A hook knife. The tip of the knife is bent at a right angle. The length of hook part is 1.3 mm and that of the arm part is 4.5 mm. The knife is hosted within an outer sheath. The tip of the sheath has a hood like shape that allows the hook of the knife to be retracted within it

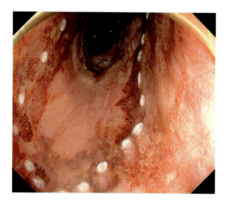

Fig. 2 Marks should be placed 2 or 3 mm away from the edge of the lateral extension of the cancer. The hook knife is a useful device to place the marks safely. The tip of hook knife can be retracted within the sheath, and a sharp mark can be placed when the tip of hook knife makes contact with the mucosa. We use soft coagulation (effect 4, 20 W) for the esophagus

4.2 Marking and Submucosal Injection

The lateral extension of SCC could be diagnosed easily after 0.75–1 % iodine dying. Marks should be placed 2 or 3 mm away from the edge of the unstained area that represents the cancer. The esophageal wall is thinner than that of stomach. Therefore, perforation can occur during marking if a needle knife is used. The hook knife is a useful device to place the marks safely. The tip of hook knife could be retracted within the sheath, and a sharp mark could be placed when the tip of hook knife was contacted with the mucosa, and coagulated by soft coagulation (effect 4, 20 W) (Fig. 2). Next, Glyceol® (CHUGAI Pharmaceutical Co., LTD., Tokyo, Japan) was injected into the submucosal layer to separate the mucosa from the proper muscular layer. This solution includes 10 % glycerin.

4.3 Mucosal incision

Basically, the mucosal incision is performed from oral side. At first, the backside of the hook knife was contacted with the mucosa, and a hole was made by Endo

Fig. 3 We initially place the backside of the hook knife in contact with the mucosa after submucosal injection, and then make a mucosal defect using Endo cut I mode (Effect 3)

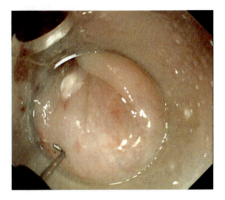

Fig. 4 After that, we insert the tip of hook knife into submucosal layer, and hook and cut the mucosa with the hook part of the knife

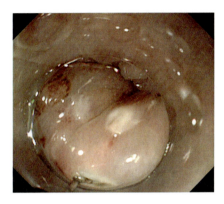

cut I mode (Effect 3) (Fig. 3). After that, the tip of hook knife was inserted into submucosal layer, and mucosa was hooked and cut with the hook part of the knife (Fig. 4). It is an important point to prevent perforation.

The arm part of the hook knife is used for longitudinal mucosal incision. The direction of the hook knife is turned to the esophageal lumen, and the knife was inserted into the submucosal layer by sliding the back side. Then the mucosa is captured by the arm part of the knife (Fig. 5); finally, the mucosa was cut by the combination of Spray coagulation (Effect 2, 60 W) and Endo cut mode (Effect 3, duration 2, and interval 2). It is important procedure to prevent bleeding during mucosal incision. The submucosal vessels could not be observed by endoscopy. Sometimes they are cut unexpected, and bleeding occurs during mucosal incision. The initial spray coagulation can coagulate submucosal vessel; therefore, such unexpected bleeding could be prevent with initial spray coagulation.

Deeper cut of submucosal fibers was performed after mucosal incision. The hook knife was inserted into submucosal layer, and submucosal fibers were hooked and cut. Then the lesion shrank by the contraction of muscularis mucosa (Fig. 6). After that, the mucosal incision and deeper cut of the other side was performed and a circumferential incision was completed.

Fig. 5 The arm part of the hook knife is used for longitudinal mucosal incision. We then direct the hook knife to the lumen, and insert it into the submucosal layer by sliding the back of the knife. Then the mucosa is elevated to the lumen by the arm part of the knife

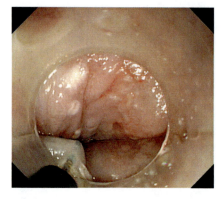

Fig. 6 Deeper cut of submucosal fibers is performed following mucosal incision. We insert the hook knife into the submucosal layer, and move it to the lumen side in order to hook the submucosal fibers

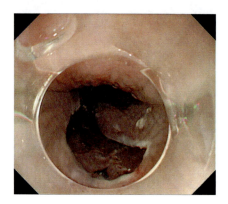

4.4 Submucosal Dissection

Submucosal dissection was performed from oral to anal side. There are two strategies for submucosal dissection. In one strategy, dissection of the submucosal layer is performed sequentially from the oral side to the anal side. The hook knife should be held parallel with the proper muscle, and submucosal fibers could be cut with spray coagulation mode (effect 2, 60 W) (Fig. 7).

The resected part may cause gradual inversion of the lesion, leading to insufficient counter traction of the submucosal layer, that can make residual dissection difficult. Therefore, if the circumference is half or more, a tunnel method is better (Oyama et al. 2006). A local injection is added after a circumferential incision followed by a tunnel-shaped dissection of the center of the lesion, Tunnel-shaped dissection of the central part enables counter traction using a transparent hood, providing more efficient dissection. Finally, the fibers on both sides are dissected.

Sometimes the dissected part was turned to anal side, and enough counter traction could not be gained in this situation. "Clip with line" method is useful in this situation (Oyama et al. 2002; Oyama 2011). This method utilizes a modified clip with a line. A clip with a line is loaded to the clip placement device. The attached string is kept outside of the scope and inserted with the scope into the

Fig. 7 Submucosal fibers was hooked using the hook part of the knife, and cut by spray coagulation (effect 2, 60 W)

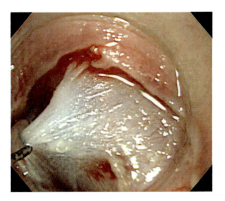

Fig. 8 Clip with line method. The clip is released to grasp the lesion for intended counter traction

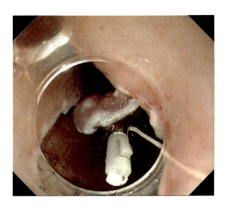

Fig. 9 The clipped site is gently pulled with a traction line to provide counter traction to facilitate submucosal dissection

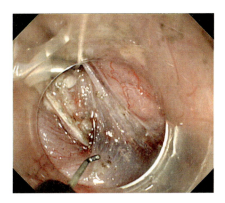

esophageal lumen. The clip is released to grasp the lesion to make counter traction (Fig. 8). The clipped site is gently pulled with a traction line to provide counter traction to facilitate submucosal dissection (Fig. 9).

The most severe complication during submucosal dissection is perforation. Therefore, the operator should check the upper level of the proper muscular layer, and take care not to injure the proper muscular layer.

4.5   Hemostasis

Bleeding makes the visual field worse; therefore hemostasis should be performed as soon as possible. When bleeding occurs during mucosal incision or dissection, the area should be flushed using a water jet system to find the origin of bleeding. Minor bleeding could be stopped using knife. However, a hemostatic forceps (coagrasper, FD-410LR, Olympus, Tokyo) should be selected for more severe bleeding.

4.5.1   Hemostasis Using Knife

Hemostasis using the endo knife is useful for controlling oozing bleeds. The tip of knife is brought close to the origin, and electrical discharge is done with Spray mode to obtain hemostasis (effect 2, 60 W). Since prolonged electrical discharge may cause perforation, electrical discharge should be performed momentarily. Therefore, it is important to maintain optimal distance using a transparent hood (Oyama et al. 2006).

A water jet system must be used to confirm the precise origin of the bleeding. A scope equipped with a water jet should be selected for esophageal ESD.

4.5.2   Hemostatic Procedures Using a Hemostatic Forceps

A hemostatic forceps FD-410LR (Olympus, Tokyo, Japan) is useful in cases of more active or spurting bleeding. After flushing with a water jet to clear the origin of bleeding, the origin is grasped accurately with the hemostatic forceps. After that, re-flushing with a water jet enables us to determine whether the origin is grasped accurately. Then, the forceps are elevated a little to separate forceps from the proper muscular layer followed by electrical discharge with soft coagulation (effect 5, 40 W) momentarily to obtain hemostasis.

For hemostatic procedures using hemostatic forceps, an accurate grasp is the most important factor. An accurate grasp of the bleeding point may provide reliable hemostasis, while an inaccurate grasp will not provide hemostasis by electrical discharge. Unnecessary electrical discharge may cause delayed perforation, so an accurate grasp should be ensured. Since the wall of the esophagus is thinner than that of the stomach, to prevent delayed and other types of perforation, care should be taken.

4.6   Prevention of Bleeding

Bleeding may worsen the visual field, leading to a higher risk of accidents. Inadvertent coagulation may cause coagulation of the blood, which creates an impaired field of vision. Incision and dissection with preventing bleeding are more desirable than hastily attempting hemostasis after bleeding starts. There are many vessels in the deep submucosal layer. A small vessel 1 mm or less could be cut using the hook knife without bleeding, when spray coagulation mode was used (effect 2, 60 W) (Figs. 10, 11). However, if the size of the vessel was 1 mm or larger, pre cut coagulation should be performed to prevent bleeding (Fig. 12). The large vessel was grasped by the hemostatic forceps, and was coagulated by soft

Fig. 10 Oozing was found during submucosal dissection

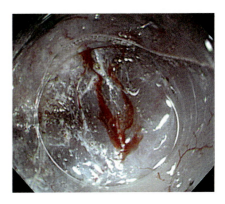

Fig. 11 Such minor bleeding could be stopped by spray coagulation (effect 2, 60 W) using the back side of the hook knife

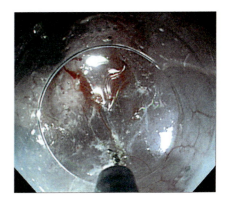

coagulation effect 5, 60 W. After that, the vessel could be cut using the hook knife and spray coagulation (effect 2, 60 W) without bleeding.

En-bloc resection for this large lesion was completed (Fig. 13). The patient could eat soft food 2 days after ESD. The resected specimen was 72 × 47 mm and the cancer was 54 × 38 mm in area (Fig. 14). Pathological diagnosis was squamous cell carcinoma, 0-IIc type, invasion depth was proper mucosal layer (T1a LPM), without lymphatic and venous involvement, and the lateral and vertical margin was negative.

5   Complications of Esophageal EMR/ESD

The major complication of EMR/ESD is perforation, bleeding, and aspiration pneumonia. Perforations may cause mediastinal emphysema, which increases the mediastinal pressure crushing the esophageal lumen, leading to difficulty in securing the visual field. Severe mediastinal emphysema may be complicated by pneumothorax, leading to shock; therefore, electrocardiography, arterial oxygen saturation, and blood pressure (using automated sphygmomanometer) monitoring should be conducted during ESD, as well as periodic observation for subcutaneous emphysema through palpation.

Fig. 12 When the size of vessel was 1 mm or thicker, pre-cut coagulation is useful. The vessel was grasped by hemostatic forceps, and coagulated using soft coagulation (effect 3, 60 W)

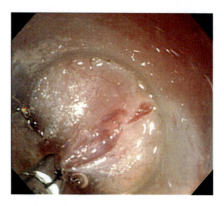

Fig. 13 En bloc resection was completed. There were no perforation and bleeding

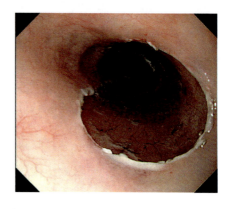

Since the esophagus has no serous membrane and the intramediastinal pressure is lower than that of the esophageal lumen, mediastinal emphysema may appear without perforation. Dissection immediately above the proper muscular layer may damage the proper muscular layer during electrical discharge, which often causes mediastinal emphysema. Therefore, it is important to dissect the submucosal layer leaving the lowest one-third without exposure of the proper muscular layer.

Under intubation general anesthesia, the mediastinal pressure is higher than the intraesophageal pressure, enabling prevention of mediastinal emphysema and/or subcutaneous emphysema. Therefore, intubation general anesthesia is preferable for the large lesion that is expected to take two or more hours to complete the resection of the lesion.

Perforation rate caused by esophageal EMR has been reported as 0–2.4 % (Makuuchi 1996; Yoshida T 2004; Inoue et al. 1993; Pech et al. 2004) and that of ESD has been reported as 0–6.4 % (Oyama et al. 2005; Fujishiro et al. 2006; Ishihara et al. 2008; Hiroaki et al. 2010). The shape and size of perforation caused by EMR is different from that caused by ESD. 1 cm or larger proper muscle was removed by EMR and sometimes closure by clips is difficult. On the other hand, the shape of perforation caused by ESD is linier without defect of proper muscle. Therefore, usually closure by clips is easier than that of EMR. However,

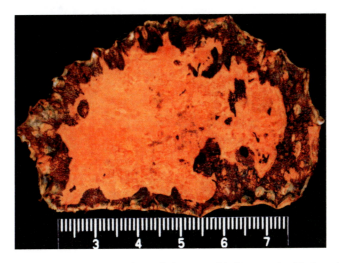

Fig. 14 The resected specimen showed a well demarcated iodine unstained lesion with enough cut margin

sometimes the clip may injure remaining proper muscle and make the perforation larger. Therefore, the operator should be skilled clipping.

Usually, such perforation can be treated by fast, insertion of nasoesophageal tube and intravenous antibiotics without surgical operation.

The water jet is useful for the detection of bleeding point. However, sometimes water reflex cases aspiration pneumonia. A flexible overtube® (Sumitomo Bakelite, Akita, Japan) is a useful device to prevent aspiration pneumonia. General anesthesia with tracheal intubation is necessary for the cervical esophageal ESD, because the risk of aspiration pneumonia is high.

References

Fujishiro M, Yahagi N, Kakushima N, Kodashima S, Muraki Y, Ono S et al (2006) Endoscopic submucosal dissection of esophageal squamous cell neoplasms. Clin Gastroenterol Hepatol 4:688–694

Hiroaki T, Yoshiaki A, Hosokawa M et al (2010) Endoscopic submucosal dissection is superior to conventional endoscopic resection as a curative treatment for early squamous cell carcinoma, of the esophagus. Gastrointest Endosc 71:255–264

Inoue H, Takeshita K, Hori H, Muraoka Y, Yoneshima H, Endo M (1993) Endoscopic mucosal resection with a cap-fitted panendoscope for esophagus, stomach and colon mucosal lesions. Gastrointest Endosc 39:58–62

Ishihara R, Iishi H, Uedo N, Takeuchi Y, Yamamoto S, Yamada T (2008) Comparison of EMR and endoscopic submucosal dissection for en bloc resection of early esophageal cancers in Japan. Gastrointest Endosc 68:1066–1072

Kuwano H, Nishimura Y, Ohtsu A, Kato H, Kitagawa Y, Tamai S, Toh Y, Matsubara H (2008) Guidelines for diagnosis and treatment of carcinoma of the esophagus April 2007 edn, edited by the Japan Esophageal Society, Esophagus 5: 61–73

Makuuchi H (1996) Endoscopic mucosal resection for early esophageal cancer indication and techniques. Dig Endosc 8:175–179

Momma K (2007) Endoscopic treatment of esophageal mucosal carcinomas: indications and outcomes. Esophagus 4:93–98

Oyama T (2011) Endoscopic submucosal dissection using a hook knife. Tech Gastrointest Endosc 13:70–73

Oyama T, Kikuchi Y (2002) Aggressive endoscopic mucosal resection in the upper GI tract—hook knife EMR method. Min Invas Ther Alied Technol 11:291–295

Oyama T, Miyata Y, Shimatani S, Tomori A, Hotta K, Yoshida M (2002a) Lymph nodal metastasis of m3, sm1 esophageal cancer (in Japanese with English abstract). Stomach Intest (Tokyo) 37:71–74

Oyama T, Yuichi Kikuchi, Shimaya S, Tomori A, Hotta K, Miyata Y, Yamada S (2002) Endoscopic Mucosal Resection using a Hooking Knife—Intra gastric lesion lifting method. Stomach Intestine 37: 1155–1161. Japanese with English summary

Oyama T, Tomori A, Hotta K, Morita S, Kominato K, Tanaka M et al (2005) Endoscopic submucosal dissection of early esophageal cancer. Clin Gastroenterol Hepatol 3:S67–S70

Oyama T, Tomori A, Hotta K, Morita S, Tanaka M, Furutachi S et al. (2006) ESD with a Hook knife for Early Esophageal Cancer. Stomach Intestine 41:491-97. Japanese with English summary

Oyama T, Akihisa T, Hotta K, Miyata Y (2006b) Hemostasis with hook knife during endoscopic submucosal dissection. Dig Endosc 18:S128–S130

Pech O, Gossner L, May A, Stolte M, Ell C (2004) Endoscopic resection of superficial esophageal squamous-cell carcinomas: western experience. Am J Gastroenterol 99:1226–1232

Kodama M, Kakegawa T (1998) Treatment of superficial cancer of the esophagus: a summary of responses to a questionnaire on superficial cancer of the esophagus in Japan. Surgery (St. Louis) 123:432–9

Makuuchi H, Yoshida T, EII C (2004) Four-Step endoscopic esophageal mucosal resection tube method of resection for early esophageal cancer. Endoscopy 36:1013–1018

Open or Minimally Invasive Resection for Oesophageal Cancer?

Christophe Mariette and William B. Robb

Abstract

Oesophagectomy is one of the most challenging surgical operations. Potential for morbidity and mortality is high. Minimally invasive techniques have been introduced in an attempt to reduce postoperative complications and recovery times. Debate continues over whether these techniques decrease morbidity and whether the quality of the oncological resection is compromised. Globally, minimally invasive oesophagectomy (MIO) has been shown to be feasible and safe, with outcomes similar to open oesophagectomy. There are no controlled trials comparing the outcomes of MIO with open techniques, just a few comparative studies and many single institution series from which assessments of the current role of MIO have been made. The reported improvements of MIO include reduced blood loss, shortened time in high dependency care and decreased length of hospital stay. In comparative studies there is no clear reduction in respiratory complications, although larger series suggest that MIO may have a benefit. Although MIO approaches report less lymph node retrieval compared with open extended lymphadenectomy, MIO cancer outcomes are comparable. MIO will be a major component of the future oesophageal surgeons' armamentarium, but should continue to be carefully assessed.

C. Mariette (✉) · W. B. Robb
Department of Digestive and Oncological Surgery,
University Hospital Claude Huriez, Lille, France
e-mail: christophe.mariette@chru-lille.fr

C. Mariette
University of Lille 2, Lille, France

C. Mariette
Inserm, UMR837, Team 5 Mucins, epithelial differentiation and carcinogenesis, JPARC,
Rue Michel Polonovski, 59045 Lille cedex, France

F. Otto and M. P. Lutz (eds.), *Early Gastrointestinal Cancers*,
Recent Results in Cancer Research 196, DOI: 10.1007/978-3-642-31629-6_10,
© Springer-Verlag Berlin Heidelberg 2012

Randomized trials comparing MIO versus open resection in oesophageal cancer are urgently needed: two phase III trials are recruiting, the TIME and the MIRO trials.

Contents

1 Introduction 156
2 MIO Techniques 157
3 Results 158
4 MIO Learning Curve 163
5 Comments and Future 164
References 165

1 Introduction

With increasing experience and skills at performing laparoscopic and thoracoscopic surgery in the past decade, minimally invasive oesophagectomy (MIO) is increasingly being used for surgical management of oesophageal cancer (OC). By the early 1990s, some surgeons had developed and used protocols for thoracoscopic oesophagectomy, initially restricting its use to T1 and T2 OC without neoadjuvant chemoradiation (Akaishi et al. 1996; Gossot et al. 1993). However, with time, indications for thoracoscopic oesophagectomy were expanded to include more advanced OC, irrespective of neoadjuvant treatment. The techniques in MIO vary from totally minimally invasive to hybrid procedures where one stage of the operation is performed either by thoracoscopy or laparoscopy. Unlike other minimally invasive procedures, to date, MIO has not been broadly adopted. It is still considered one of the most complex gastrointestinal surgical operations, and many questions remain unanswered as to the real advantages of applying minimally invasive techniques, particularly in a disease which is frequently locally advanced and highly lethal. Mortality, morbidity, oncological radicality, reproducibility and the cost of the procedure are some of the topics under debate. Recent reviews (Butler et al. 2011; Gemmill and McCulloch 2007; Nagpal et al. 2010; Sgourakis et al. 2010) focusing on the role of MIO have emphasized that the benefits of this approach are controversial due to the complexity involved. Several comparative studies have been conducted between MIO and open oesophagectomy, but uncertainty about the advantages of one technique over the other persists due to the absence of published randomized trials. The question about the best approach for oesophagectomy in OC is consequently still to be resolved.

Table 1.1 Minimally invasive oesophagectomy techniques for oesophageal cancer

With thoracoscopic approach	
Thoracoscopic/laparoscopic oesophagectomy with cervical anastomosis	MIO
Thoracoscopic/laparoscopic oesophagectomy with thoracic anastomosis	MIO
Thoracoscopic oesophageal mobilization with laparotomy and cervical anatomosis (hybrid)	Hybrid
Without thoracoscopic approach	
Laparoscopic gastric mobilization with thoracotomy and intrathoracic anastomosis (hybrid)	Hybrid
Total laparoscopic transhiatal oesophagectomy	MIO

2 MIO Techniques

As there has never been a consensus regarding the superiority of any of the various open oesophagectomy techniques, it is not surprising that there is no agreement on the best MIO approach either. Minimally invasive adapatations of every conceivable approach to oesophageal resection have been reported (Table 1.1).

Transhiatal MIO utilizes laparoscopic abdominal dissection and preparation of the gastric conduit followed by a cervical anastomosis created via a traditional open approach in the neck. Mediastinal dissection of perioesophageal lymph nodes, including those in the subcarinal station, can be assessed through the hiatus using the lighting and magnifications afforded by the laparoscopic technology (Swanstrom and Hansen 1997). The oesophageal specimen can be removed through the neck incision. Some surgeons prefer to combine the laparoscopic tranhiatal approach with a mini-laparotomy to facilitate gastric tube creation as well as to remove the specimen. Finally, the oesophagus can be also removed from the mediastinum via an inversion technique with or without division of the vagus nerve (Jobe et al. 2004; Peyre et al. 2007).

Many surgeons prefer a thoracoscopic approach, typically performed through the right chest, with patients positioned in lateral decubitus or prone positions (Dapri et al. 2008; Fabian et al. 2008). Thoracoscopy can be used as a part of a 3 stage MIO, where the procedure begins in the chest and ends with laparoscopy and a cervical anastomosis, or as part of the Ivor- Lewis oesophagectomy where the oesophagogastric anastomosis resides in the chest. In this procedure the specimen is removed through a mini-thoracotomy, and the anastomosis is created at the apex of the chest (Bonavina et al. 2003).

Combinations of open and minimally invasive techniques are also an option, such as laparoscopy with thoracotomy (Briez et al. 2012) or thoracoscopy with laparotomy. These so-called hybrid techniques are applied for a variety of reasons, such as an oncological requirement, prior surgery in either cavity, surgeon experience, comfort level or surgeon preference.

Although the goal of MIO is to perform an equivalent operation to the open procedure without omitting any critical steps, some aspects considered as routine for open oesophagectomy have fallen out of favour, such as the performance of a pyloroplasty, jejunostomy placement or removal of the azygos vein.

3 Results

The primary goal of MIO is to decrease surgical morbidity associated with the open approach. No direct comparative trials have been published so far between open and MIO, but results for the TIME (Biere et al. 2011) and the MIRO (Briez et al. 2011) trials are urgently awaited. At present, the data shows that mortality rates and the incidence of complications reported are essentially equivalent for both techniques (Table 1.2). It is likely that any benefit of MIO is overshadowed by the persistent rate of complications independent of the approach, such as anastomotic leaks. It seems conceivable that, in the absence of such complications, patients with a minimal access approach enjoy quicker recovery, quicker return to normal activities and decreased long-term pain when compared to patients with similarly uncomplicated open procedures. This, however, has yet to be proven. MIO has been demonstrated as feasible for OC resection, but the oncologic value and safety is often questioned especially following neoadjuvant chemoradiation. The debate over the optimal surgical approach for OC, regardless of the technique, continues despite accumulating evidence in support of radical lymphadenectomy (Mariette and Piessen 2012). Few MIO series report lymph node retrieval and long-term results (Table 1.3).

Results coming from 3 meta-analyses published, based on non randomized comparative data, are contradictory. Two did not find significant differences between the MIO and the open approaches (Biere et al. 2009; Sgourakis et al. 2010). The third suggests that patients undergoing MIO had better operative and postoperative outcomes with no compromise in oncological outcomes (as assessed by lymph node retrieval) (Nagpal et al. 2010). Patients receiving MIO had significantly lower blood loss, and shorter postoperative ICU and hospital stay. There was a 50 % decrease in total morbidity in MIO group. Subgroup analysis of comorbidities demonstrated significantly lower incidence of respiratory complications after MIO; however, other postoperative outcomes such as anastomotic leak, anastomotic stricture, gastric conduit ischemia, chyle leak, vocal cord palsy, and 30 days mortality were comparable between the two techniques. The benefit of even one endoscopic stage in hybrid MIO (thoracoscopy with laparotomy or laparoscopy with thoracotomy) was noted, and blood loss and respiratory complications were still found to be lower, consistent with open versus totally MIO analysis, thus highlighting the advantage of applying a minimally invasive approach to oesophagectomy. It should be noted that few studies were matched for tumour stage, location or perioperative treatments. This fact could have introduced some bias, as for example patients with more advanced stages may have undergone open surgery.

Table 1.2 Postoperative surgical outcomes after minimally invasive oesophagectomy compared to open resections: literature study results

Authors Year	n	Approaches	Mortality (%)	Overall morbidity (%)	Pneumonia (%)	Cardiac arrhythmia (%)	Anastomotic leak (%)	Graft ischemia (%)	Chylothorax (%)
Law et al. (1997)	22	MIO (TSO)	0	18 (81.8 %)	3 (13.6 %)	3 (13.6 %)	0	NR	NS
	63	Open	0	63 (100 %)	11 (17.5 %)	14 (22.2 %)	2 (3.2 %)	NR	NS
Nguyen et al. (2000)	18	MIO (TLSO)	0	7 (38.9 %)	2 (11.1 %)	NR	2	0	0
	36	Open	0	19 (52.8 %)	6 (16.7 %)	NR	(11.1 %) 4 (11.1 %)	1 (2.8 %)	1 (2.8 %)
Nguyen et al. (2000)	77	MIO (VATS)	0	31 (40.3 %)	12 (15.6 %)	1 (1.3 %)	1 (1.3 %)	0	3 (3.9 %)
	72	Open	0	32 (44.4 %)	14 (19.4 %)	3 (4.2 %)	2 (2.8 %)	0	0
Kunisaki et al. (2004)	15	MIO (VATS + HALS)	0	NR	0	NR	2 (13.3 %)	NR	NS
	30	Open	0	NR	1 (3.3 %)	NR	1 (3.3 %)	NR	NS
Van den Broek et al. (2004)	25	MIO (THO)	0	14 (70 %)	2 (8 %)	NR	2 (8 %)	0	2 (8 %)
	20	Open	0	18 (72 %)	2 (10 %)	NR	3 (15 %)	0	0
Bresadola et al. (2006)	14	MIO (THO and TLSO)	0	8 (57.1 %)	1 (7.1 %)	NR	1 (7.1 %)	NR	0
	14	Open	0	6 (42.9 %)	2 (14.2 %)	NR	2 (14.2 %)	NR	0
Bernabe et al. (2005)	17	MIO (THO)	0	NR	NR	NR	NR	NR	NS
	14	Open	0	NR	NR	NR	NR	NR	NS
Shiraishi et al. (2006)	116	MIO (TLSO)	3 (2.6 %)	NR	25 (21.6 %)	3 (2.6 %)	13 (11.2 %)	NR	NS
	37	Open	3 (8.1 %)	NR	12 (32.4 %)	4 (10.8 %)	9 (24.3 %)	NR	NS

(continued)

Table 1.2 (continued)

AuthorsYear	n	Approaches	Mortality (%)	Overall morbidity (%)	Pneumonia (%)	Cardiac arrhythmia (%)	Anastomotic leak (%)	Graft ischemia (%)	Chylothorax (%)
Braghetto et al. (2006)	47	MIO (VATS/LSO)	3 (6.3 %)	18 (38.2 %)	7 (14.8 %)	NR	3 (6.4 %)	0	1 (2.1 %)
	119	Open	13 (10.9 %)	72 (60.5 %)	22 (18.5 %)	NR	17 (14.3 %)	1 (0.8 %)	0
Smithers et al. (2007)	332	MIO (TLSO)	7 (2.1 %)	207 (62.3 %)	87 (26.2 %)	55 (16.6 %)	18 (5.4 %)	5 (1.5 %)	17 (5.1 %)
	114	Open	3 (2.6 %)	76 (66.7 %)	35 (27.8 %)	21 (18.4 %)	10 (8.7 %)	2 (1.7 %)	7 (6.1 %)
Fabian et al. (2008)	22	MIO (TLSE)	1 (4.5 %)	15 (68.2 %)	1 (4.5 %)	4 (18.2 %)	3 (13.6 %)	1 (4.5 %)	0
	43	Open	4 (9.8 %)	31 (72.1 %)	10 (23.3 %)	8 (18.6 %)	3 (7.0 %)	0	2 (4.7 %)
Zingg et al. (2009)	56	MIO (TLSO)	2 (3.6 %)	19 (34.5 %)	17 (30.9 %)	NR	NR	NR	NR
	98	Open	6 (6.1 %)	20 (23.5 %)	33 (38.8 %)	NR	NR	NR	NR
Perry et al. (2009)	21	MIO (LIO)	0 1	13	1 (5 %)2	4	4 (19 %)	NR	NR
	21	Open	(5 %)	(62 %) 17 (81 %)	(10 %)	(19 %) 7 (33 %)	6 (29 %)	NR	NR
Parameswaran et al. (2009)	50	MIO (TLSO)	1 (2 %)	24 (48 %)	4 (8 %)	NR	4 (8 %)	5 (16 %)	3 (6 %)
	30	Open	1 (3 %)	15 (50 %)	2 (7 %)	NR	1 (3 %)	2 (10 %)	1 (3 %)
Pham et al. (2010)	44	MIO (TLSO)	3 (6.8 %)	NR	11 (25 %)	NR	4 (9 %)	1 (2 %)	NS
	46	Open	2 (4.3 %)	NR	7 (15 %)	NR	5 (11 %)	1 (2 %)	NS
Schoppmann et al. (2010)	31	MIO (TLSO)	0	11 (35.5 %)	2 (6.2 %)	NR	1 (3.2 %)	0	2 (6.4 %)
	31	Open	0	23 (74.2 %)	11 (35.5 %)	NR	8 (25.8 %)	1 (3.2 %)	1 (3.2 %)

(continued)

Table 1.2 (continued)

Authors/Year	n	Approaches	Mortality (%)	Overall morbidity (%)	Pneumonia (%)	Cardiac arrhythmia (%)	Anastomotic leak (%)	Graft ischemia (%)	Chylothorax (%)
Singh et al. (2011)	33	MIO (TLSO)	Values NR	Values NR	NR	NR	NR	NR	NR
	31	Open	$p = 0.34$	$P = 0.06$	NR	NR	NR	NR	NR
Mamidanna et al. (2012)	1155	MIO (TLSO,,HMIO)	46 (4.0 %)	NR	230 (19.9 %)	102 (8.8 %)	NR	NR	NR
	6347	Open	274 (4.3 %)	NR	1181 (18.6 %)	611 (9.6 %)	NR	NR	NR
Ben-David et al. (2012)	100	MIO (TLSO)	1 (1 %)	NR	9 (9 %)	8 (8 %)	5 (5 %)	NR	3 (3 %)
	32	Open	2 (5 %)	NR	5 (15.6 %)	R	4 (12.5 %)	NR	NR
Briez et al. (2012)		MIO (HMIO)	2.1	35.7	15.7	NR	5.7	0.7	NR
		Open	12.9	59.3	42.9	NR	4.3	0.0	NR

MIO minimally invasive oesophagectomy; *VATS* video-assisted thoracoscopic oesophagectomy; *HMIO* hybrid MIO; *HALS* hand-assited laparoscopic oesophagectomy; *TSO* thoracoscopic –assisted oesophagectomy; *TLSO* thoracolaparoscopic oesophagectomy; *LIO* laparoscopic inversion oesophagectomy; *LSO* laparoscopic oesophagectomy; *NR* not reported

Table 1.3 Oncological outcomes after minimally invasive oesophagectomy compared to open resections: literature study results

Authors (Year)	n	Approaches	Number of lymph nodes retrieved (median)	R0 resection rate (%)	3-year survival (%)
Law et al. (1997)	22	MIO (TSO)	7 (2–13)	10	62 (2 years)
	63	Open	13 (5–34)	NR	63 (2years)
Nguyen et al. (2000)	18	MIO (TLSO)	10.8 ± 8.4	18	NR
	36	Open	6.6 ± 5.8	NR	NR
Osugi et al. 2003 (2003)	77	MIO (VATS)	33.9 ± 12	NR	70
	72	Open	32.8 ± 14	NR	60
Kunisaki et al. 2004 (2004)	15	MIO (VATS + HALS)	24.5 ± 10	NR	NR
	30	Open	26.6 ± 10.4	NR	NR
Van den Broek et al. (2004)	25	MIO (THO)	7 ± 4.9	21 (84 %)	60 % (f/u 17 ± 11 months)
	20	Open	6.5 ± 4.9	18 (90 %)	50 % (f/u 54 ± 16 months)
Bresadola et al. (2006)	14	MIO (THO/ TLSO)	22.2 ± 12	NR	NR
	14	Open	18.6 ± 13.4	NR	NR
Bernabe et al. (2005)	17	MIO (THO)	9.8 (NR)	NR	NR
	14	Open	8.7 (NR)	NR	NR
Shiraishi et al. (2006)	116	MIO (TLSO)	31.8 (NR)	NR	NR
	37	Open	30.1 (NR)	NR	NR
Braghetto et al. (2006)	47	MIO (VATS/ LSO)	NS	NR	45.5 %
	119	Open	NS	NR	32.5 %
Smithers et al. (2007)	332	MIO (TLSO)	17 (9–33)	263	42 %
	114	Open	16 (1–44)	90	30 %
Fabian et al. (2008)	22	MIO (TLSE)	15 ± 6	22 (100 %)	NR
	43	Open	8 ± 7	NR	NR
Zingg et al. (2009)	56	MIO (TLSO)	5.7 ± 0.4	NR	Median survival— 35 months MIO and 29 months open
	98	Open	6.7 ± 0.5	NR	
Perry et al. (2009)	21	MIO (LIO)	10 (4–12)	NR	NR
	21	Open	3 (0–7)	NR	NR

(continued)

Table 1.3 (continued)

Authors (Year)	n	Approaches	Number of lymph nodes retrieved (median)	R0 resection rate (%)	3-year survival (%)
Parameswaran et al. (2009)	50	MIO (TLSO)	23 (7–49)	NR	74 % (2 year survival)
	30	Open	10 (2–23)	NR	58 % (2 year survival)
Pham et al. (2010)	44	MIO (TLSO)	13 (9–15)	NR	NR
	46	Open	8 (3–14)	NR	NR
Schoppman et al. (2010)	31	MIO (TLSO)	17.9 ± 7.7	29 (93.5 %)	64 %
	31	Open	20.5 ± 12.6	30 (96.8 %)	46 %
Singh et al. (2011)	33	MIO (TLSO)	14 (6–16)	30	55 % (2 year survival)
	31	Open	8 (3–14)	30	32 % (2 year survival)
Mamidanna et al. (2012)	1155	MIO (TLSO/ HMIO)	NR	NR	NR
	6347	Open	NR	NR	NR
Ben-David et al. (2012)	100	MIO (to be detailed)	NR	1 (1 %)	NR
	32	Open	NR	0	NR
Briez et al. (2012)		MIO (HMIO)	22 (8–53)	85.7	58 (2 year survival)
		Open	22 (6–56)	87.9	57 (2 year survival)

MIO minimally invasive oesophagectomy; *VATS* video-assisted thoracoscopic oesophagectomy; *HMIO* hybrid MIO; *HALS* hand-assisted laparoscopic oesophagectomy; *TSO* thoracoscopic – assisted oesophagectomy; *TLSO* thoracolaparoscopic oesophagectomy; *LIO* laparoscopic inversion oesophagectomy; *LSO* laparoscopic oesophagectomy; *f/u* follow up; *NR* not reported

From a technical and biological standpoint, the outcomes of open and MIO for cancer should be equivalent. Improved lighting and visibility, along with the magnification afforded by minimally invasive equipment, may prove superior for meticulous dissection and lymph node harvest. However, until large series report long-term survival by stage or results of large randomized trials are published, the true oncologic value of MIO will remain controversial.

4 MIO Learning Curve

As with all procedures, there are inherent technical challenges faced when applying a new technique. Oesophagectomy is a complex, technically challenging procedure fraught with potential pitfalls in nearly every step of the procedure. Many of the largest open series discuss the fact that morbidity and mortality decrease with experience (Hofstetter et al. 2002; Mariette et al. 2004). Technical complication rates have also been shown to negatively impact cancer specific survival (Rizk et al. 2004). As such, oesophagectomy has been designated an operation best left in the hands of experts at high-volume centers. Little is written regarding the learning for MIO directly, but is has been suggested that it may be more than 50 procedures (Bizekis et al. 2006; Decker et al. 2009). It appears that a hybrid procedures, especially using a laparoscopic and open thoracic approach may have a short learning curve and less oncological drawbacks (Briez et al. 2012).

Ideally, MIO should be performed by surgeons experienced in both advanced laparoscopy/thoracoscopy and surgical oncology for OC. Dedication to mastery of several MIO techniques allows the operation to be tailored to the individual patient using the less invasive approach matched to the pathology at hand. Certainly the extent of the oncologic resection should be based on the tumour, not the technique, and should be the primary goal.

5 Comments and Future

Open oesophagectomy remains the most effective treatment for OC with 5 year survival rates of approximatively 50 % being reported in several selected series, especially in combination with neoadjuvant chemoradiation (Bonavina et al. 2003; Mariette et al. 2008; Portale et al. 2006). This is a dramatic improvement, with survival rates several decades ago being consistently less than 20 %. Whereas endoscopic mucosal resection or radiofrequency ablation can cure OC that have not penetrated the muscularis mucosa, open oesophagectomy remains the gold standard treatment for the disease (Mariette et al. 2011). Improvements in chemoradiation protocols have been reported as effective adjuncts in surgical therapy (Mariette et al. 2007). Today, a multimodality approach to OC is common and preferred for tumours extending beyond the submucosa or with suspected lymph node involvement.

MIO has been gaining popularity since the first reports nearly two decades ago. Similar to open surgery, several techniques exist including totally laparoscopic transhiatal or transthoracic resection, as well as combinations, or hybrid techniques. Much as with open OC surgery, no consensus has been reached regarding the superiority of any particular MIO adaptation. Currently, no significant decrease in operative morbidity has been proven for MIO compared to its open counterpart, even if some large comparative studies suggest a significantly better postoperative course without compromising oncological outcomes (Briez et al. 2012; Osugi et al. 2003; Shiraishi et al. 2006; Smithers et al. 2007). Most reports of MIO for locally advanced cancers include a thoracic dissection. The role for MIO in these cancer stages is controversial but will become more defined as the procedures mature beyond their steep learning curves and long-term outcome data becomes available.

Randomized trials may be difficult due to the wide variety of techniques available, the heterogeneity in surgeons' preferences, the relative low number of procedures performed, the complexity of such surgery, and the variety of postoperative complications after oesophagectomy. Even if no direct comparative trials have been published so far between open and MIO, results of two well-known randomized

Open or Minimally Invasive Resection for Oesophageal Cancer? 165

trials, the TIME (Biere et al. 2011) and the MIRO (Briez et al. 2011) trials are keenly awaited. The TIME trial aims at comparing over 120 patients, the approach to the MIO includes a right thoracosocpy and laparoscopy. The primary endpoint are postoperative respiratory complications within the first two postoperative weeks, whereas secondary endpoints are duration of the operation, blood loss, conversion to the open procedure, morbidity, quality of life and hospital stay. The MIRO trial will test, in over 200 patients randomised, the impact of laparoscopic gastric conduit creation with open thoracotomy (hybrid procedure) on major 30-day postoperative morbidity, especially on pulmonary complications. Secondary objectives are to assess the overall 30-day morbidity, 30-day mortality, disease-free and overall survival, quality of life and medico-economic analysis. It is hypothetized that hybrid MIO would decrease major postoperative morbidity without compromising onco-logical outcomes through an easily reproducible surgical procedure.

To conclude, there are many variations of MIO with combinations of tho-racoscopic and laparoscopic approaches with and without open approaches to the abdomen or chest. Data coming from non randomized studies suggest MIO is safe, with similar outcomes to open resection for both the surgical and the oncological outcomes. Data from meta-analyses suggest that MIO may show improvement with less blood loss, less time in ICU, less pulmonary complications and shorter hospital stay. However, the effect of MIO on quality of life and return to normal activity has not been assessed. Medico-economic analyses are required. Results from two randomized trials (Biere et al. 2011; Briez et al. 2011) will soon be published to offer higher level evidence of this highly debated procedure.

References

Akaishi T, Kaneda I, Higuchi N, Kuriya Y, Kuramoto J, Toyoda T, Wakabayashi A (1996) Thoracoscopic en bloc total esophagectomy with radical mediastinal lymphadenectomy. J Thorac Cardiovasc Surg 112:1533–1540 (discussion 1540–1541)

Ben-David K, Sarosi GA, Cendan JC, Howard D, Rossidis G, Hochwald SN (2012) Decreasing morbidity and mortality in 100 consecutive minimally invasive esophagectomies. Surg Endosc 26:162–167

Bernabe KQ, Bolton JS, Richardson WS (2005) Laparoscopic hand-assisted versus open transhiatal esophagectomy: a case-control study. Surg Endosc 19:334–337

Biere SS, Cuesta MA, van der Peet DL (2009) Minimally invasive versus open esophagectomy for cancer: a systematic review and meta-analysis. Minerva Chir 64:121–133

Biere SS, Maas KW, Bonavina L, Garcia JR, van Berge Henegouwen MI, Rosman C, Sosef MN, de Lange ES, Bonjer HJ, Cuesta MA, van der Peet DL (2011) Traditional invasive vs. minimally invasive esophagectomy: a multi-center, randomized trial (TIME-trial). BMC Surg 11:2

Bizekis C, Kent MS, Luketich JD, Buenaventura PO, Landreneau RJ, Schuchert MJ, Alvelo-Rivera M (2006) Initial experience with minimally invasive Ivor lewis esophagectomy. Ann Thorac Surg 82:402–406 (discussion 406–407)

Bonavina L, Via A, Incarbone R, Saino G, Peracchia A (2003) Results of surgical therapy in patients with Barrett's adenocarcinoma. World J Surg 27:1062–1066

Braghetto I, Csendes A, Cardemil G, Burdiles P, Korn O, Valladares H (2006) Open transthoracic or transhiatal esophagectomy versus minimally invasive esophagectomy in terms of morbidity, mortality and survival. Surg Endosc 20:1681–1686

Bresadola V, Terrosu G, Cojutti A, Benzoni E, Baracchini E, Bresadola F (2006) Laparoscopic versus open gastroplasty in esophagectomy for esophageal cancer: a comparative study. Surg Laparosc Endosc Percutan Tech 16:63–67

Briez N, Piessen G, Bonnetain F, Brigand C, Carrere N, Collet D, Doddoli C, Flamein R, Mabrut JY, Meunier B, Msika S, Perniceni T, Peschaud F, Prudhomme M, Triboulet JP, Mariette C (2011) Open versus laparoscopically-assisted oesophagectomy for cancer: a multicentre randomised controlled phase III trial—the MIRO trial. BMC Cancer 11:310

Briez N, Piessen G, Torres F, Lebuffe G, Triboulet JP, Mariette C (2012) Hybrid minimally invasive surgery in oesophageal cancer decreases major postoperative pulmonary complications without compromising oncological outcomes. Br J Surg (in press)

Butler N, Collins S, Memon B, Memon MA (2011) Minimally invasive oesophagectomy: current status and future direction. Surg Endosc 25:2071–2083

Dapri G, Himpens J, Cadiere GB (2008) Minimally invasive esophagectomy for cancer: laparoscopic transhiatal procedure or thoracoscopy in prone position followed by laparoscopy? Surg Endosc 22:1060–1069

Decker G, Coosemans W, De Leyn P, Decaluwe H, Nafteux P, Van Raemdonck D, Lerut T (2009) Minimally invasive esophagectomy for cancer. Eur J Cardiothorac Surg 35:13–20 (discussion 20–21)

Fabian T, Martin JT, McKelvey AA, Federico JA (2008) Minimally invasive esophagectomy: a teaching hospital's first year experience. Dis Esophagus 21:220–225

Gemmill EH, McCulloch P (2007) Systematic review of minimally invasive resection for gastro-oesophageal cancer. Br J Surg 94:1461–1467

Gossot D, Fourquier P, Celerier M (1993) Thoracoscopic esophagectomy: technique and initial results. Ann Thorac Surg 56:667–670

Hofstetter W, Swisher SG, Correa AM, Hess K, Putnam JB Jr, Ajani JA, Dolormente M, Francisco R, Komaki RR, Lara A, Martin F, Rice DC, Sarabia AJ, Smythe WR, Vaporciyan AA, Walsh GL, Roth JA (2002) Treatment outcomes of resected esophageal cancer. Ann Surg 236:376–384 (discussion 384–385)

Jobe BA, Reavis KM, Davis JJ, Hunter JG (2004) Laparoscopic inversion esophagectomy: simplifying a daunting operation. Dis Esophagus 17:95–97

Kunisaki C, Hatori S, Imada T, Akiyama H, Ono H, Otsuka Y, Matsuda G, Nomura M, Shimada H (2004) Video-assisted thoracoscopic esophagectomy with a voice-controlled robot: the AESOP system. Surg Laparosc Endosc Percutan Tech 14:323–327

Law S, Fok M, Chu KM, Wong J (1997) Thoracoscopic esophagectomy for esophageal cancer. Surgery 122:8–14

Mamidanna R, Bottle A, Aylin P, Faiz O, Hanna GB (2012) Short-term outcomes following open versus minimally invasive esophagectomy for cancer in England: a population-based national study. Ann Surg 255:197–203

Mariette C, Piessen G (2012) Oesophageal cancer: how radical should surgery be? Eur J Surg Oncol 38:210–213

Mariette C, Piessen G, Briez N, Gronnier C, Triboulet JP (2011) Oesophagogastric junction adenocarcinoma: which therapeutic approach? Lancet Oncol 12:296–305

Mariette C, Piessen G, Briez N, Triboulet JP (2008) The number of metastatic lymph nodes and the ratio between metastatic and examined lymph nodes are independent prognostic factors in esophageal cancer regardless of neoadjuvant chemoradiation or lymphadenectomy extent. Ann Surg 247:365–371

Mariette C, Piessen G, Triboulet JP (2007) Therapeutic strategies in oesophageal carcinoma: role of surgery and other modalities. Lancet Oncol 8:545–553

Mariette C, Taillier G, Van Seuningen I, Triboulet JP (2004) Factors affecting postoperative course and survival after en bloc resection for esophageal carcinoma. Ann Thorac Surg 78:1177–1183

Nagpal K, Ahmed K, Vats A, Yakoub D, James D, Ashrafian H, Darzi A, Moorthy K, Athanasiou T (2010) Is minimally invasive surgery beneficial in the management of esophageal cancer? A meta-analysis. Surg Endosc 24:1621–1629

Nguyen NT, Follette DM, Wolfe BM, Schneider PD, Roberts P, Goodnight JE Jr (2000) Comparison of minimally invasive esophagectomy with transthoracic and transhiatal esophagectomy. Arch Surg 135:920–925

Osugi H, Takemura M, Higashino M, Takada N, Lee S, Kinoshita H (2003) A comparison of video-assisted thoracoscopic oesophagectomy and radical lymph node dissection for squamous cell cancer of the oesophagus with open operation. Br J Surg 90:108–113

Parameswaran R, Veeramootoo D, Krishnadas R, Cooper M, Berrisford R, Wajed S (2009) Comparative experience of open and minimally invasive esophagogastric resection. World J Surg 33:1868–1875

Perry KA, Enestvedt CK, Pham T, Welker M, Jobe BA, Hunter JG, Sheppard BC (2009) Comparison of laparoscopic inversion esophagectomy and open transhiatal esophagectomy for high-grade dysplasia and stage I esophageal adenocarcinoma. Arch Surg 144:679–684

Peyre CG, DeMeester SR, Rizzetto C, Bansal N, Tang AL, Ayazi S, Leers JM, Lipham JC, Hagen JA, DeMeester TR (2007) Vagal-sparing esophagectomy: the ideal operation for intramucosal adenocarcinoma and barrett with high-grade dysplasia. Ann Surg 246:665–671 (discussion 671–674)

Pham TH, Perry KA, Dolan JP, Schipper P, Sukumar M, Sheppard BC, Hunter JG (2010) Comparison of perioperative outcomes after combined thoracoscopic-laparoscopic esophagectomy and open Ivor-Lewis esophagectomy. Am J Surg 199:594–598

Portale G, Hagen JA, Peters JH, Chan LS, DeMeester SR, Gandamihardja TA, DeMeester TR (2006) Modern 5-year survival of resectable esophageal adenocarcinoma: single institution experience with 263 patients. J Am Coll Surg 202:588–596 (discussion 596–598)

Rizk NP, Bach PB, Schrag D, Bains MS, Turnbull AD, Karpeh M, Brennan MF, Rusch VW (2004) The impact of complications on outcomes after resection for esophageal and gastroesophageal junction carcinoma. J Am Coll Surg 198:42–50

Schoppmann SF, Prager G, Langer FB, Riegler FM, Kabon B, Fleischmann E, Zacherl J (2010) Open versus minimally invasive esophagectomy: a single-center case controlled study. Surg Endosc 24:3044–3053

Sgourakis G, Gockel I, Radtke A, Musholt TJ, Timm S, Rink A, Tsiamis A, Karaliotas C, Lang H (2010) Minimally invasive versus open esophagectomy: meta-analysis of outcomes. Dig Dis Sci 55:3031–30340

Shiraishi T, Kawahara K, Shirakusa T, Yamamoto S, Maekawa T (2006a) Risk analysis in resection of thoracic esophageal cancer in the era of endoscopic surgery. Ann Thorac Surg 81:1083–1089

Shiraishi T, Shirakusa T, Hiratsuka M, Yamamoto S, Iwasaki A (2006b) Video-assisted thoracoscopic surgery lobectomy for c-T1N0M0 primary lung cancer: its impact on locoregional control. Ann Thorac Surg 82:1021–1026

Singh RK, Pham TH, Diggs BS, Perkins S, Hunter JG (2011) Minimally invasive esophagectomy provides equivalent oncologic outcomes to open esophagectomy for locally advanced (stage II or III) esophageal carcinoma. Arch Surg 146:711–714

Smithers BM, Gotley DC, Martin I, Thomas JM (2007) Comparison of the outcomes between open and minimally invasive esophagectomy. Ann Surg 245:232–240

Swanstrom LL, Hansen P (1997) Laparoscopic total esophagectomy. Arch Surg 132:943–947 (discussion 947–949)

Van den Broek WT, Makay O, Berends FJ, Yuan JZ, Houdijk AP, Meijer S, Cuesta MA (2004) Laparoscopically assisted transhiatal resection for malignancies of the distal esophagus. Surg Endosc 18:812–817

Zingg U, McQuinn A, DiValentino D, Esterman AJ, Bessell JR, Thompson SK, Jamieson GG, Watson DI (2009) Minimally invasive versus open esophagectomy for patients with esophageal cancer. Ann Thorac Surg 87:911–919

Choosing the Best Treatment for Esophageal Cancer
Criteria for Selecting the Best Multimodal Therapy

A. H. Hölscher and E. Bollschweiler

Abstract

The best multimodal therapy in esophageal cancer comprises neoadjuvant radiochemotherapy in patients with adenocarcinoma or squamous cell carcinoma whereas neoadjuvant chemotherapy is only appropriate for patients with adenocarcinoma. However, the 2-year survival benefit by this induction therapy compared to surgery alone is only 5–9 %. Targeted drugs seem to be promising in order to improve the response rate. The choice of the best multimodal therapy by response prediction seems only to be possible in patients during chemotherapy for adenocarcinoma, whereas during neoadjuvant radiochemotherapy a response prediction by FDG–PET is not possible. The principle item of multimodal therapy is still transthoracic en bloc esophagectomy which should be performed in high volume centers in order to guarantee stable and good results.

Contents

1	Introduction	170
2	Postoperative Mortality	170
3	R0-Resection	171
4	Lymphadenectomy	171
5	Multimodal Treatment	172
6	Adjuvant Therapy	172
7	Neoadjuvant Radiotherapy	172
8	Neoadjuvant Chemotherapy or Radiochemotherapy	173

A. H. Hölscher (✉) · E. Bollschweiler
Department of General, Visceral and Cancer Surgery,
University of Cologne, Kerpener Straße 62, 50937 Köln, Germany
e-mail: Arnulf.Hoelscher@uk-koeln.de

F. Otto and M. P. Lutz (eds.), *Early Gastrointestinal Cancers*,
Recent Results in Cancer Research 196, DOI: 10.1007/978-3-642-31629-6_11,
© Springer-Verlag Berlin Heidelberg 2012

9 Response Prediction 174
10 Targeted Drugs in Multimodal Therapy.. 174
References.. 175

1 Introduction

Multimodal therapy is a combination of different treatment modalities for one disease. In esophageal cancer therapy with curative intent, surgery is still the principle item whereas chemotherapy and/or radiotherapy are additional treatment modalities. If the best treatment for esophageal cancer should be chosen it is obvious that primarily the best surgery has to be applied. This is characterized by

- low perioperative morbidity and mortality,
- high rate of R0 resection,
- adequate lymphadenectomy,
- appropriate type of reconstruction with high quality of life and
- surgery performed in high volume centers.

Surgery after neoadjuvant treatment is difficult because of scar and adhesions in the dissection plains due to shrinkage of the primary tumor or destruction and fibrosis of the lymph nodes.

2 Postoperative Mortality

The latest metaanalysis by Sjöquist shows a range of postoperative mortality after neoadjuvant radiochemotherapy from 13 studies with 1,932 patients between 0 and 17 % compared to the control groups with surgery alone between 0 and 19 %. Postoperative mortality after induction chemotherapy based on the same metaanalysis of 10 studies with 2,062 patients was between 2 and 15 % in the intervention group compared to 0–10 % in the group with surgery alone (Sjöquist 2011). The comparison of the mortality rates between the intervention group and the control group in this metaanalysis shows no clear difference between both strategies. Our own data in 655 patients with transthoracic en bloc esophagectomy for cancer with gastric pull-up and high intrathoracic esophagogastrostomy show the results of Table 1.

During the performance of cis-Platin 5 FU-based chemotherapy severe (grade 3) or life threatening (grade 4) toxicities were observed in 31 % and preoperative mortality in 1–2 % of the treated patients (Urschel 2002; Malthaner and Fenlon 2003). Some metaanalysis about neoadjuvant radiochemotherapy, however, showed an elevated postoperative morbidity and mortality (Urschel 2003; Kaklamanos 2003; Malthaner 2004; Fiorica 2004; Grear 2005; Gebski 2007; Jin 2009). In these metaanalysis especially, an elevated rate of pulmonary complications and anastomotic insufficiency was reported and by this an increased mortality. In this context, the single dosage and also the total dosage of radiotherapy are of great importance. Postoperative mortality was no more significantly elevated if radiotherapy studies

Table 1 Own results of 655 patients with esophagectomy for cancer (radiochemotherapy (RTX/CTX)): 5-FU-Cisplatin

	Without RTX/CTX	With RTX/CTX
T category	pT1–pT3	cT3
n	286	362
morbidity	34 %	35 %
30-day mortality	2.7 %	2.2 %
R0-resection	94 %	94 %

with single dose of more than 2 Gy were excluded (Fiorica 2004). The total dosage of preoperative radiotherapy should be limited to 45 Gy as a higher dose can lead to an increased rate of complications and mortality (Semrau 2009). However, the latest published metaanalysis of Sjöquist did not show an elevated postoperative mortality after neoadjuvant radiochemotherapy (Sjöquist 2011). In our own group of 362 patients after neoadjuvant radiochemotherapy and esophagectomy, the postoperative mortality was also not elevated compared to surgery alone (Table 1).

The time interval between neoadjuvant therapy and surgery is also important. Mostly an interval of 4–6 weeks is used. In case of an earlier operation, disadvantages can develop because of the remaining edema or inflammation of the tissue or not completely established regression of the tumor. If the time interval between neoadjuvant therapy and surgery is too extended a new onset of cancer growth can develop and surgical dissection can be difficult by the fibrosis after radiation. Ruol showed in a retrospective analysis that an interval of up to 90 days after neoadjuvant therapy of squamous cell carcinoma of the thoracic esophagus does not lead to a prognostic disadvantage (Ruol 2010).

3 R0-Resection

Another important issue for defining best surgery is a high rate of R0 resection.

The rate of R0 resection in our patient group with neoadjuvant radiochemotherapy was 94 % which was not different to the patient group with surgery alone. (Table 1) Our results compare favorably with the literature which f. e. in the metaanalysis of Jin showed a R0-resection rate of only 77 % (Jin 2009).

4 Lymphadenectomy

The extent of lymphadenectomy has important consequences on prognosis. We could show in an analysis of several international centers of esophageal surgery in 2,166 patients without induction therapy and more than 5-year follow-up that the prognosis is correlating with the number of resected lymph nodes (Peyre 2008). This is not only true for patients with infiltrated lymph nodes but also for patients with N0 category. In our own analysis of pN0 patients, the number of resected lymph nodes also had an effect on survival (Bollschweiler 2006). This is probably due to an effect on micrometastasis. The favorable effect of adequate lymphadenectomy is also demonstrated by the comparison of the less radical transhiatal esophagectomy versus radical transthoracic esophagectomy in adenocarcinoma of the esophagus. Omloo reported from the Dutch prospective randomized trial comparing both kinds of surgery a significant survival benefit for the group of patients with radical transthoracic esophagectomy (Omloo 2007). Therefore, best surgery in the frame of multimodal treatment should include an adequate abdominal and thoracic lymphadenectomy.

5 Multimodal Treatment

Our own data on patients with pT3 esophageal carcinoma and R0 resection without neoadjuvant treatment show a 5-year survival rate of 20 % which is similar to the results of the literature. As this outcome is not satisfying, it is agreed today that patients with cT3 or resectable cT4 esophageal cancer should receive neoadjuvant treatment. However, if the survival curves of patients with pT2 and also pT1 sm3 esophageal adenocarcinomas are considered, these are also not completely satisfying. The 5-year survival rate of patients with pT1 sm3 and pT2 were both 50 % (Hölscher et al. 2011). This is due to the high rate of lymph node metastasis which in pT1 sm3 carcinoma was already 56 %. Therefore, there is a current discussion on the indication for multimodal therapy. Considering the mentioned data, it could be appropriate to favor induction therapy also in patients with pT2 or even pT1 sm3 carcinoma.

The best type of surgery has been defined above. As for multimodal therapy also the best additional modalities should be applied. This means the question if the therapy should be performed in a neoadjuvant or adjuvant setting and if this modality should be radiotherapy, chemotherapy, or combined radiochemotherapy.

6 Adjuvant Therapy

Adjuvant treatment after R0 resection of esophageal carcinoma could not show a survival benefit in randomized studies for locally advanced esophageal cancer by radiotherapy alone, chemotherapy alone, or radiochemotherapy. The same is true for additive therapy after R1 or R2 resection. For these reasons, currently there is no indication for adjuvant or additive therapy after esophagectomy.

7 Neoadjuvant Radiotherapy

Neoadjuvant radiotherapy alone followed by esophagectomy in locally advanced esophageal cancer has been analyzed in six randomized trials (Fok 1993; Launois 1981; Gignoux 1987; Wang 1989; Nygard 1992; Arnott 1992). A clinical response on induction therapy was only found in one-third of the patients. Only in one of six

Choosing the Best Treatment for Esophageal Cancer 173

studies a significant survival benefit could be achieved. Two studies even showed an inferior survival of the patients after neoadjuvant radiotherapy. A metaanalysis of 1,147 patients of five randomized studies mostly with squamous cell carcinoma reported a non-significant survival benefit of only 4 % after 5 years (Arnott 1992). Because of these reasons neoadjuvant radiotherapy alone is not appropriate for advanced esophageal carcinoma.

8 Neoadjuvant Chemotherapy or Radiochemotherapy

To answer this question it is most appropriate to report the results of the latest metaanalysis of Sjöquist from 2011 (Sjöquist 2011). This analysis comprised ten randomized controlled trials with the comparison between neoadjuvant chemotherapy plus surgery versus surgery alone. This trial included 2,062 patients. Further 13 randomized controlled trials comparing neoadjuvant radiochemotherapy plus surgery versus surgery alone, with a total of 1,932 patients were analyzed. Concerning neoadjuvant chemotherapy the result of the metaanalysis is a 2-year overall-survival benefit of 5.1 % after induction therapy which is significant. The difference for patients with squamous cell carcinoma was not significant whereas the benefit for those with adenocarcinoma was significant. Concerning neoadjuvant radiochemotherapy plus surgery this group showed a significant 2-year overall-survival benefit of 8.7 % compared to surgery alone. The prognostic advantage was similar for patients with adenocarcinoma or squamous cell carcinoma.

Because of these results the choice of neoadjuvant treatment has to be differentiated between patients with squamous cell carcinoma or adenocarcinoma. In squamous cell carcinoma only radiochemotherapy is effective. In adenocarcinoma, neoadjuvant chemotherapy and also neoadjuvant radiochemotherapy are effective. There are no sufficiently large randomized trials with a direct comparison of both treatment modalities. Smaller studies like the one from Stahl and from Burmeister show a higher effectiveness of neoadjuvant radiochemotherapy compared to neoadjuvant chemotherapy in adenocarcinoma of the esophagus (Stahl 2009; Burmeister 2011). Based on the latest metaanalysis of Sjöquist no definitive advantage for neoadjuvant radiochemotherapy compared to chemotherapy is evident for adenocarcinoma. However, in patients with squamous cell carcinoma neoadjuvant radiochemotherapy should be performed as chemotherapy alone is not sufficiently effective.

Our own study showed that the histological type of esophageal cancer might affect the response to neoadjuvant radiochemotherapy and subsequent prognosis (Bollschweiler 2009). This study comprised 297 patients with cT3 or resectable cT4 esophageal cancer. A total of 154 had squamous cell carcinoma and 143 adenocarcinoma. The rate of radiochemotherapy was 65 %. All patients had transthoracic esophagectomy with a median number of resected lymph nodes of 27. The 30-day mortality rate was 3.2 % in patients with squamous cell carcinoma and 2.8 % in those with adenocarcinoma. The rate of response was defined by the percentage of residual vital tumor cells according to histology (Schneider 2008). Minor response was more than 10 % vital tumor cells and major response less than 10 % vital tumor cells. The first interesting result was that in patients with squamous cell carcinoma the relation between minor and major response was 49–51 % whereas in adenocarcinoma this was 71–29 % ($p = 0,01$). This means that patients with adenocarcinoma had a less good response of only one-third compared to squamous cell carcinoma with about half of the patients. However, those patients with squamous cell carcinoma and major response had a 5-year survival rate of only 30 % compared to the patients with adenocarcinoma and major response of about 70 %.

The best results can be achieved in those patients with complete response. According to our own multicenter trial these patients with ypT0 N0 M0 R0 have a 5-year overall-survival rate of 55 % and a disease free survival rate of 70 % (Vallböhmer 2010).

9 Response Prediction

The survival benefit for patients after neoadjuvant therapy is only approved for patients with good response to induction therapy. Non-responder have not only no survival benefit but also an unnecessary investment of time and can suffer from side effects by treatment. In our own studies, we could show that lymph node status and histomorphologic tumor regression are very important prognostic factors after radiochemotherapy of esophageal carcinoma (Schneider et al. 2008; Bollschweiler 2010). Because of this background great efforts were started to predict the response to neoadjuvant therapy. Clinical examinations like endoscopy with biopsy, endosonography, and computed tomography have only a minor significance in response prediction after neoadjuvant therapy (Schneider 2008). A response prediction by FDG-PET two weeks after start of induction therapy seems to be possible after neoadjuvant chemotherapy of esophageal adenocarcinoma (Lordick 2007). In neoadjuvant radiochemotherapy, however, an early prediction of response during the induction therapy is not possible (Vallböhmer 2009; van Heijl 2011). Concerning response prediction by biomarkers from biopsy only retrospective results are currently available. Prospective studies are urgently needed.

10 Targeted Drugs in Multimodal Therapy

In order to select the best multimodal therapy targeted drugs have been applied. These drugs block specific tumor signal transduction pathways and have been analyzed in the treatment of adenocarcinomas of the esophagus (Bang 2010). In a prospective multicentric phase I/II study, it was shown that the monoclonal EGFR antibody Cetuximab which is added to the conventional neoadjuvant radiochemotherapy can affect a significant increase of histopathologic response (Ruhstaller 2011). In this study, the induction therapy was tolerated very well. However, another phase II study with addition of Cetuximab to neoadjuvant radiochemotherapy of locally advanced adenocarcinoma had to be stopped because of a high rate of side

Choosing the Best Treatment for Esophageal Cancer

effects (Gibson et al. 2010). Because of these controversial results targeted drugs currently should only be applied in prospective studies. The amplification of MET Proto-Oncogen defines a small aggressive subgroup of adenocarcinoma of the esophagus and the gastroesophageal junction with evidence for a good response on the MET inhibitor Crizotinib (Lennerz 2011). Therefore, targeted drugs seem to be promising in order to contribute to the selection of the best multimodal therapy.

References

Arnott SJ, Duncan W, Kerr GR, Walbaum PR, Cameron E, Jack WJ, Mackillop WJ (1992) Low dose preoperative radiotherapy for carcinoma of the oesophagus: results of a randomized clinical trial. Radiother Oncol 24:108–113

Bang YJ, Van Cutsem E, Feyereislova A, Chung HC, Shen L, Sawaki A, Lordick F, Ohtsu A, Omuro Y, Satoh T, Aprile G, Kulikov E, Hill J, Lehle M, Rüschoff J, Kang YK (2010) Trastuzumab in combination with chemotherapy versus chemotherapy alone for treatment of HER2-positive advanced gastric or gastro-oesophageal junction cancer (ToGA): a phase 3, open-label, randomised controlled trial. Lancet 376(9742):687–697

Bollschweiler E, Metzger R, Drebber U, Baldus S, Vallböhmer D, Kocher M, Hölscher AH (2009) Histological type of esophageal cancer might affect response to neo-adjuvant radiochemotherapy and subsequent prognosis. Ann Oncol 20:231–238

Bollschweiler E, Baldus S, Schroder W, Schneider P, Hölscher A (2006) Staging of esophageal carcinoma: length of tumor and number of involved regional lymph nodes. Are these independent prognostic factors? J Surg Oncol 94:355–363

Bollschweiler E, Besch S, Drebber U, Schröder W, Mönig SP, Vallböhmer D, Baldus SE, Metzger R, Hölscher AH (2010) Influence of neoadjuvant chemoradiation on the number and size of analyzed lymph nodes in esophageal cancer. Ann Surg Oncol 17:3187–3194

Burmeister TH, Thomas JM, Burmeister EA, Walpole ET, Harvey JA, Thomson DB, Barbour AP, Gotley DC, Smithers BM (2011) Is concurrent radiation therapy required in patients receiving preoperative chemotherapy for adenocarcinoma of the oesophagus? A randomised phase II trial. Eur J Cancer 47:354–360

Fiorica F, Di Bona D, Schepis F et al (2004) Preoperative chemoradiotherapy for oesophageal cancer: a systematic review and meta-analysis. Gut 53:925–930

Fok M, Sham JS, Choy D, Cheng SW, Wong J (1993) Postoperative radiotherapy for carcinoma of the esophagus: a prospective, randomized controlled study. Surgery 113(2):138–147

Gebski V, Burmeister B, Smithers BM, Foo K, Zalcberg J, Simes J (2007) Survival benefits from neoadjuvant chemoradiotherapy or chemotherapy in esophageal carcinoma: a meta-analysis. Lancet Oncol 8:226–234

Gibson MK, Catalano PJ, Kleinberg L (2010) E2205: a phase II study to measure response rate and toxicity of neoadjuvant chemoradiotherapy (CRT) with oxaliplatin (OX) and infusional 5-flourouracil (5-FU) plus cetuximab (C) followed by postoperative docetaxel (DT) and C in patients with operable adenocarcinoma of the esophagus. J Clin Oncol 28:15s (abstract 4064)

Gignoux M, Roussel A, Paillot B, Gillet M, Schlag P, Dalesio O, Buyse M, Duez N (1987) The value of preoperative radiotherapy in esophageal cancer: results of a study of the E.O.R.T.C. World J Surg 11:426–432

Greer SE, Goodney PP, Sutton JE, Birkmeyer JD (2005) Neoadjuvant chemoradiation for esophageal carcinoma: a meta-analysis. Surgery 137:172–179

Hölscher AH, Bollschweiler E, Schröder W, Metzger R, Gutschow C, Drebber U (2011) Prognostic impact of upper, middle, and lower third mucosal or submucosal infiltration in early esophageal cancer. Ann Surg 254(5):802–807 (discussion 807–808)

Jin HL, Zhu H, Ling TS, Zhang HJ, Shi RH (2009) Neoadjuvant chemoradiotherapy for respectable esophageal carcinoma: a meta-analysis. World J Gastroenterol 15:5983–5991

Kaklamanos IG, Walker GR, Ferry K, Franceschi D, Livingstone AS (2003) Neoadjuvant treatment for resectable cancer of the esophagus and the gastroesophageal junction: a meta-analysis of randomized clinical trials. Ann Surg Oncol 10:754–761

Launois B, Delarue D, Campion JP, Kerbaol M (1981) Perioperative radiotherapy for carcinoma of the esophagus. Surg Gynecol Obstet 153:690–692

Lennerz JK, Kwak EL, Ackerman A, Michael M, Fox SB, Bergethon K, Lauwers GY, Christensen JG, Wilner KD, Haber DA, Salgia R, Bang YJ, Clark JW, Solomon BJ, Lafrate AJ (2011) MET amplification identifies a small and aggressive subgroup of esophagogastric adenocarcinoma with evidence of responsiveness to crizotinib. J Clin Oncol 29(36):4803–4810

Lordick FL, Hölscher AH (2007) Chirurgische und internistische Diagnostik und Therapie des Oesophaguskarzinom. Gastroenterologie up 2 date 2007. 3:293–319

Malthaner R, Fenlon D (2003) Preoperative chemotherapy for resectable thoracic esophageal cancer the cochrane database of systematic reviews 4: CD001556. DOI: 10.1002/14651858.CD001556

Malthaner R, Wong R, Rumble R, Zuraw L (2004) Neoadjuvant or adjuvant therapy for resectable esophageal cancer: a systematic review and meta-analysis. BMC Med 2:35

Nygard K, Hagen S, Hansen HS (1992) Preoperative radiotherapy prolongs survival in operable esophageal carcinoma: a randomized multicenter study of preoperative radiotherapy and chemotherapy. The second scandinavian trial in esophageal cancer. World J Surg 16:1104–1109

Omloo JM, Lagarde SM, Hulscher JB, Reitsma JB, Focken P, van Dekken H, Ten Kate FJ, Obertop H, Tilanus HW, van Lanschot JJ (2007) Extended transthoracic resection compared with limited transhiatal resection for adenocarcinoma of the mid/distal esophagus. Five-year survival of a randomized clinical trial. Ann Surg 246:992–1001

Peyre C, Hagen J, De Meester S, Altorki N, Ancona E, Griffin S, Hölscher A, Lerut T, Law S, Rice T, Ruol A, van Lanschot J, Wong J, De Meester T (2008) The number of lymph nodes removed predicts survival in esophageal cancer: an international study on the impact of extent of surgical resection. Ann Surg 248:549–556

Ruhstaller T, Pless M, Dietrich D, Kranzbuehler H, von Moos R, Moosmann P, Montemurro M, Schneider PM, Rauch D, Gautschi O, Mingrone W, Widmer L, Inauen R, Brauchli P, Hess V (2011) Cetuximab in combination with chemoradiotherapy before surgery in patients with resectable, locally advanced esophageal carcinoma: a prospective, multicenter phase IB/II Trial (SAKK 75/06). J Clin Oncol 29:626–639

Ruol A, Rizzetto C, Castoro C, Cagol M, Alfieri R, Zanchettin G, Cavallin F, Michieletto S, Da Dalt G, Sileni VC, Corti L, Mantoan S, Zaninotto G, Ancona E (2010) Interval between neoadjuvant chemoradiotherapy and surgery for surgery for squamous cell cancer of the thoracic esophagus. Ann Surg 252:788–796

Schneider PM, Metzger R, Schaefer H, Baumgarten F, Vallbohmer D, Brabender J, Wolfgarten E, Bollschweiler E, Baldus SE, Dienes HP, Hoelscher AH (2008) Response evaluation by endoscopy, rebiopsy, and endoscopic ultrasound does not accurately predict histopathologic regression after neoadjuvant chemoradiation for esophageal cancer. Ann Surg 248:902–908

Semrau R, Vallböhmer D, Hölscher AH, Müller RP (2009) Neoadjuvant therapy of adenocarcinomas of the upper gastrointestinal tract. Status of radiotherapy. Chirurg 80:1035–1041

Sjoquist KM, Burmeister BH, Smithers BM et al (2011) Survival after neoadjuvant chemotherapy or chemoradiotherapy for resectable oesophageal carcinoma: an updated meta-analysis. Lancet Oncol 12:681–692

Stahl M, Walz MK, Stuschke M et al (2009) Phase III comparison of preoperative chemotherapy compared with chemoradiotherapy in patients with locally advanced adenocarcinoma of the esophagogastric junction. J Clin Oncol 27:851–856

Urschel JD, Vasan H, Blewett CJ (2002) A meta-analysis of randomized controlled trials that compared neoadjuvant chemotherapy and surgery to surgery alone for resectable esophageal cancer. Am J Surg 183:274–279

Urschel JD, Vasan H (2003) A meta-analysis of randomised controlled trials that compared neoadjuvant chemoradiation and surgery alone for resectable esophageal cancer. Am J Surg 185:538–543

Vallböhmer D, Hölscher AH, DeMeester S, DeMeester T, Salo J, Peters J, Lerut T, Swisher SG, Schröder W, Bollschweiler E, Hofstetter W (2010) A multicenter study of survival after neoadjuvant radiotherapy/chemotherapy and esophagectomy for ypT0N0M0R0 esophageal cancer. Ann Surg 252:744–749

Vallböhmer D, Hölscher AH, Dietlein M, Bollschweiler E, Baldus SE, Mönig SP, Metzger R, Schicha H, Schmidt M (2009) [^{18}F]-Fluorodeoxyglucose-positron emission tomography for the assessment of histopathologic response and prognosis after completion of neoadjuvant chemoradiation in esophageal cancer. Ann Surg 250:888–894

van Heijl M, Omloo JM, van Berge Henegouwen MI, Hoekstra OS, Boellaard R, Bossuyt PM, Busch OR, Tilanus HW, Hulshof MC, van der Gaast A, Nieuwenhuijzen GA, Bonenkamp HJ, Plukker JT, Cuesta MA, Ten Kate FJ, Pruim J, van Dekken H, Bergman JJ, Sloof GW, van Lanschot JJ (2011) Fluorodeoxyglucose positron emission tomography for evaluating early response during neoadjuvant chemoradiotherapy in patients with potentially curable esophageal cancer. Ann Surg 253:56–63

Wang M, Gu XZ, Yin WB, Huang GJ, Wang LJ, Zhang DW (1989) Randomized clinical trial on the combination of perioperative irradiation and surgery in the treatment of esophageal carcinoma: report on 206 patients. Int J Radiat Oncol Biol Phys 16:325–327

Part V
Multimodal Therapy of GEJ Cancer

Multimodal Therapy of GEJ Cancer: When is the Definitive Radiochemotherapy the Treatment of Choice?

Michael Stahl

Abstract

Today, patients with localized gastroesophageal junction adenocarcinomas (AC) should be considered for combined modality therapy, at least when they have locally advanced (T3–T4 category) or lymph node positive tumors. But what about patients unable or unwilling to undergo surgical resection? Unlike esophageal squamous cell carcinoma (SCC), we have no randomized data to consider definitive radiochemotherapy without surgery as accepted treatment option in these patients. Retrospective results from an US surveillance epidemiology and end results (SEER) analysis state that the results of definitive or preoperative radio(chemo)therapy are equal or even improved for adenocarcinoma compared to SCC. Other retrospective data using the method of matched-pair analysis showed that median overall survival appears not different between AC and SCC after definitive radiochemotherapy. Nevertheless, since prospective randomized results are lacking, definitive radiochemotherapy cannot be considered as treatment standard in GEJ cancer, and therefore should be restricted to patients with increased operation risk.

Contents

1 Introduction	182
2 Standard Treatment Options in Localized Disease	182
2.1 Perioperative Therapy	182
2.2 Definitive Chemoradiotherapy	182
3 Conclusion	184
References	184

M. Stahl (✉)
Department of Medical Oncology and Hematology, Kliniken Essen-Mitte,
Henricistr 92, 45136 Essen, Germany
e-mail: m.stahl@kliniken-essen-mitte.de

F. Otto and M. P. Lutz (eds.), *Early Gastrointestinal Cancers*,
Recent Results in Cancer Research 196, DOI: 10.1007/978-3-642-31629-6_12,
© Springer-Verlag Berlin Heidelberg 2012

1 Introduction

Adenocarcinomas (AC) of the gastro-esophageal junction (GEJ) reflect a tumor entity with aggressive biology. In the Western countries, most of the patients present with advanced tumor stage at time of diagnosis. In this situation, the prognosis is poor and a minority of patients will survive 3 years even after complete primary tumor resection in experienced centers (Pyre et al. 2008). Among other reasons this comes from the fact that most of the locally advanced tumors (T3–T4 category) have spread to regional lymph nodes. Interestingly, even in lymph node negative tumors, the risk of systemic recurrence increases with T-category rising up to 70 % in completely resected pT3pN0 tumors (Pyre et al. 2008).

2 Standard Treatment Options in Localized Disease

2.1 Perioperative Therapy

A plenty of studies investigated multimodal therapy with the goal for improving the prognosis, in particular the cure rate of the patients. Based on a couple of meta-analyses in esophageal carcinoma (Table 1), most recent guidelines are recommending trimodal therapy, e.g., chemoradiation followed by surgery at least for those patients with locally advanced tumors (Moehler et al. 2011). With this respect, it appears most useful to combine all treatment options available, e.g., chemotherapy, radiotherapy, and surgery to optimize treatment results.

2.2 Definitive Chemoradiotherapy

So, why should we discuss the role of definitive radiochemotherapy without surgery? First of all, because some of our patients present with severe comorbidities which will unacceptably increase the risk for postoperative mortality. This risk will increase with the need for transthoracic instead of transhiatal esophagectomy, and therefore is higher in patients with tumors clearly centered in the esophagus (type I cancer according to Sievert) (Hulscher et al. 2002). However, it is easily spoken and hardly done to properly define inoperability of a patient, and the scarce data we have from treatment centers worldwide are somewhat different in their numbers of patients to be excluded from surgery. Secondly, because there are always patients who deny surgery because they want to keep their esophagus und stomach preserved. No doubt this will be the most appropriate way to safe life quality. But is definitive radiochemotherapy a treatment with curative potency in this tumor entity?

Multimodal Therapy of GEJ Cancer

Table 1 Metaanalyses of preoperative chemoradiotherapy versus surgery for esophageal cancer

Author/year	HR (95 % CI) for overall survival	Log rank p value
Urschel and Vasan (2002)	0.66 (0.47–0.92)	0.02
Fiorica (2004)	0.53 (0.31–0.89)	0.03
Malthaner (2004)	0.87 (0.80–0.96)	<0.05
Greer (2005)	0.86 (0.74–1.01)	0.07
Gebski (2007)	0.81 (0.70–0.93)	0.002
Kranzfelder (2011)	0.81 (0.70–0.95)	0.008

HR hazard ratio; *CI* confidence interval

2.2.1 Results in Squamous Cell Carcinomas of the Esophagus

Three randomized trials involving patients with locally advanced SCC compared outcome after definitive chemoradiation (CRT) with neoadjuvant CRT followed by surgery (Bedenne et al. 2007; Stahl et al. 2005), or surgery alone (Chiu et al. 2005). Definitive RCT based on cisplatin/5-FU combinations was applied with radiation doses of 50–66 Gy. One of the studies selected patients with tumor response to induction CRT, only (Bedenne et al. 2007). Overall, compliance with definitive RCT was higher than with preoperative RCT + surgery (89 vs. 83 %). The trials demonstrated no significant difference in survival with preoperative and definitive CRT (HR 0.83–0.89). A recent meta analysis (Kranzfelder et al. 2011) on these trials proved that mortality risk to be lower with definitive CRT (HR 7.60, 1.76–32.88, $p = 0.007$) due to postoperative mortality risk ranging from 5 to 8 % after preoperative CRT. The rate of local recurrence was significantly lower with trimodal therapy. Therefore, the ESMO clinical recommendations consider definitive CRT with salvage surgery only for selected patients with local tumor progression, a treatment option in locally advanced SCC of the esophagus (Stahl et al. 2010).

2.2.2 Results in GEJ Cancer

Unlike squamous cell carcinomas (SCC), we have no prospectively randomized studies investigating definitive radiochemotherapy in AC of the GEJ, so far.

From an US surveillance epidemiology and end results (SEER) analysis including more than 4,700 patients treated between 1973 and 2004 we know that the results of definitive or preoperative radio(chemo)therapy are equal or even improved for AC compared to SCC of the esophagus with a 3-year survival rate after definitive radiotherapy of 20 % in both histologies. Moreover, a French matched-pair analysis showed that despite clinical complete response to definitive radiochemotherapy was observed significantly more often in SCC (70 vs. 46 %, $p = 0.01$), local recurrence in responders to CRT was significantly more frequent in SCC, and therefore median overall survival was not different between SCC and AC.

In contrary, a recent Dutch retrospective analysis on patients with localized esophageal cancer treated with radiotherapy ($n = 172$) or RCT ($n = 106$) revealed a significant advantage for SCC compared to AC (e.g. EGJ cancer) by multivariate analysis (Smit et al. 2012). The overall survival after 5 years was 11 % for SCC patients, whereas no patient with AC survived 5 years. Although it can be suggested that these poor results reflect the advanced tumor stage and the risk situation of the patients, these data question a relevant curative potency of definitive RCT in unselected patients with AC. So, it may be helpful to better select patients for definitive therapy without surgery. An US group published data on patients with localized GEJ cancer who should receive trimodal therapy but did not proceed to surgery because of poor performance status (Taketa et al. 2012). All these patients had reached a clinical complete response (negative biopsy and normal PET) to CRT. This group accounted for 32 out of 599 patients with intended trimodal therapy, only. The survival rate after 3 years was 65 % and recurrence free survival reached 38 % in this highly selected patient group.

3 Conclusion

Definitive radiochemotherapy cannot be regarded as standard treatment in GEJ cancer. However, it is an option for patients who are not operable or who deny surgery, particulary if they showed major clinical response to CRT. Since randomized data are lacking true curative potency of definitive CRT in EGJ cancer remains unclear.

References

Bedenne L, Michel P, Bouche O et al (2007) Chemoradiation followed by surgery compared with chemoradiation alone in squamous cancer of the esophagus: FFCD 9102. J Clin Oncol 25:1160–1168

Chiu PW, Chan AC, Leung SF et al (2005) Multicenter prospective randomized trial comparing standard esophagectomy with chemoradiotherapy for treatment of squamous esophageal cancer: early results from the Chinese University Research Group for Esophageal Cancer (CURE). J Gastrointest Surg 9:794–802

Fiorica F, Di Bona D, Schepis F et al (2004) Preoperative chemoradiotherapy for oesophageal cancer: a systematic review and meta-analysis. Gut 53:925–930

Gebski V, Burmeister B, Smithers B et al (2007) Survival benefits from neoadjuvant chemoradiotherapy or chemotherapy in oesophageal carcinoma: a meta-analysis. Lancet Oncol 8:226–234

Greer S, Goodney P, Sutton J et al (2005) Neoadjuvant chemoradiotherapy for esophageal carcinoma: a meta-analysis. Surgery 137:172–177

Hulscher J, van Sandick J, de Boer A et al (2002) Extended transthoracic resection compared with limited transhiatal resection for adenocarcinoma of the esophagus. N Engl J Med 347:1662–1669

Kranzfelder M, Schuster T, Geinitz H et al (2011) Meta-analysis of neoadjuvant treatment modalities and definitive non-surgical therapy for oesophageal squamous cell cancer. Br J Surg 98:768–783

Malthaner R, Wong R, Rumble R et al (2004) Neoadjuvant or adjuvant therapy for resectable esophageal cancer: a systematic review and meta-analysis. BMC Med 2:35–52

Möhler M, Al-Batran S, Andus T et al (2011) German S3-guideline "diagnosis and treatment esophagogastric cancer". Z Gastroenterol 49:461–531

Peyre C, Hagen J, DeMeester S et al (2008) The number of lymph nodes removed predicts survival in esophageal cancer: an international study on the impact of extent of surgical resection. Ann Surg 248:549–556

Smit JK, Muijs CT, Paul R et al. (2012) Definitive (chemo)radiotherapy in patients with esophageal cancer: a population-based study in northeast Netherlands. J Clin Oncol 30(suppl. 4), abstract 83

Stahl M, Stuschke M, Lehmann N et al (2005) Chemoradiation with and without surgery in patients with squamous cell carcinoma of the esophagus. J Clin Oncol 23:2310–2317

Stahl M, Budach W, Meyer HJ, Cervantes A (2010) Esophageal cancer: clinical recommendations for diagnosis, treatment and follow-up. Ann Oncol 21(suppl 5):v46–v49

Taketa T, Correa AM, Suzuki A et al. (2012) Outcome of trimodality-eligible esophago-gastric cancer patients who declined surgery after preoperative chemoradiation. J Clin Oncol 30(suppl. 4), abstract 6

Urschel J, Vasan H (2002) A meta-analysis of randomized controlled trials that compared neoadjuvant chemoradiation and surgery to surgery alone for resectable esophageal cancer. Am J Surg 185:538–543

Radiotherapy of Gastroesophageal Junction Cancer

Florian Sterzing, Lars Grenacher and Jürgen Debus

Abstract

Adenocarcinomas of the gastroesophageal junction (GEJ) require multimodal treatment approaches to accomplish good local control and overall survival. While early T1/2 N0 tumors are treated with surgery alone, they are only found in a small subset of patients due to the lack of symptoms at this stage. Most of the tumors are detected in locally advanced stage where surgery alone results in disappointing outcome. Chemotherapy and/or chemoirradiation in the neoadjuvant setting are used to improve conditions for oncological surgery. They aim to achieve a downsizing with a pathological complete remission in the optimal case, improve R0 rates, and upfront treat microscopic metastatic tumor cells. The optimal neoadjuvant treatment approach—chemotherapy, chemoirradiation, or a multiphase approach of both—is yet unclear. Chemoirradiation can improve local control after incomplete surgery and is an important option for patients unfit for surgery. In addition, it enables symptom relief in a palliative setting, namely dysphagia, pain, or bleeding. While target volumes are very much standardized, new technologies as image-guided intensity-modulated radiotherapy (IG-IMRT) and particle therapy have the potential to improve the therapeutic window by minimizing toxicity. Challenges of the present and the future will be the combination of radiotherapy with other cytostatic drugs and modern targeted therapies. This should ideally be integrated into a multimodal setting that is able to identify risk groups according to predictive markers and tumor response, altogether leading to a personalized oncological approach.

F. Sterzing (✉) · J. Debus
Department of Radiation Oncology, INF 400, 69120 Heidelberg, Germany
e-mail: florian.sterzing@med.uni-heidelberg.de

L. Grenacher
Department of Radiology, INF 110, 69120 Heidelberg, Germany

F. Otto and M. P. Lutz (eds.), *Early Gastrointestinal Cancers*,
Recent Results in Cancer Research 196, DOI: 10.1007/978-3-642-31629-6_13,
© Springer-Verlag Berlin Heidelberg 2012

Contents

1	Background	188
2	Diagnostic Workup	189
3	Early Stage Disease	189
4	Locally Advanced Disease	189
5	Neoadjuvant Therapy	190
6	Response-Guided Therapy	191
7	Definitive Chemoirradiation	193
8	Adjuvant Therapy	193
9	Salvage Radiotherapy	194
10	Palliative Radiotherapy	195
11	New Radiation Technologies	195
12	New Combination Possibilities	196
13	Conclusions	197
References		197

1 Background

Times have changed in the treatment of upper gastrointestinal cancers. Some time ago, the choice was either surgery or radiotherapy or chemotherapy. In the past decades, therapy moved toward sophisticated stage-dependant multimodal approaches involving two or three of the mentioned disciplines (Bystricky et al. 2011). In addition, all three columns of therapy were improved by marked innovations—new surgical methods, new combinations of cytostatic drugs and targeted agents, and new radiation technology. This is accompanied by excellent diagnostic workup in endoscopy and radiology including CT, MRI, and PET-CT. The latter also has an evolving role in determining metabolic treatment response and tailoring the sequence of therapeutic steps.

For esophageal cancer the role of radiotherapy within the multimodal setting is supported by many trials and summarized in very recent meta-analyses (Kranzfelder et al. 2011; Sjoquist et al. 2011). Determining the role of radiotherapy for gastroesophageal junction (GEJ) tumors, however, presents a more difficult challenge and leaves a lot more unanswered questions. This is due to the fact that GEJ tumors have often been subgroups in either esophageal or gastric cancer trials, some of them including both adeno- and squamous cell carcinomas. In addition, the exclusive GEJ trials have been frequently underpowered to prove clear advantages of different approaches. A third factor is the heterogeneity of the used doses and fractionation schemes. This led to huge differences in various parts of the world with more frequent use of chemoirradiation in the US and more perioperative chemotherapy in Europe (Okines and Cunningham 2010).

This chapter describes the role of radiotherapy in the multimodal treatment of GEJ tumors. It reviews neoadjuvant, adjuvant, and definitive settings; it deals with radiation techniques, the combination with chemotherapy and targeted therapy, treatment response and brings up open questions that should be the basis for upcoming trials.

2 Diagnostic Workup

Sophisticated stage-adapted therapy requires excellent tools to determine local tumor situation, lymph node involvement, and distant metastases (Jamil et al. 2008; Lordick et al. 2010, 2011). It allows the assessment of tumor extension and prognostic evaluation (Blank et al. 2012). Many trials we rely our decisions on only used barium swallow and thorax X-ray. Today, modern endoscopy including endoscopic ultrasound helps to quantify infiltration depth and with clip marks at the tumor ends enables more precise target definition than CT alone.

In neoadjuvant therapy, exact staging is necessary to adapt the treatment field to the appropriate areas while dose is the same in the entire target volume. In the setting of definitive radiochemotherapy, precise localization of tumor borders and involved lymph nodes is of additional importance for a tailor-made definition of boost areas and selective dose escalation.

3 Early Stage Disease

GEJ tumors stage Ia/b is sufficiently treated with mucosal resection or surgery alone and do not benefit from multimodal approaches (Greer et al. 2005). This, however, represents only a small subgroup of patients since patients rarely have symptoms during this stage. For patients unfit or unwilling to undergo surgery, chemoirradiation is an excellent alternative (Sjoquist et al. 2011). For small superficial tumors, brachytherapy is an excellent radiotherapy option to minimize dose exposure to surrounding tissues (Muijs et al. 2012).

4 Locally Advanced Disease

In locally advanced disease, surgery alone results in poor outcome and intensified multimodal therapy approaches are necessary (Allum et al. 2011). Positive resection margins and positive lymph node involvement are known to correlate with markedly lower survival. Perioperative strategies aim to achieve a down-sizing and increase R0 resection rates (Lordick et al. 2011). But these treatments are often problematic, since patients are frequently in their 7th or 8th decade and due to their often heavy smoking history can have severe comorbidities. There is no clear consent on the optimal perioperative treatment, both chemotherapy and chemoirradiation are used.

5 Neoadjuvant Therapy

Not only are perioperative treatment strategies associated with a better survival in patients in locally advanced disease, this approach also allows an assessment of therapy response that can guide adjuvant therapy (Lv et al. 2009; Power and Ilson 2009).

The UK medical research adjuvant gastric infusional chemotherapy (MAGIC) study changed clinical practice across Europe with three cycles of ECF (epirubicin, cisplatin, and continuous infusion fluorouracil) chemotherapy delivered before and after surgery for patients with operable adenocarcinoma of the lower esophagus, OGJ, or stomach (Cunningham et al. 2006). Five-year survival in the surgery alone arm was 23 %, it was increased to 36 % with the addition of perioperative chemotherapy (HR 0.75, 95 % CI 0.60–0.93, $P = 0.009$). Similar to this the FNCLCC and FFCD multicenter phase III trial demonstrated a 14 % increase of 5 year survival using perioperative fluorouracil plus cisplatin (Ychou et al. 2011).

Trials comparing perioperative chemotherapy and chemoirradiation failed to show an advantage of either modality in terms of survival (Stahl et al. 2009; Burmeister et al. 2011). Stahl et al. found an improvement of 3 year survival in the chemoirradiation group (47.4 versus 27.7 %) which was just not significant with a p value of 0.07.

For neoadjuvant chemoirradiation, there are published guidelines by the EORTC for the extent of elective lymph node irradiation according to tumor localisation and stage to enable a standardized radiotherapy practice (Matzinger et al. 2009). For distal esophageal cancer the inclusion of lymph node regions paracardial, in the lower mediastinum, along the lesser curvature, around the celiac artery and at the hiatus is recommended. For AEG II and III tumors, the addition of nodes along the splenic artery to the hilum is suggested. A total dose of 45 Gy in conventional fractionation of 5 9 1.8 Gy per week is recommended by the authors.

The recently published CROSS study shows the potential of neoadjuvant chemoirradiation (van Hagen et al. 2012) 368 patients were randomly assigned toeither surgery alone or neoadjuvant combined chemoirradiation followed by operation. The neoadjuvant regimen consisted of radiotherapy with a dose of 41.4Gy in 23 fractions with concurrent carboplatin and paclitaxel. R0 rate in the surgery only group was 69 % whilst it was 92 % in the combined group. Medianoverall survival was significantly higher in the combined modality group (49 months versus 24 months).

The literature shows that using this or similar regimens is a safe way to improve the situation for surgery and has less impact on perioperative morbidity than factors like age and body mass index (Fujitani et al. 2007). Some authors, however, describe slightly increased morbidity rates especially due to pulmonary complications (Fiorica et al. 2004). Usually, a radiation plan where 20 % of the lung volume receives 20 Gy or more is regarded as safe. But there are reports that in this setting even more than 20 % of the lung receiving more than 10 Gy can be associated with higher lung toxicity, special care has to be taken on this in radiotherapy planning (Leibl et al. 2011).

To make the choice of the optimal neoadjuvant strategy even more complex, there are a couple of studies combining the two modalities in a sequence of induction chemotherapy plus radiochemotherapy followed by surgery (Ajani et al. 2001).

The quest for the optimal neoadjuvant strategy is still ongoing. In the attempt to intensify chemotherapy approaches with multiple cytostatic agents and target drugs, one fact is often neglected. There is a drug available that can be selectively delivered to the tumor, that can be selectively dosed according to macroscopic or microscopic tumor cell spread, that has little harm to the rest of the body, and that has been refined in its application during the last 100 years—the X-ray.

Until prospective randomized trials answer this question, it is justified to say that for patients with the main part of the tumor in the esophagus there is a stronger rationale for neoadjuvant chemoirradiation, while predominantly gastric tumors can rather be treated with chemotherapy alone. The higher the risk for positive resection margins is the more radiochemotherapy could be of benefit with the higher chances of significant downsizing. But, especially these tumors which are bigger and have a more advanced infiltration of surrounding tissues might have a higher risk of developing distant metastasis, therefore might need early systemic therapy.

Future strategies will most likely not ask either one or the other, it will rather include a combination of both to unite maximal local effect and early systemic treatment.

6 Response-Guided Therapy

Patients with response to neoadjuvant therapies show a better overall survival (Lordick et al. 2010, 2011; Wieder et al. 2004). This has been used by Lordick and colleagues to tailor therapy for every patient according to metabolic response as detected in FDG PET CT. In the Municon I trial, nonresponders were directly referred to surgery instead of continuing a nonefficient chemotherapy (Lordick et al. 2007). In the Municon II trial, nonresponders underwent additional chemoirradiation before surgery. But a hyperfractionated radiotherapy of 32 Gy failed to improve the prognosis of these nonresponding patients. The question remains if nonresponding patients might benefit from a conventionally fractionated treatment with alternative drugs like taxanes (Fig 1).

What is the optimal method to assess treatment response in these patients? While some patients quickly show clinical improvement under therapy with the diminished dysphagia, some need imaging methods to assess tumor size or metabolism. While there are more data available for metabolic response measurements using the FDG-PET, there are new trials that demonstrated the capacity of diffusion-weighted MRI using the apparent diffusion coefficient (ADC) that correlates with tumor response and is a surrogate for a better prognosis (Aoyagi et al. 2011; Sun et al. 2011). An example of MRI with diffusion imaging before and after chemoirradiation is displayed in Fig. 2.

Outside of clinical trials, the literature data does not justify to alter therapeutic strategies for our patients today.

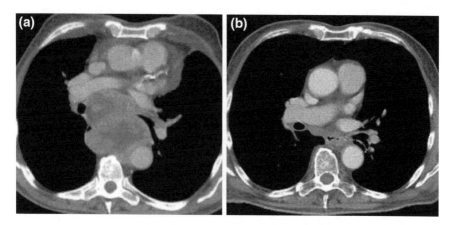

Fig. 1 Illustrates the case of a large AEG type I that has shown no response to chemotherapy with ECF. **a** After chemoirradiation with 45 Gy and cisplatin, 5FU restaging revealed excellent response, **b** pathological evaluation showed a complete pathological remission

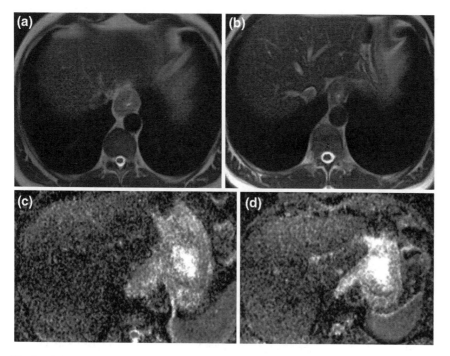

Fig. 2 Displays MRI response of an AEG tumor type I in T2-weighted sequences before and after neoadjuvant chemotherapy (**a** and **b**) and ADC maps before and after chemotherapy (**c** and **d**)

It is possible now to visualize treatment response, but the appropriate consequences are to be established: immediate surgery, intensified chemoirradiation with other substances? On the other hand, especially the responders might have a tumor biology that is positively affected by additional chemoirradiation.

7 Definitive Chemoirradiation

Many patients with GEJ tumors suffer from severe comorbidities and are unfit for surgery. For these patients, definitive chemoirradiation is an alternative with local control and survival rates very close to multimodal therapy including surgery (Sjoquist et al. 2011).

Sjoquist et al. and Kranzfelder et al. (2011) showed in their meta analysis that this can be achieved with less mortality and morbidity than in the surgical approaches. It is beyond the scope of this article to give a thorough overview of the different trials here. Figure 3 visualizes the possibilities of modern radiotherapy for an AEG tumor type I with celiac lymph node metastasis.

Clinical reality frequently reveals a different practice. In many cases the relatively young and fit patients undergo surgery, while old patients with a lot of comorbidities are referred to radiotherapy. But with equivalent oncological results and favorable morbidity radiation is a lot more than the last sheet anchor. However, in case of a relapse after radiation, salvage therapy is associated with high complications. Salvage radiotherapy after surgery, in contrast, can be done more safely.

8 Adjuvant Therapy

The largest trial testing the value of adjuvant chemoirradiation is the intergroup 0116 trial which predominantly included gastric cancer patients. However, 49 of 556 patients had tumors located in the cardia (Macdonald et al. 2001). This trial was often criticized for the quality of surgery and the extent of lymph node resection. Nevertheless, it showed survival benefit for patients treated with postoperative chemoirradiation compared to those treated with surgery alone. The data give the rationale to irradiate patients in an adjuvant setting if no preoperative chemotherapy was given, and high risk of locoregional relapse is present due to lymph node involvement or positive resection margins. Strauss et al. evaluated almost 2,000 patients at the age of 65 or older treated in the US between 1991 and 2002, either with surgery only or with surgery and adjuvant chemoirradiation (Strauss et al. 2010). Seventeen percent of these patients had cardia carcinoma. They could show that this treatment was associated with mild toxicity even in an elderly population. In this retrospective analysis, they could reproduce the survival benefit for patients in stage II and higher.

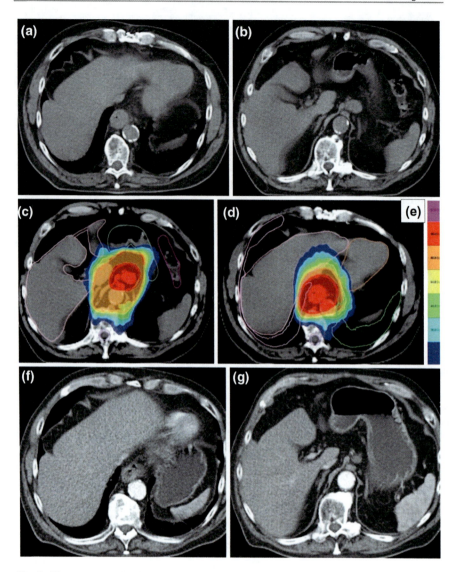

Fig. 3 Shows a case of definitive radiochemotherapy of an AEG tumor type I. **a** and **b** display the primary tumor and celiac lymph node metastasis before treatment, **c**, **d** and **e** an intensity-modulated radiotherapy plan, **f** and **g** the complete response after a follow up of 6 months

9 Salvage Radiotherapy

Radiotherapy plays an important role in the treatment of locoregional relapse. Fakhrian et al. (2012) reported a series of 54 patients treated with radiotherapy for recurrent esophageal cancer after surgery. They demonstrated an improvement of symptoms in 68 % of the patients and a survival of 55, 29, and 19 % after 1, 2, and 3 years.

The advantage of initial surgery is that in the case of locoregional relapse, radiochemotherapy can be offered as salvage therapy. After chemoirradiation, a salvage surgery procedure is associated with markedly higher complication rates.

10 Palliative Radiotherapy

Radiotherapy can also play an important role in a palliative setting. In cases of systemic disease, palliative chemotherapy regimens are of course treatment of choice. However, if this fails to improve local problems and systemic tumor burden is not the leading problem, radiotherapy as a local therapy might still be indicated. In cases of diffuse tumor bleeding, pain, or dysphagia significant improvement can be achieved with positive impact on patients' quality of life.

11 New Radiation Technologies

The discipline of radiation oncology has experienced a remarkable evolution during the last years. Radiotherapy has moved from opposing beam techniques with full dose to all tissues in the entry and exit areas to conformal CT-based multifield treatments and individually tailored irradiations. Additionally, the introduction of imaging modalities to the treatment unit itself has improved the precision of applying tailor-made dose distributions in the highest possible precision (Xing et al. 2006; Jensen et al. 2009). That way surrounding radiosensitive organs at risk can be spared in a matter that was not possible before. So, to judge the quality and toxicity of a radiotherapy course, it is not only about the question 45 Gy yes or no. A more subtle evaluation of dose exposure to different organs is necessary.

In the definitive setting, a selective adaptation of radiation doses to the macroscopic primary tumor or involved lymph nodes is possible, called a simultaneous integrated boost concept (Welsh et al. 2012). In earlier days with older techniques, a dose escalation ment higher dose to all surrounding tissues. With image-guided intensity-modulated radiotherapy (IG-IMRT) this can be accomplished in a more selective manner. The clinical toxicity data, however, are still missing.

An open question is whether this sort of treatment intensification is an option in a neoadjuvant setting to improve response and increase the number of pathological complete remissions and R0 resections. With a known dose–response-relationship of tumor cells a higher dose should be associated with higher remission rates. But higher radiation doses can possibly result in more fibrosis and difficulties for surgical procedures. In addition, it is not clear if a higher remission rate achieved by selective dose escalation translates into better local control or survival. The histopathological response is only a surrogate marker for prognosis. If an improvement of 20 % pCR after 45 Gy to 30 % pCR after 55 Gy is possible, safety and consequence to the patient is unknown. A selective dose escalation to visible tumor areas might technically be feasible, but in many cases these areas are not the site of positive resection margins. This often occurs in areas of "invisible" microscopic tumor spread.

Similar to the impact of new photon radiotherapy techniques, the potential of particle therapy (proton and carbon ion irradiation) for esophageal cancer or GEJ tumors is unclear. This technology has both physical advantages in terms of better treatment conformity and biological advantages (for carbon ions) due to differences in DNA damage and possibilities to overcome radioresistance (Welsh et al. 2011). But besides these theoretical advantages, there are no clinical data available currently that supports the use of particles for these tumors outside of trials.

12   New Combination Possibilities

What is the best cytostatic agent in the combination with X-rays? Most trials involved a combined therapy with cisplatin and 5FU (Sjoquist et al. 2011). With the current trend in multiagent chemotherapy regimens toward including topoisomerase inhibitors or taxanes, there might also be an advantage of these substances in a combined modality.

Ilson et al. (2011) found no additional effect when they introduced irinotecan into neoadjuvant radiochemotherapy in combination with cisplatin. The combination of oxaliplatin, docetaxel, and capecitabine in combination with 45 Gy irradiation in a phase I/II trial showed a 2-year DFS and OS of 45.1 and 52.2 %, respectively.

Ruhstaller et al. performed a phase I/II trial evaluating a combination of cisplatin, docetaxel, and cetuximab together with 45 Gy irradiation in a neoadjuvant setting. They demonstrated no effect on perioperative mortality due to the addition of the antiEGFR antibody, while an impressive rate of 68 % of complete or near complete pathological remissions was found (Ruhstaller et al. 2011). Several trials are currently recruiting patients into protocols involving cetuximab. The UK SCOPE-1 trial is investigating the addition of cetuximab to definitive CRT with cisplatin and capecitabine in patients with esophageal and OGJ adenocarcinoma or SCC, the German Leopard II trial is using a similar approach together with cisplatin and 5FU.

Besides this, the her2 status has moved into the focus of therapy, since the expression status is associated with prognosis (Yoon et al. 2012). It remains to be shown that this intensified approach is not at the cost of increased cardiac toxicity.

To evaluate the role of antiangiogenesis, protocols involving perioperative ECX+- bevacizumab before and after surgery are being tested. In addition, a trial in the US is open for recruitment evaluating neoadjuvant bevacizumab, cisplatin, irinotecan as chemoradiation followed by surgery and adjuvant bevacizumab. These new combination strategies have an enormous potential to improve outcome, and in junction with a translational research program might help to identify subgroups with certain molecular markers that benefit from different individualized approaches, a swith of agents in nonresponders or those that rather benefit from X-rays or chemotherapy (Bain and Petty 2010).

13 Conclusions

A combination of excellent endoscopic and radiological workup, radiotherapy, systemic therapy, and state-of-the-art surgery is mandatory for the successful treatment of advanced GEJ tumors. Radiotherapy together with chemotherapy improves local control and overall survival for patients with locally advanced disease. The optimal choice of the two in the neoadjuvant setting has yet to be determined in upcoming trials.

In addition, radiation is an excellent treatment for patients that are unfit or unwilling to undergo surgery. It can provide palliation of pain, dysphagia, and tumor bleeding.

The potential of new therapy methods as IG-IMRT and particle therapy and the possibilities of new combined approaches have to be evaluated. Further trials are urgently needed to enable personalized multimodal approaches according to predictive markers and treatment response.

References

Ajani JA, Komaki R, Putnam JB et al (2001) A three-step strategy of induction chemotherapy then chemoradiation followed by surgery in patients with potentially resectable carcinoma of the esophagus or gastroesophageal junction. Cancer 92:279–286

Allum WH, Blazeby JM, Griffin SM, Cunningham D, Jankowski JA, Wong R (2011) Guidelines for the management of oesophageal and gastric cancer. Gut 60:1449–1472

Aoyagi T, Shuto K, Okazumi S, Shimada H, Kazama T, Matsubara H (2011) Apparent diffusion coefficient values measured by diffusion-weighted imaging predict chemoradiotherapeutic effect for advanced esophageal cancer. Dig Surg 28:252–257

Bain GH, Petty RD (2010) Predicting response to treatment in gastroesophageal junction adenocarcinomas: combining clinical, imaging, and molecular biomarkers. Oncologist 15:270–284

Blank S, Blaker H, Schaible A et al (2012) Impact of pretherapeutic routine clinical staging for the individualization of treatment in gastric cancer patients. Langenbecks Arch Surg 397:45–55

Burmeister BH, Thomas JM, Burmeister EA et al (2011) Is concurrent radiation therapy required in patients receiving preoperative chemotherapy for adenocarcinoma of the oesophagus? A randomised phase II trial. Eur J Cancer 47:354–360

Bystricky B, Okines AF, Cunningham D (2011) Optimal therapeutic strategies for resectable oesophageal or oesophagogastric junction cancer. Drugs 71:541–555

Cunningham D, Allum WH, Stenning SP et al (2006) Perioperative chemotherapy versus surgery alone for resectable gastroesophageal cancer. N Engl J Med 355:11–20

Fakhrian K, Gamisch N, Schuster T, Thamm R, Molls M, Geinitz H (2012) Salvage radiotherapy in patients with recurrent esophageal carcinoma. Strahlenther Onkol 188:136–142

Fiorica F, Di Bona D, Schepis F et al (2004) Preoperative chemoradiotherapy for oesophageal cancer: a systematic review and meta-analysis. Gut 53:925–930

Fujitani K, Ajani JA, Crane CH et al (2007) Impact of induction chemotherapy and preoperative chemoradiotherapy on operative morbidity and mortality in patients with locoregional adenocarcinoma of the stomach or gastroesophageal junction. Ann Surg Oncol 14:2010–2017

Greer SE, Goodney PP, Sutton JE, Birkmeyer JD (2005) Neoadjuvant chemoradiotherapy for esophageal carcinoma: a meta-analysis. Surgery 137:172–177

Ilson DH, Minsky BD, Ku GY et al. (2011) Phase 2 trial of induction and concurrent chemoradiotherapy with weekly irinotecan and cisplatin followed by surgery for esophageal cancer. Cancer

Jamil LH, Gill KR, Wallace MB (2008) Staging and restaging of advanced esophageal cancer. Curr Opin Gastroenterol 24:530–534

Jensen AD, Grehn C, Nikoghosyan A et al (2009) Catch me if you can—the use of image guidance in the radiotherapy of an unusual case of esophageal cancer. Strahlenther Onkol 185:469–473

Kranzfelder M, Schuster T, Geinitz H, Friess H, Buchler P (2011) Meta-analysis of neoadjuvant treatment modalities and definitive non-surgical therapy for oesophageal squamous cell cancer. Br J Surg 98:768–783

Leibl BJ, Vitz S, Schafer W, Alfrink M, Gschwendtner A, Grabenbauer GG (2011) Adenocarcinoma of the esophagogastric junction: neoadjuvant radiochemotherapy and radical surgery: early results and toxicity. Strahlenther Onkol 187:231–237

Lordick F, Ott K, Krause BJ et al (2007) PET to assess early metabolic response and to guide treatment of adenocarcinoma of the oesophagogastric junction: the Municon phase II trial. Lancet Oncol 8:797–805

Lordick F, Ott K, Krause BJ (2010) New trends for staging and therapy for localized gastroesophageal cancer: the role of PET. Ann Oncol 21(Suppl 7):294–299

Lordick F, Ott K, Krause BJ (2011a) Positron emission tomography—current role in the diagnosis and treatment of upper gastrointestinal carcinomas. Dtsch Med Wochenschr 136:1061–1066

Lordick F, Ott K, Sendler A (2011b) Gastric cancer and adenocarcinoma of the esophagogastric junction: principles of neoadjuvant therapy. Chirurg 82:968–973

Lv J, Cao XF, Zhu B, Ji L, Tao L, Wang DD (2009) Effect of neoadjuvant chemoradiotherapy on prognosis and surgery for esophageal carcinoma. World J Gastroenterol 15:4962–4968

Macdonald JS, Smalley SR, Benedetti J et al (2001) Chemoradiotherapy after surgery compared with surgery alone for adenocarcinoma of the stomach or gastroesophageal junction. N Engl J Med 345:725–730

Matzinger O, Gerber E, Bernstein Z et al (2009) EORTC-ROG expert opinion: radiotherapy volume and treatment guidelines for neoadjuvant radiation of adenocarcinomas of the gastroesophageal junction and the stomach. Radiother Oncol 92:164–175

Muijs CT, Beukema JC, Mul VE, Plukker JT, Sijtsema NM, Langendijk JA (2012) External beam radiotherapy combined with intraluminal brachytherapy in esophageal carcinoma. Radiother Oncol 102:303–308

Okines AF, Cunningham D (2010) Multimodality treatment for localized gastro-oesophageal cancer. Ann Oncol 21 Suppl 7:vii286–vii293

Power DG, Ilson DH (2009) Integration of targeted agents in the neo-adjuvant treatment of gastro-esophageal cancers. Ther Adv Med Oncol 1:145–165

Ruhstaller T, Pless M, Dietrich D et al (2011) Cetuximab in combination with chemoradiotherapy before surgery in patients with resectable, locally advanced esophageal carcinoma: a prospective, multicenter phase IB/II Trial (SAKK 75/06). J Clin Oncol 29:626–631

Sjoquist KM, Burmeister BH, Smithers BM et al (2011) Survival after neoadjuvant chemotherapy or chemoradiotherapy for resectable oesophageal carcinoma: an updated meta-analysis. Lancet Oncol 12:681–692

Stahl M, Walz MK, Stuschke M et al (2009) Phase III comparison of preoperative chemotherapy compared with chemoradiotherapy in patients with locally advanced adenocarcinoma of the esophagogastric junction. J Clin Oncol 27:851–856

Strauss J, Hershman DL, Buono D et al (2010) Use of adjuvant 5-fluorouracil and radiation therapy after gastric cancer resection among the elderly and impact on survival. Int J Radiat Oncol Biol Phys 76:1404–1412

Sun YS, Cui Y, Tang L et al (2011) Early evaluation of cancer response by a new functional biomarker: apparent diffusion coefficient. AJR Am J Roentgenol 197:W23–W29 van Hagen P, Hulshof MC, van Lanschot JJ et al (2012) Preoperative chemoradiotherapy for esophageal or junctional cancer. N Engl JMed 366:2074–2084

Welsh J, Gomez D, Palmer MB et al (2011) Intensity-modulated proton therapy further reduces normal tissue exposure during definitive therapy for locally advanced distal esophageal tumors: a dosimetric study. Int J Radiat Oncol Biol Phys 81:1336–1342

Welsh J, Palmer MB, Ajani JA et al (2012) Esophageal cancer dose escalation using a simultaneous integrated boost technique. Int J Radiat Oncol Biol Phys 82:468–474

Wieder HA, Brucher BL, Zimmermann F et al (2004) Time course of tumor metabolic activity during chemoradiotherapy of esophageal squamous cell carcinoma and response to treatment. J Clin Oncol 22:900–908

Xing L, Thorndyke B, Schreibmann E et al (2006) Overview of image-guided radiation therapy. Med Dosim 31:91–112

Ychou M, Boige V, Pignon JP et al (2011) Perioperative chemotherapy compared with surgery alone for resectable gastroesophageal adenocarcinoma: an FNCLCC and FFCD multicenter phase III trial. J Clin Oncol 29:1715–1721

Yoon HH, Shi Q, Sukov WR et al (2012) Association of HER2/ErbB2 expression and gene amplification with pathologic features and prognosis in esophageal adenocarcinomas. Clin Cancer Res 18:546–554

Optimizing Neoadjuvant Chemotherapy Through the Use of Early Response Evaluation by Positron Emission Tomography

Florian Lordick

Abstract

Metabolic imaging and early response assessment by positron emission tomography (PET) may guide treatment of localized esophageal cancers. The most consistent and validated results have been obtained during neoadjuvant treatment of adenocarcinoma of the esophago-gastric junction (AEG). It was demonstrated that 18F-Fluorodeoxyglucoe (FDG)-PET is highly accurate for identifying non-responding tumors within 2 weeks after the initiation of neoadjuvant chemotherapy when a quantitative threshold for metabolic response is used. In consecutive phase II studies the metabolic activity, defined by the standardized uptake (SUV) of 18-FDG before and during chemotherapy, was measured. Significant decreases of the SUV after only two weeks of induction chemotherapy were observed. A drop of >35 % 2 weeks after the start of chemotherapy revealed as an accurate cut-off value to predict response after a 12-week course of preoperative chemotherapy. This cut-off was recently confirmed in a US study, where investigators did follow-up PET not 14 days but 6 weeks after initiation of chemotherapy. It was further noticed that the metabolic response to induction chemotherapy revealed as an independent prognostic factor in locally advanced AEG. Therefore, PET could be used to tailor treatment according to the sensitivity of an individual tumor. This concept was realized in the MUNICON-1 and -2 trials. These trials prospectively confirmed that responders to induction chemotherapy can be identified by early metabolic imaging using FDG-PET. Continuing neoadjuvant chemotherapy in the responding population resulted in a favorable outcome. Moreover, MUNICON-1 showed that chemotherapy can be

---

F. Lordick (✉)
University Cancer Center Leipzig (UCCL), University of Leipzig,
Liebigstr.21, 04103 Leipzig, Germany
e-mail: florian.lordick@medizin.uni-leipzig.de

F. Otto and M. P. Lutz (eds.), *Early Gastrointestinal Cancers*,
Recent Results in Cancer Research 196, DOI: 10.1007/978-3-642-31629-6_14,
© Springer-Verlag Berlin Heidelberg 2012

discontinued at an early stage in metabolic non-responders without compromising the patients' prognosis, but saving time and reducing side effects and costs. MUNICON-2 showed that the addition of neoadjuvant radiation therapy in metabolic nonresponders did not lead to an improvement of their poor prognosis, thus showing that early metabolic nonresponse indicates dismal tumor biology. Future studies need to validate the prognostic and predictive value of PET in multicenter settings and in conjunction with different neoadjuvant chemotherapy and chemo-immunotherapy regimens.

Contents

1 Introduction 202
2 PET Tracers 203
3 PET for Staging 203
4 PET and Prognosis 204
5 PET and Treatment Response 205
    5.1 Post-Therapeutic Response Assessment 205
    5.2 Pre-Therapeutic Assessment 206
    5.3 Early Metabolic Response 207
6 Conclusions 208
References 209

1 Introduction

Progress has been made in the treatment of locally advanced esophageal cancer. With the introduction of more sophisticated surgical techniques, standardized perioperative care and the introduction of active preoperative chemotherapy, with or without radiation, we have moved toward a more effective and stage-specific approach for every patient.

Novel imaging techniques may enhance the accuracy of clinical staging and thereby improve the estimation of the patients' prognosis. Molecular imaging may also be of value to predict and assess the response to neoadjuvant therapy.

Positron emission tomography (PET) in combination with computed tomography (CT) in a hybrid imaging modality (PET/CT) offers the unique chance of combining anatomic and functional information of the tumor. PET/CT has been widely investigated in oncology. Some centers routinely use PET imaging when assessing esophageal cancers. However, in some countries, PET is not refunded for this indication as prospective studies are scarce and a positive impact on prognosis by applying this technique has not yet been proven.

This chapter reviews the current literature and attempts to define the role of PET scanning in the management of esophageal cancer. Future clinical research directions in this field are delineated.

2 PET Tracers

The most widely used tracer for PET in oncology is 18F-Fluordeoxyglucose (FDG), which is a glucose analog. It is avidly taken up and retained by most esophageal cancers. About 83–95 % esophageal cancers are FDG avid and therefore can be accurately detected (Flamen et al. 2000; Räsänen et al. 2003).

Other tracers have also been investigated: $3'$-deoxy-$3'$-(18)F-fluorothymidine (FLT) has been reported as stable tracer which accumulates in proliferating tissues and malignant disease (Shields et al. 1998; Shields 2012). A disadvantage of FLT is its high accumulation in the liver which limits its ability to detect liver metastases (Hermann et al. 2007). In a study undertaken in esophageal cancer, uptake of 18F-FDG was shown to be significantly higher compared to 18F-FLT uptake. 18F-FLT scans showed more false-negative findings on the one hand but fewer false-positive findings than 18F-FDG scans on the other hand. Disappointingly, neither uptake of 18F-FDG nor 18F-FLT did correlate with proliferation measured by Ki-67 expression on histopathology (van Westreenen et al. 2005).

3 PET for Staging

Several studies have looked at how PET imaging can improve tumor staging. Due to its physically determined limitations in spatial resolution, PET is per se not a good tool for defining the T category in esophageal cancer where the definition of the T stage is based on the depth of penetration into the esophageal wall. In contrast, PET may add information with regard to N- and M-stage. In a systematic review it was shown that the sensitivity and specificity for CT and PET in lymph node staging (N category) is 51 and 84 %, respectively. For the detection of distant metastases (M category) the corresponding numbers are 67 and 91 %, respectively (van Westreenen et al. 2004). In a more recent meta-analysis the authors come to the conclusion that EUS, CT, and FDG-PET each play a distinctive role in the detection of metastases in esophageal cancer. For the detection of regional lymph node metastases, EUS is the most sensitive investigation, while CT and FDG-PET are more specific. For the assessment of distant metastases, FDG-PET has probably a higher sensitivity than CT. Its combined use could however be of clinical value, with FDG-PET detecting possible metastases and CT confirming or excluding their presence and precisely determining their location (van Vliet et al. 2008). An expert panel recently recommended the use of FDG-PET for the detection of distant metastases in esophageal cancer (Fletcher et al. 2008).

In view of its limited accuracy one may conclude that PET-based treatment decisions have to be taken with some caution. The chance of a false-negative result on FGD-PET is not negligible; therefore, it is recommended that radiation volumes and resection fields should not be downsized based on a negative FDG-PET finding. However, due to the relatively high specificity of FDG-PET enlarging irradiated volumes or extending resections based on positive FDG-PET findings,

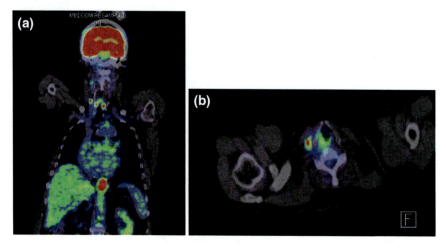

Fig. 1 It shows a positive FDG-PET in the right neck region of a patient presenting with a distal esophageal cancer. In case of a lymph node metastasis this would constitute a distant metastasis (cM1) and esophagectomy would not be indicated. In this particular case histology revealed a lymph node metastasis of a follicular thyroid micro-carcinoma and the patient underwent curative resection of two separate malignant diseases

e.g., in a region without suspected lymph node involvement on CT and/or EUS should be considered (Vrieze et al. 2004).

Of note, the specificity of PET is still limited and false-positive findings are reported in up to 20 % of cases. Therefore, treatment decisions should not be based on PET results alone. Positive findings in PET which would lead to relevant treatment limitations need to be confirmed by other methods, especially by histopathology. Figure 1 gives the example of a positive FDG-PET in the right neck region of a patient who had localized distal esophageal cancer. In case of a lymph node metastasis this finding would define a distant metastasis (cM1). In this particular case histology revealed a lymph node metastasis of a thyroid follicular micro-carcinoma and the patient underwent curative resection for both diseases.

4 PET and Prognosis

Prognosis is linked with the tumor stage on the hand. But an additional question is if the quantification of FDG-uptake gives independent prognostic information.

The standardized uptake value (SUV) is often used for (semi-)quantitative analysis of dynamic data (Schomburg et al. 1996). The SUV is calculated either pixel-wise or over a region of interest (ROI) for each image of a dynamic series at time points (t) as the ratio of tissue radioactivity concentration (e.g. in MBq/kg = kBq/g) at time t, $c(t)$, and injected dose (e.g. in MBq) at the time of injection ($t = 0$) divided by body weight (e.g. in kg). Some authors prefer to use the lean body weight or the body surface area instead of the body weight. Also, for $c(t)$ either the maximum or the mean value of a ROI is taken (Boellard et al. 2004).

In the newer literature, a change from region of Interest-based SUV calculation to volume of Interest-based SUV calculation can be observed (Boellard et al. 2008).

Investigators from New York analyzed 40 patients with esophageal cancer who had undergone FDG-PET scanning prior to primary tumor resection without any neoadjuvant treatment. The median SUV in their patients was found to be 4.5. Patients with a higher SUV had a significantly worse prognosis than patients with a SUV of less than 4.5 (Rizk et al. 2006). The survival advantage of the SUVmax 4.5 or less group was also seen in clinically early-stage patients (defined as no adenopathy on CT and PET, and by EUS (T1-2 N0)), as well as in patients with pathologically early-stage disease (T1-2 N0). This publication indicates that PET may help to identify patients who are usually no candidates for perioperative treatment because their tumor stage is considered as "early" but who might need neoadjuvant chemotherapy or chemoradiation, because their prognosis is worse than expected. This hypothesis would merit to be tested in a prospective trial.

5 PET and Treatment Response

Conventional imaging techniques like CT and endoscopy are of limited value in assessing response to preoperative treatment in esophageal cancer, especially following chemoradiation. Particularly, the discrimination of vital tumor tissue from scar is difficult. Clinical evaluation of dysphagia scores was shown to be meaningless with regard to histopathologic response (Ribi et al. 2009). Even post-treatment cytology and biopsies failed to accurately assess response to preoperative treatment, because residual tumor is often located at the outward areas of the tumor and not within its accessible luminal parts (Peng et al. 2009; Sarkaria et al. 2009).

Recently, PET response criteria in solid tumors (PERCIST 1.0) have been advocated (Wahl et al. 2009). The authors argued that anatomic imaging alone using standard World Health Organization (WHO) criteria, and response criteria in solid tumors (RECIST) have important limitations, particularly in assessing the activity of newer cancer therapies that stabilize disease rather than shrink it. FDG-PET appears particularly valuable in such cases. The proposed PERCIST 1.0 criteria should serve as a starting point for use in clinical trials and in structured quantitative clinical reporting. According to the authors, subsequent revisions and enhancements are to be expected as validation studies are ongoing in several diseases and during different forms of treatment.

5.1 Post-Therapeutic Response Assessment

The value of resection has been called into question in squamous cell cancer of the cervical and intrathoracic esophagus. Being able to predict the true response and prognosis following chemoradiation would be of major importance in order to refine the selection of patients who require surgery.

Table 1 Predictive and prognostic impact of FDG-PET imaging following preoperative chemoradiotherapy in patients with esophageal cancer

Author and year	Tumor	n	Correlation with response	Correlation with prognosis
			p value	p value
Monjazeb et al. (2010)	AC/SCC	163	0.18	0,01
Javeri et al. (2009)	AC	151	0.06	0.01
Vallböhmer et al. (2009)	AC/SCC	119	0.056	n.s.
Kim et al. (2007)	SCC	62	n.d.	0.033
Levine et al. (2006)	AC/SCC	64	0.004	n.d.
Wieder (2004)	SCC	38	0.011	n.d.
Swisher et al. (2004)	AC/SCC	83	0.03	0.01
Downey et al. (2003)	AC/SCC	39	n.d.	0.088
Flamen et al. (2002)	AC/SCC	36	0.001	0.002
Brücher et al. (2001)	SCC	27	0.001	0.001

AC adenocarcinoma; *n* number; *n.d.* not determined; *n.s.* not significant; *SCC* squamous cell cancer

Numerous studies have investigated post-therapeutic PET scanning in order to define the predictive and prognostic value of the test (Table 1). In summary, most studies show a clear correlation of metabolic response as assessed by FDG-PET on the one hand and response and survival on the other hand. One recent study even indicated a relatively strong concordance of 71 % between histopathologic and metabolic complete response (Kim et al. 2007). However, cut-off values that may indicate a correlation with histopathologic complete response have never been validated in prospective studies. Multicenter experience from prospective studies is lacking. Finally, the positive predictive value of the test (i.e., the ability of PET to predict complete histopathologic response) does not seem to be high enough to justify treatment decisions against surgery.

5.2 Pre-Therapeutic Assessment

In an ideal scenario, we would use one pre-therapeutic PET to complement staging and to predict response to any preoperative treatment (chemotherapy or chemoradiation). Some investigators examined the value of pre-therapeutic FDG tumor uptake and treatment response (Table 2). In summary, results are conflicting. While some investigators found a correlation between higher SUV's and response

Table 2 Predictive impact of FDG-PET imaging prior to preoperative chemo- or chemoradiotherapy in patients with esophageal cancer

Author and year	Tumor	n	SUV	Correlation with response
Rizk et al. (2009)	AC	189	Absolute	$P = 0.02$
Javeri et al. (2009)	AC	161	Absolute	$P = 0.06$
Lordick et al. (2007)	AC	110	Median	$P = 0.018$
Levine et al. (2006)	AC/SCC	64	Absolute	$P = 0.005$
Ott et al. (2006)	AC	65	Median	$P = 0.16$
Swisher et al. (2004)	AC/SCC	56	Absolute	$P = 0.56$
Wieder et al. (2004)	SCC	33	Absolute	$P = 0.23$

AC adenocarcinoma; *n* number; *SCC* squamous cell cancer; *SUV* standard uptake value

to subsequent chemo- or chemoradiotherapy, some others did not. Prospective validation studies confirming specific techniques and cut-offs are lacking.

5.3 Early Metabolic Response

Early metabolic response assessment during neoadjuvant chemotherapy of AEG has been intensively studied; cut-offs have been prospectively validated and have also been used in an interventional clinical study (Fig. 2). In consecutive phase II studies the metabolic tumor activity was quantified, defined by the SUV before and during chemotherapy. It was observed that only after 2 weeks of induction chemotherapy significant decreases of SUV were measured. A drop of ≥ 35 % measured after 2 weeks of chemotherapy revealed as the most accurate cut-off value to predict the clinical and histopathological response that was found after 12 weeks of preoperative chemotherapy. Weber et al. first established the cut-off decrease in a retrospective study. Ott et al. performed a prospective validation study of this cut-off (Weber et al. 2001; Ott et al. 2006). The validated cut-off was used in subsequent studies. It was further noticed that the metabolic response to induction chemotherapy was an independent and important prognostic factor in case of locally advanced adenocarcinoma of the oesophago-gastric junction (Ott et al. 2006). Metabolic changes measured by PET were shown to be much more sensitive in detecting response early in the course of chemotherapy as compared to morphologic changes measured by high resolution CT (Wieder et al. 2005). This suggested that PET could be used to tailor treatment according to the chemoresponsiveness of tumors. This concept was realized in the MUNICON trial (Lordick et al. 2007) (Fig. 3). This trial prospectively confirmed that responders to induction chemotherapy can be identified by early metabolic imaging using FDG-PET. The rate of major histopathologic remissions in PET responders was 58 %. The continuation of chemotherapy in the responding population resulted in a favorable outcome: after a follow-up 28 months the median overall survival was

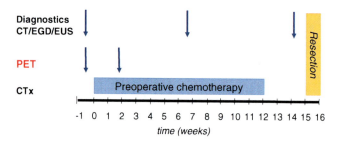

Fig. 2 Schema of the explorative and validation studies for the early metabolic response assessment by PET during neoadjuvant chemotherapy of AEG (Lordick et al. 2007; Ott et al. 2006; Weber et al. 2001). *CT* computed tomography, *CTx* chemotherapy, *EGD* esophago-gastroduodenoscopy, *EUS* endoscopic ultrasound, *PET* positron emission tomography

not reached in PET responders as compared to 26 months in nonresponders. In patients with metabolic nonresponse, chemotherapy could be discontinued at an early stage, thereby saving time, and reducing side effects and costs. Compared to patients from previous studies one can delineate that the outcome of metabolic nonresponders was at least not compromised by the early discontinuation of preoperative treatment. Investigators from the United States validated the −35 % SUV cut-off for patients receiving neoadjuvant chemotherapy. In contrast to the German investigators they did a second PET after having finished induction chemotherapy (which is 6 weeks after its start) and before commencing neoadjuvant chemoradiation (Ilson et al. 2011).

Of note, the concept of early response evaluation was successfully studied in patient receiving chemotherapy without radiation. In contrast, in patients treated with chemotherapy plus radiation therapy, metabolic response assessment during treatment failed to accurately predict tumor response (Gillham et al. 2006; Klaeser et al. 2009; van Heijl et al. 2011). This indicates that cell death induced by radiation therapy may follow different mechanisms and time lines than chemotherapy-induced apoptosis. In addition, radiation induces inflammatory reactions and other phenomena leading to false-positive and false-negative features. Therefore, step-by-step implementation of cut-off values is required when metabolic thresholds for response monitoring are implemented into clinical practice.

6 Conclusions

Current data indicate that FDG-PET ameliorates the staging accuracy in esophageal cancer. The main indication is the exclusion of distant metastases which has an important impact on treatment decisions. Whether PET may serve as a basis for tailoring radiation volumes or defining the extent of surgery should be further studied. In the light of the limited sensitivity of PET in detecting locoregional lymph nodes, the risk of reducing treatment radicality must be carefully weighed against the increased morbidity and mortality associated with surgery and large radiation volumes in the preoperative setting.

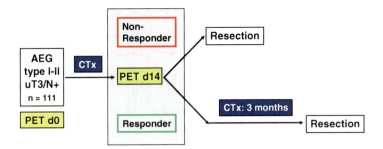

Fig. 3 Design of the MUNICON study (Lordick et al. 2007), *AEG* adenocarcinoma of the esophago-gastric junction, *CTx* chemotherapy, *n* number, *PET* positron emission tomography

High FDG uptake values may indicate a critical prognosis of patients presenting with localized esophageal cancer. This finding may guide the decision for multimodality treatment. This is even more true, as some studies show that patients with FDG-avid tumors have a better response and benefit more from neoadjuvant chemo- or chemoradiotherapy. But cut-off values are not clear at this stage and prospective multicenter studies need to be performed.

Post-therapeutic FDG uptake values have a prognostic impact and correlate with histologic response. However, the limited positive predictive value for complete pathologic response does not allow to taking decisions against surgical resection. But this point certainly merits further investigation, especially in patients presenting with proximal esophageal squamous cell cancer, where the operative risk following chemoradiation is high.

The most exciting use of FDG-PET in the management of esophageal cancer is the early assessment of metabolic response during neoadjuvant chemotherapy. This approach may allow for modifications of the treatment plan in patients who do not respond to chemotherapy. However, it must be taken into account that all data are derived from single-center studies, many data have been gathered with older generations of PET machines (before the era of combined PET-CT) and therefore the multicenter validation of cut-off values and quality control is of major importance. The European organization of research and treatment of cancer (EORTC) is currently planning an international validation trial of the MUNICON findings, using a central imaging platform and central quality assurance of PET and pathologic response criteria (Lordick et al. 2008).

References

Boellaard R, Krak NC, Hoekstra OS et al (2004) Effects of noise, image resolution, and ROI definition on the accuracy of standard uptake values: a simulation study. J Nucl Med 45:1519–1527

Boellaard R, Oyen WJ, Hoekstra CJ et al (2008) The Netherlands protocol for standardisation and quantification of FDG whole body PET studies in multi-centre trials. Eur J Nucl Med Mol Imaging 35:2320–2333

Brücher BL, Weber W, Bauer M et al (2001) Neoadjuvant therapy of esophageal squamous cell carcinoma: response evaluation by positron emission tomography. Ann Surg 233:300–309

Downey RJ, Akhurst T, Ilson D et al (2003) Whole body 18FDG-PET and the response of esophageal cancer to induction therapy: results of a prospective trial. J Clin Oncol 21:428–432

Flamen P, Lerut A, Van Cutsem E et al (2000) Utility of positron emission tomography for the staging of patients with potentially operable esophageal carcinoma. J Clin Oncol 18:3202–3210

Flamen P, Van Cutsem E, Lerut A et al (2002) Positron emission tomography for assessment of the response to induction radiochemotherapy in locally advanced oesophageal cancer. Ann Oncol 13:361–368

Fletcher JW, Djulbegovic B, Soares HP et al (2008) Recommendations on the use of 18F-FDG PET in oncology. J Nucl Med 49:480–508

Gillham CM, Lucey JA, Keogan M et al (2006) (18)FDG uptake during induction chemoradiation for oesophageal cancer fails to predict histomorphological tumour response. Br J Cancer 95:1174–1179

Herrmann K, Ott K, Buck AK et al (2007) Imaging gastric cancer with PET and the radiotracers 18F-FLT and 18F-FDG: a comparative analysis. J Nucl Med 48:1945–1950

Ilson DH, Minsky BD, Ku GY et al (2011) Phase 2 trial of induction and concurrent chemoradiotherapy with weekly irinotecan and cisplatin followed by surgery for esophageal cancer. Cancer. doi: 10.1002/cncr.26591. (Epub ahead of print)

Javeri H, Xiao L, Rohren E et al (2009) The higher the decrease in the standardized uptake value of positron emission tomography after chemoradiation, the better the survival of patients with gastroesophageal adenocarcinoma. Cancer 115:5184–5192

Kim MK, Ryu JS, Kim SB et al (2007) Value of complete metabolic response by (18)F-fluorodeoxyglucose-positron emission tomography in oesophageal cancer for prediction of pathologic response and survival after preoperative chemoradiotherapy. Eur J Cancer 43:1385–1391

Klaeser B, Nitzsche E, Schuller JC et al (2009) Limited predictive value of FDG-PET for response assessment in the preoperative treatment of esophageal cancer: results of a prospective multi-center trial (SAKK 75/02). Onkologie 32:724–730

Levine EA, Farmer MR, Clark P et al (2006) Predictive value of 18-fluoro-deoxy-glucose-positron emission tomography (18F-FDG-PET) in the identification of responders to chemoradiation therapy for the treatment of locally advanced esophageal cancer. Ann Surg 243:472–478

Lordick F, Ott K, Krause BJ et al (2007) PET to assess early metabolic response and to guide treatment of adenocarcinoma of the oesophagogastric junction: the MUNICON phase II trial. Lancet Oncol 8:797–805

Lordick F, Ruers T, Aust DE et al (2008) European organisation of research and treatment of cancer (EORTC) gastrointestinal group: workshop on the role of metabolic imaging in the neoadjuvant treatment of gastrointestinal cancer. Eur J Cancer 44:1807–1819

Monjazeb AM, Riedlinger G, Aklilu M et al (2010) Outcomes of patients with esophageal cancer staged with [^{18}F] fluorodeoxyglucose positron emission tomography (FDG-PET): can postchemoradiotherapy FDG-PET predict the utility of resection. J Clin Oncol 28(31):4714–4721

Ott K, Weber WA, Lordick F et al (2006) Metabolic imaging predicts response, survival, and recurrence in adenocarcinomas of the esophagogastric junction. J Clin Oncol 24:4692–4698

Peng HQ, Halsey K, Sun CC et al (2009) Clinical utility of postchemoradiation endoscopic brush cytology and biopsy in predicting residual esophageal adenocarcinoma. Cancer Cytopathol 117:463–472

Räsänen JV, Sihvo EI, Knuuti MJ et al (2003) Prospective analysis of accuracy of positron emission tomography, computed tomography, and endoscopic ultrasonography in staging of adenocarcinoma of the esophagus and the esophagogastric junction. Ann Surg Oncol 10:954–960

Ribi K, Koeberle D, Schuller JC et al (2009) Is a change in patient-reported dysphagia after induction chemotherapy in locally advanced esophageal cancer a predictive factor for pathological response to neoadjuvant chemoradiation? Support Care Cancer 17:1109–1116

Rizk N, Downey RJ, Akhurst T et al (2006) Preoperative 18[F]-fluorodeoxyglucose positron emission tomography standardized uptake values predict survival after esophageal adenocarcinoma resection. Ann Thorac Surg 81:1076–1081

Rizk NP, Tang L, Adusumilli PS et al (2009) Predictive value of initial PET-SUVmax in patients with locally advanced esophageal and gastroesophageal junction adenocarcinoma. J Thorac Oncol 4:875–879

Sarkaria IS, Rizk NP, Bains MS et al (2009) Post-treatment endoscopic biopsy is a poor-predictor of pathologic response in patients undergoing chemoradiation therapy for esophageal cancer. Ann Surg 249:764–767

Schomburg A, Bender H, Reichel C et al (1996) Standardized uptake values of fluorine-18 fluorodeoxyglucose: the value of different normalization procedures. Eur J Nucl Med 23:571–574

Shields AF (2012) PET imaging of tumor growth: not as easy as it looks. Clin Cancer Res 18:1189–1191

Shields AF, Grierson JR, Dohmen BM et al (1998) Imaging proliferation in vivo with [F-18]FLT and positron emission tomography. Nat Med 4:1334–1336

Swisher SG, Erasmus J, Maish M et al (2004) 2-Fluoro-2-deoxy-D-glucose positron emission tomography imaging is predictive of pathologic response and survival after preoperative chemoradiation in patients with esophageal carcinoma. Cancer 101:1776–1785

Vallböhmer D, Hölscher AH, Dietlein M et al (2009) [18F]-Fluorodeoxyglucose-positron emission tomography for the assessment of histopathologic response and prognosis after completion of neoadjuvant chemoradiation in esophageal cancer. Ann Surg 250:888–894

van Heijl M, Omloo JM, van Berge Henegouwen MI (2011) Fluorodeoxyglucose positron emission tomography for evaluating early response during neoadjuvant chemoradiotherapy in patients with potentially curable esophageal cancer. Ann Surg 253(1):56–63

van Vliet EP, Heijenbrok-Kal MH, Hunink MG et al (2008) Staging investigations for oesophageal cancer: a meta-analysis. Br J Cancer 98:547–557

van Westreenen HL, Cobben DC, Jager PL et al (2005) Comparison of 18F-FLT PET and 18F-FDG PET in esophageal cancer. J Nucl Med 46:400–404

van Westreenen HL, Westerterp M, Bossuyt PM et al (2004) Systematic review of the staging performance of 18F-fluorodeoxyglucose positron emission tomography in esophageal cancer. J Clin Oncol 22:3805–3812

Vrieze O, Haustermans K, De Wever W et al (2004) Is there a role for FGD-PET in radiotherapy planning in esophageal carcinoma? Radiother Oncol 73:269–275

Wahl RL, Jacene H, Kasamon Y, Lodge MA (2009) From RECIST to PERCIST: evolving considerations for PET response criteria in solid tumors. J Nucl Med 50(Suppl 1):122S–150S

Weber WA, Ott K, Becker K et al (2001) Prediction of response to preoperative chemotherapy in adenocarcinomas of the esophagogastric junction by metabolic imaging. J Clin Oncol 19:3058–3065

Wieder HA, Beer AJ, Lordick F et al (2005) Comparison of changes in tumor metabolic activity and tumor size during chemotherapy of adenocarcinomas of the esophagogastric junction. J Nucl Med 46:2029–2034

Part VI
Gastric Cancer

Optimal Surgery for Gastric Cancer: Is More Always Better?

William H. Allum

Abstract

The extent of surgical resection for carcinoma of the stomach has been debated for many years. The aims of surgery are to obtain complete histopathological clearance of all possible sites of disease based on oncological principles. This has included radical resection of the primary site with combined organ resection as required and resection of associated lymph nodes. Detailed understanding of the natural history of gastric cancer has resulted in the Pichlmayr total gastrectomy "en principe" approach being super-ceded by a tailored approach according to tumour and patient characteristics. Careful tumour staging is fundamental to the selection of surgical intervention. Endoscopic therapy is recommended for well differentiated, mucosal cancers less than 2 cm in size as the risk of nodal disease is 0–3 %. Recently, these criteria have been extended to include some larger and ulcerated cancers. Although extended lymphadenectomy has formed the basis of radical surgery, Japanese experience has also confirmed that for early gastric cancer involving the submucosa limited nodal resection can achieve the same outcome as standardised D2 lymphadenectomy. The approach to locally advanced T2, T3 and some T4 cancers has been defined by the Japanese rules specifying proximal and distal margins as well as extent of lymph node resection. Translation of Japanese results to Western patients has not been straightforward. Two randomised controlled trials have shown limited or no benefit over conventional limited nodal dissection. However, these studies have not been without criticism and individual specialist practice in the West now preferentially includes D2 lymphadenectomy in suitable patients. Extending conventional D2 lymphadenectomy has been evaluated but the results are not conclusive. Japanese

W. H. Allum (✉)
Royal Marsden NHS Foundation Trust, London, UK
e-mail: William.Allum@rmh.nhs.uk

F. Otto and M. P. Lutz (eds.), *Early Gastrointestinal Cancers*,
Recent Results in Cancer Research 196, DOI: 10.1007/978-3-642-31629-6_15,
© Springer-Verlag Berlin Heidelberg 2012

RCTs have not shown an advantage but in selected cases several groups have reported a benefit. Historically, radical gastric surgery in the West was associated with significant morbidity and mortality reflecting the comorbidity of the patient groups. Perioperative approaches have shown that outcome approaching that of radical surgery can be achieved with multimodal therapies for high-risk patient groups for whom radical surgery would be contraindicated. Surgery for gastric cancer needs to be determined by a multidisciplinary team to ensure appropriate procedure selection for an individual patient. This allows all relevant information to be considered and to provide the best chance for high-quality patient outcome.

Contents

1	Introduction	216
2	Surgical Anatomy	216
3	Characteristics of the Primary Tumour	218
	3.1 T1 Disease	219
	3.2 T2 and T3 Disease	221
	3.3 T4 Disease	222
	3.4 Extended Lymphadenectomy	223
	3.5 Metastatic Disease	224
4	Patient Factors	225
5	Conclusions	225
	References	226

1 Introduction

The aims of surgery for carcinoma of the stomach are to obtain complete histopathological clearance of all possible sites of disease based on oncological principles. This includes radical resection of the primary site with combined organ resection as required and resection of associated lymph nodes. A "potentially curative" (R0) resection is defined as a surgical procedure in which there is no evidence of macroscopic residual tumour in the tumour bed, lymph nodes and/or distant sites with microscopic negative resection margins (Hermanek 1995). Careful tumour staging is fundamental to the selection of surgical intervention. In addition, detailed histopathological features now define the most appropriate operative treatment ranging from endoscopic resection to limited gastric resection to extended gastric resection and extended lymphadenectomy (D2). This discussion addresses the evidence for treatment selection and places it in the context of non-surgical treatments and patient factors.

2 Surgical Anatomy

The inclusion of appropriate lymphadenectomy has been the key factor in loco-regional control and associated improved outcome in gastric cancer surgery. Autopsy and reoperation series (McNeer et al. 1951; Gunderson and Sosin 1982)

Optimal Surgery for Gastric Cancer

Table 1 Nodal stations to be excised according to extent of gastrectomy

	D1	D1+	D2
Total gastrectomy	1, 2, 3, 4sa, 4sb, 4d, 5,6, 7	8a, 9, 11p	10, 11d, 12a
Distal gastrectomy	1, 3, 4sb, 4d, 5, 6,7	8a, 9	11p, 12a

studies clearly demonstrated the high risk of recurrence within the gastric bed following limited gastrectomy and related this to residual lymph node disease. It is essential therefore to appreciate the anatomy of lymphatic drainage of the stomach in planning strategy for gastric cancer surgery.

Detailed electron microscopy has demonstrated networks of lymphatics in the layers of the submucosa, the muscularis propria and the subserosa which connect to extramural perigastric lymph nodes. Cancer cells gain access to the lymphatics and are carried by lymphatic flow to the regional nodes. Extended systematic nodal dissection is aimed to resect involved nodes and microscopic metastatic disease which may have spread beyond the range of detectable gross disease. There is evidence of natural regression of isolated tumour cells by natural killer cell activity but also proliferation of micrometastases from in vivo gastric cell line studies (Yokoyama et al. 2006).

These meticulous studies, which have been incorporated into the Japanese classification of gastric cancer (JCGC) (2011), have defined the pattern of lymph node spread according to tumour site and classified the associated tiers of lymph nodes. This approach has been based on the incidence of metastases to individual lymph node stations and the proportion of long-term survivors with metastases in those stations. A prerequisite to this evidence is the nodal dissection according to the anatomical nodal stations. The Japanese rules have defined the nodal stations to be included in a specific level of dissection, the most frequent being D2. Latterly, however, the focus on the anatomical stations has shifted as the main prognostic factor is the number of nodes involved by metastasis. The current TNM Classification (7th Edition, Sobin et al 2009) for gastric cancer describes nodal staging according to the number involved and defines that a minimum of 15 nodes should be examined for adequate staging. This has limitations because such a number may be insufficient to include nodes with microscopic metastatic foci. A surrogate for a formal D2 dissection has been the recommendation to resect a minimum of 25 nodes. This may be achieved without necessarily performing a lymphadenectomy radical enough to include the at risk nodal stations. The JCGC (2011) has defined which nodal stations should be excised according to the type of gastrectomy (Table 1). Despite these recommendations, it is still relevant to appreciate which anatomical groups are relevant in the context of a particular tumour site (Table 2).

The JCGC has divided the stomach into thirds, upper (C), middle (M) and lower (A). This division designates the associated lymph node stations and can be the sole site or a combination. The anatomical distribution of regional lymph nodes can be considered in three groups: around the left gastric artery, around the splenic

Table 2 Nodal tiers according to site of tumour

	N1	N2	N3	M
Upper third	1, 2, 3, 4sa, 4sb	4d, 7, 8a, 9, 10, 11p, 11d,	5, 6, 12a, 16	14v
Upper/middle third	1, 2, 3, 4sa, 4sb, 4d, 5, 6	7, 8a, 9, 10, 11p, 11d, 12a	14v, 16	
Middle/lower third	1, 3, 4sb, 4d, 5, 6	7, 8a, 9, 11p, 12a	2, 4sa, 19, 11d, 14v, 16	
Lower third	3, 4d, 5, 6	1, 7, 8a, 9, 11p, 12a, 14v	4sb, 16	2, 10, 11d

artery and around the common hepatic artery. Those around the left gastric artery drain lymphatics from the pericardial nodes and the lesser curve nodes including anterior and posterior aspects of the upper third of the stomach. Those around the splenic artery drain the upper greater curvature principally via the short gastric vessels and the left gastro-epiploic artery, the splenic hilum and the posterior proximal stomach via the posterior gastric artery. The group around the common hepatic artery drain the distal third of the stomach via nodes associated with the right gastric artery and the right gastroepiploic artery (the supra and infra pyloric nodes respectively) and the lower greater curvature. Flow from the nodes along the hepatoduodenal ligament and the surface of the head of the pancreas also drains into the common hepatic group. These three major groups drain to the para-aortic nodes either via the coeliac axis nodes or via the superior mesenteric artery nodes or directly particularly from the splenic artery or retrohepatic and retro-pancreatic nodes.

Nodal involvement in stations distant from the stomach reflects metastatic disease, which is unlikely to be appropriate for radical surgery and associated with a poor outcome. However, absence of nodal disease in local nodes associated with small cancers supports much less invasive procedures and may exclude the need for nodal dissection completely. The results of more extended nodal dissection need to be considered in the context of patient factors, low morbidity procedures and outcome of non-surgical therapies. However, the surgical results according to the JCGC are the benchmark against which combination therapies need to be considered.

3 Characteristics of the Primary Tumour

The factors which influence treatment of the primary site include anatomical position within the stomach, tumour size, macrosopic appearance including local infiltration and microscopic histological subtype. The at risk lymph node stations and the planned lymphadenectomy are directly linked to the selection of primary excision.

Fig. 1 Classification of early gastric cancer

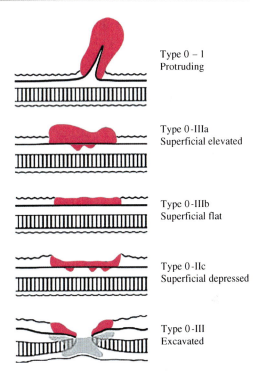

3.1 T1 Disease

The diagnosis and classification of T1 tumours is based on endoscopic appearance (Fig. 1). Additional information of the depth of penetration is possible with endoscopic ultrasound, although there can be limitations with associated ulceration and excavation. Careful histopathological examination is essential to establish detail of differentiation. Combination of these criteria allows a prediction of associated lymph node metastasis and guide the selection of endoscopic therapy.

3.1.1 Endoscopic Therapy
Tada and colleagues (2000) established the indications for endoscopic therapy are:
1. well-differentiated adenocarcinoma
2. tumour size <20 mm in elevated type
3. tumour size <10 mm in depressed type
4. no associated ulceration
5. invasion limited histologically to the mucosa

The associated lymph node metastatic risk is virtually zero for this group. Detail from large surgical series has allowed expansion of these criteria based on the absence of lymph node disease (Gotoda et al. 2000). Current criteria for endoscopic therapy are:
1. well-differentiated adenocarcinoma
2. no lymphatic or venous invasion

3. intramucosal cancer regardless of size without ulceration
4. intramucosal cancer <30 mm with ulceration
5. minute submucosal penetration (sm1) and <30 mm

Although small polypoidal lesions can be resected by mucosal resection (EMR), detail of depth of penetration of flatter lesions requires the more advanced intervention of submucosal dissection (ESD) with en bloc removal. Most series report up to 98 % completeness of resection after ESD (Oda et al. 2005) contrasting with 74–90 % after EMR (Kojima et al. 1998; Giovanni 1999). In addition, ESD provides a more complete pathological specimen as EMR can remove tumours piecemeal with potential risk to margins. Series after EMR have reported 4 % recurrence rates after up to 5-year follow-up which may be treated by repeated endoscopic resection or by resectional surgery (Ida et al. 2004).

Survival after endoscopic therapy is equivalent to surgery in this selected group of patients. Long-term survival was reported equivalent in those under 65 years (EMR 92.8 %; Surgery 91.9 %) (Fukase et al. 1994) and slightly longer in those over 65 years (EMR 80.8 %; Surgery 75 %) with better recurrence free 3-year survival after ESD (ESD 97.6 %; EMR 92.5 %) (Oda et al. 2006).

3.1.2 Surgery

T1 tumours which do not fulfil the criteria for endoscopic therapy have been traditionally treated by radical surgery. However, careful lymph node mapping has identified the lymph node groups at risk and as a result lesser procedures are now appropriate as results are the same as conventional nodal dissection. For mucosal disease lymph node dissection should include N1 tier nodes together with left gastric artery nodes (station 7) and common hepatic artery nodes (station 8) (D1 alpha). For submucosal disease inclusion of the coeliac axis (station 9) and proximal splenic artery nodes (station 11p) with D1 alpha is required (D1beta). Current interest in sentinel lymph node mapping may modify these approaches and the outcome of current trials is awaited.

The excellent outcome of treatment of early gastric cancer has also promoted approaches for lesser gastric resection to minimise the adverse effects on gastric function. Wedge excision of small tumours, pylorus preserving gastrectomy and proximal gastrectomy, are all potential options. Wedge excision is reserved for those early tumours that cannot be safely excised endoscopically and the technique can include combined endoscopic and laparoscopic approaches. A disadvantage is ensuring adequate microscopic margins and limited series have reported problems with resection margin recurrence (Nozaki et al. 2008). Pylorus preserving gastrectomy combined with vagal sparing is indicated for mid-body early gastric cancer as the associated incidence of suprapyloric lymph node involvement is very low. It is important to preserve a prepyloric cuff of 2–5 cm to prevent rapid gastric emptying. Post-prandial dumping and biliary reflux are decreased and maintenance of body weight is as good as after conventional resection with equivalent survival (Morita et al. 2008). Proximal gastrectomy is indicated for early proximal third cancers as this maintains both the gastric reservoir and pylorus function. This, however, can have the potential for significant symptomatic reflux and an anti-reflux procedure should be included with this approach.

3.2 T2 and T3 Disease

3.2.1 Extent of Lymphadenectomy

The JCGC has clearly established that resection of the stomach with an appropriate margin together with surrounding omenta and the first two nodal tiers by systematic lymph node dissection (D2 resection) is a curative procedure for gastric cancer. It has been challenging for surgeons in the West to emulate the achievements of their Japanese counterparts. Individual surgical series have shown similar outcomes (Sue-Ling et al. 1993; Siewert et al. 1993). However, adoption of D2 resection by all surgeons has been limited without the preferred evidence from randomised controlled trials (RCTs). The Dutch (Bonenkamp et al. 1999) and the UK Medical Research Council (Cuschieri et al. 1999) trials showed little difference in initial outcome between traditional D1 and D2 lymphadenectomy. Long-term follow-up of the Dutch trial, however, has reported better gastric cancer related survival after D2 (Songun et al. 2010). The apparent lack of benefit from the two European trials has been carefully considered. The high operative mortality compared to Japanese experience is a key factor and many have speculated that this reflected limited experience in the technical aspects of the surgery. The inclusion of splenectomy and excision of the tail of the pancreas was certainly shown to be an adverse factor in the UK trial despite the intention to resect splenic hilar nodes.

Subsequent experience in Europe has shown that equivalent results to the Far East can be achieved in specialist centres. Operative mortality results of less than 5 % have been reported with equivalent survival. In the UK, there has been a policy of centralisation of oesophageal and gastric cancer surgery since 2001. Recent data from a national audit have shown that 30-day mortality is now 4.2 % for gastric resection (National Oesophago-Gastric Cancer Audit 2009). The results of the Italian gastric cancer study group trial of D1 versus D2 is keenly awaited. The interim report showed a 30-day mortality for D1 of 3 % and for D2 of 2.2 % (Degiuli et al. 2010). The phase II initial study demonstrated a 5-year survival of 55 % for D2 (Degiuli et al. 2004). It would, thus, seem that Japanese results can be achieved in Western patients at least in terms of operative outcome and this is likely to reflect not only better technical ability, but also greater and more effective management of postoperative complications. Most would now accept that D2 resection is the procedure of choice in appropriate patients.

3.2.2 Extent of Gastric Resection

Detail of the position and histological subtype is important in the decision on the extent of resection. The Japanese classification stipulates a margin of 2 cm for resection of early gastric cancer. For locally advanced disease the recommendation is for 5 cm proximal clearance. If this margin includes the oesophago-gastric junction then a total gastrectomy should be performed. The outcome with diffuse and signet ring cell type cancer is poorer overall than for intestinal type reflecting submucosal permeation of cancer cells. As a result a margin of 8 cm has been advocated for diffuse type cancers. Thus, for most such cancers a subtotal resection will only be possible for very distally situated tumours.

3.2.3 Cardia and Subcardia Cancers

Proximal gastric cancers are an increasing problem with the migration of both oesophageal and gastric cancers to the oesophago-gastric junction particularly in Western countries. The approach to subcardial or Siewert type III cancers has been a source of controversy. The incidence of lower mediastinal node metastases has been variably reported from 10–40 %. The issue is how to ensure resection of these nodes and to achieve a clear margin with low morbidity particularly from anastomotic dehiscence. The Japanese clinical outcome group (JCOG) has performed a RCT including 167 patients assigned either to left thoraco-abdominal resection (LTA) or to trans-hiatal resection (TH) (Sasako et al. 2006). Perioperative mortality and morbidity were greater for LTA (Mortality: LTA—4 %; TH—0 %; Morbidity: LTA—49 %; TH—34 %). In addition, 5-year survival was less for LTA (37.7 %) compared with TH (52.3 %). Although this supports a trans-hiatal approach for these cancers with an extended total gastrectomy, there can be practical difficulties in endoscopic diagnosis differentiating cardia and subcardia cancers. In addition, there can be difficulties with submucosal cranial spread with diffuse type cancers and some have advocated formal oesophago-gastrectomy for these tumours with combined radical abdominal and mediastinal lymphadenectomy

3.2.4 Splenectomy

The European trials included splenectomy and distal pancreatectomy in the initial protocol in order to remove distal splenic artery and splenic hilar nodes. Retrospective data from Japan had shown that 20–30 % of patients with locally advanced proximal gastric cancer have splenic hilar metastases. The adverse effect of splenectomy on operative mortality in the Dutch and UK trials has prompted the Japanese Clinical Oncology Group (JCOG) to assess the role of splenectomy in patients undergoing total gastrectomy. Interim results of a RCT with 505 patients have shown similar operative mortality but greater postoperative morbidity and intraoperative blood loss in those undergoing splenectomy (Sano et al. 2010). The effect on overall survival is awaited.

3.3 T4 Disease

T4 disease is defined as tumour infiltrating or adherent to adjacent organs and/or structures with or without lymph node involvement in the absence of distant metastases. The aim of resection is to achieve microscopic clearance. The potential for microscopic clearance is frequently not possible to identify from preoperative assessment. Therefore, the rationale for multivisceral resection is that dissection between the stomach and the adjacent organs should be avoided to minimise residual microscopic disease. Thus en bloc resection of involved organs is recommended. The difficulty is the potential for postoperative complications particularly if the liver, pancreas or transverse colon are involved. Historical series have clearly shown that multivisceral resection is associated with poor outcome. However, more recently similar results in terms of early outcome have been reported for more radical procedures (Kim et al. 2009).

Long-term survival following multivisceral resection appears to be specifically related to the completeness of resection. The 5-year survival of patients undergoing an R0 resection is 23–46 % compared to 0–17.5 % for R1/2 resection (Jeong et al. 2009). There appears to be little effect with the number of organs resected nor the specific organs resected. Although extended resections are associated with increased perioperative morbidity that they are indicated in patients with good performance status, without distant metastases or peritoneal seeding and a strong likelihood of a complete R0 resection. It should be stressed that such radical surgery should only be undertaken by experienced surgeons in specialised institutions.

Linitus plastica presents a specific problem in gastric cancer surgery. The majority of cases are diffusely infiltrative with locally advanced disease at presentation for which little can be offered apart from symptomatic palliation. Some are indolent in development and radical resection is possible although the outcome is generally poor. Historically, left upper abdominal exenteration has been performed but current perioperative chemotherapy regimens in combination with surgery may be considered in specific cases as quality of life may be improved. The JCOG is currently recruiting to a trial including S-1 chemotherapy (JCOG trial 0110).

3.4 Extended Lymphadenectomy

The pattern of spread to nodal tiers beyond the first two tiers has already been described. The Japanese classification has demonstrated that the incidence of micrometastases to the para-aortic nodes varies from 10 to 30 % in T3 and T4 disease. Individual institution series have reported 5-year survival rates up to 20 % after radical resection of para-aortic nodes.

A number of studies have been undertaken to determine whether there is a role for more extended nodal dissection. Wu and colleagues (2006) reported their experience in a RCT comparing D1 with D3. This showed a clear advantage for D3 dissection (5-year survival: D3 59.5 %; D1 53.6 %. $p = 0.041$). This study, however, defined D3 dissection as a conventional D2 but including hepatoduodenal ligament nodes (station 12), retropancreatic nodes (station 13) and superior mesenteric vein nodes (station 14v).

The JCOG has reported their experience in a RCT of D2 and D2 with para-aortic node dissection (PAND) in patient with T2 ($n = 196$), T3 and T4 ($n = 326$) disease (Sasako et al. 2008). The D2 dissection included stations 12, 13 and 14v for antral cancers treated with subtotal gastrectomy and the PAND specifically included the para-aortic nodes (station 16). Patients undergoing the more radical procedure had a higher rate of surgery-related complications with a greater intraoperative blood loss. There was no difference in overall 5-year survival between the two groups (D2: 69.2 %; D2 and PAND 70.3 %). Slightly, paradoxically D2 and PAND was associated with a better survival in pathologically node negative patients (D2 78.4 %; D2 and PAND 96.8 %) contrasting with survival in node positive patients (D2 65.2 %; D2 and PAND 54.9 %). A limitation of the study is lower than the expected incidence of para-aortic nodal metastases of 8.5 %. Despite this lower incidence 5-year survival in those with para-aortic metastases was 18 %.

The Italian Research Group for Gastric Cancer has reported their experience with N3 dissection which has been introduced to routine practice (Roviello et al. 2010). Para-aortic nodal disease occurred in 13 % of 286 patients with locally advanced disease occurred in 13 %. These were most frequently observed in patients with upper third cancers. Overall 5-year survival for T2-4 cancer with R0 resection was 52 %. In patients with para-aortic nodal involvement 5-year survival was 17.1 %. This group has further defined risk groups for para-aortic node involvement (De Manzoni et al. 2011). The high risk group (42 % chance) included T3/4 cancers with mixed or diffuse histology arising from the upper third of the stomach. The low risk group (0–10 % chance) included middle and lower third cancers, T2 irrespective of histology or T3/4 with intestinal type tumours. The intermediate risk (16–30 % chance) included all other cancers. Para-aortic nodal metastases were common in the presence of metastases in stations 1, 3 and 7, but never occurred if stations 1 and 3 were both negative.

The implications of these varying data are that there is no role for prophylactic para-aortic nodal dissection. However, it does appear that there is a potential advantage in certain groups of patients. This should be considered further for careful study in the context of randomised trials but also should be considered in the context of the effect of perioperative therapies. PAND is not a procedure for the inexperienced surgeon and combination therapies may be less complicated.

3.5   Metastatic Disease

The biological behaviour of gastric cancer largely precludes surgery in the presence of metastatic disease. However, a number of studies have shown that surgery may be used with benefit in selected cases. Studies of unselected groups of patients with synchronous hepatic metastases have shown some limited benefit if strict criteria are applied. In a systematic review, Kerkar and colleagues (2010) reported from 19 studies including 436 patients and described 5-year survival of 13.4 % in highly selected patients. Ueda and colleagues (2009) reported that small size and solitary deposits with no or limited (N1) nodal disease were favourable independent prognostic factors and recommended that such patients with synchronous metastases should be considered for hepatic resection.

Surgery also has a role in selected patients with isolated metastatic disease. As part of the cohort of patients in the Dutch D1/D2 trial Hartgrink and colleagues (Hartgrink et al. 2002) have reported on the group excluded because of metastatic disease. In those with isolated peritoneal disease and small volume hepatic or distant nodal metastases resection was associated with a prolonged median survival in comparison to no resection (10.5 months versus 6.7 months). This benefit was particularly marked in those under 70 years.

4   Patient Factors

A recurrent theme in this discussion has been the associated risk of postoperative complications for patients undergoing radical gastric resection and systematic lymphadenectomy. In their initial report on the D2 and PAND trial JCOG defined risk factors for postoperative complications. In a multivariate analysis the addition of pancreatic resection, patient age and obesity was significant adverse prognostic factors. Many patients have significant cardiovascular and respiratory comorbidity. Careful assessment of comorbidity and its optimisation is essential in planning selection of surgical treatment. The use of cardio-pulmonary exercise testing has been useful in determining level of risk for an individual patient in order to discuss treatment options (Older et al. 2000). The results of perioperative therapy studies including the US Intergroup study of adjuvant chemo-radiation (McDonald et al. 2001) and the UK MAGIC trial (Cunningham et al. 2006) of perioperative chemotherapy have shown how benefit can be achieved with combination therapy. It would, thus, seem appropriate to consider these approaches in patients whose general fitness precludes radical surgery as their chances of satisfactory outcome were they to develop postoperative complications would be significantly reduced. The principle of tailoring treatments for the best benefit in individual patients should be carefully considered by the multidisciplinary team (Sano 2007).

5   Conclusions

Surgical treatment of gastric cancer combines a series of options depending on the pre-operative stage with emphasis on the likelihood of lymph node metastasis. Early gastric cancer can be treated endoscopically or by limited gastric resection and lymph node dissection. Locally, advanced disease requires radical resection with lymphadenectomy according to the predicted pattern of lymph node spread. Perioperative therapies should be considered in these patients. Proximal gastric cancer is preferentially managed as an abdominal transhiatal procedure. Evidence for more extended lymph node dissection is not sufficiently robust to recommend as a standard, although there may be subgroups for whom it should be considered. In advanced and metastatic disease surgery should be carefully considered in very selected patients and should be combined with neoadjuvant and adjuvant therapies.

References

Bonenkamp JJ, Hermans J, Sasako M et al (1999) Extended lymph-node dissection for gastric cancer. N Engl J Med 340:908–914

Cunningham D, Allum WH, Stenning SP et al (2006) Perioperative chemotherapy versus surgery alone for resectable gastroesophageal cancer. N Engl J Med 355:11–20

Cuschieri A, Weeden S, Fielding J et al (1999) Patient survival after D1 and D2 resections for gastric cancer: long-term results of the MRC randomized surgical trial. Surgical co-operative group. Br J Cancer 79:1522–1530

De Manzoni G, Di Leo A, Roviello F et al (2011) Tumour site and perigastric nodal status are the most important predictors of para-aortic nodal involvement in advanced gastric cancer. Ann Surg Oncol 18:2273–2280

Degiuli M, Sasako M, Ponti A, Calvo F (2004) Survival results of a multicentre phase II study to evaluate D2 gastrectomy for gastric cancer. Br J Cancer 90:1727–1732

Degiuli M, Sasako M, Ponti A (2010) Morbidity and mortality in the Italian gastric cancer study group randomized clinical trial of D1 versus D2 resection for gastric cancer. Br J Surg 97:643–649

Fukase K, Matsuda T, Suzuki M et al (1994) Evaluation of the efficacy of endoscopic treatment of gastric cancer considered in terms of long term prognosis. A comparison with surgical treatment. Dig Endosc 6:241–247

Giovannini M, Berrardini D, Moutardier V et al (1999) Endoscopic mucosal resection (EMR): results and prognostic factors in 21 patients. Endoscopy 31:698–701

Gotoda T, Yanagisawa A, Sasako M et al (2000) Incidence of lymph node metastasis from early gastric cancer: estimation with a large number of cases at 2 centres. Gastric Cancer 3:219–225

Gunderson L, Sosin H (1982) Adenocarcinoma of the stomach: areas of failure in a reoperation series (second or symptomatic look) clinicopathological correlation and implications for adjuvant therapy. Int J Radiat Oncol Biol Phys 8:1–11

Hartgrink HH, Putter H, Klein Kranenbarg E (2002) Value of palliative resection in gastric cancer. Br J Surg 89:1438–1443

Hermanek P (1995) pTNM and residual classifications: problems of assessment and prognostic significance. World J Surg 19:184–190

Ida K, Kakazawa S, Yoshino J et al (2004) Multicentre collaborative prospective study of endoscopic treatment of early gastric cancer. Dig Endosc 16:295–302

Japanese Gastric Cancer Association (2011) Japanese classification of gastric carcinoma—3rd English edition. Gastric Cancer 14:101–112

Jeong O, Choi WY, Park YK (2009) Appropriate selection of patients for combined organ resection in cases of gastric carcinoma invading adjacent organs. J Surg Oncol 100:115–120

Kerkar SO, Kemp CD, Avital I (2010) Liver resections in metastatic gastric cancer HPB 12: 589–596

Kim JH, Jang YJ, Park SS et al (2009) Surgical outcomes and prognostic factors for T4 gastric cancers. Asian J Surg 32:198–204

Kojima T, Parra-Blanco A, Takahashi H, Fujita R (1998) Outcome of endoscopic resection for early gastric cancer: review of the Japanese literature. Gastrointestinal Endosc 48:550–555

Macdonald JS, Smalley SR, Benedetti J et al (2001) Chemoradiotherapy after surgery compared with surgery alone for adenocarcinoma of the stomach or gastroesophageal junction. N Engl J Med 345:725–730

McNeer G, Vandenberg H, Donn FY, Bowden LA (1951) A critical evaluation of subtotal gastrectomy for the cure of cancer of the stomach. Ann Surg 134:2–7

Morita S, Katai H, Saka M et al (2008) Outcome of pylorus-preserving gastrectomy for early gastric cancer. Br J Surg 95:1131–1135

National Oesophago-Gastric Cancer Audit (2009) Second annual report. The NHS Information Centre, UK

Nozaki I, Kubo Y, Kurita A et al (2008) Long term outcome after laparoscopic wedge resection for early gastric cancer. Surg Endosc 22:2665–2669

Oda I, Gotada T, Hamanaka H et al (2005) Endoscopic mucosal dissection for early gastric cancer: technical feasibility, operation time and complications from a large consecutive series. Dig Endosc 17:54–58

Oda I, Saito D, Tada M et al (2006) A multicentre retrospective study of endoscopic resection for early gastric cancer. Gastric Cancer 9:262–270

Older P, Smith R, Hall A et al (2000) Preoperative cardiopulmonary risk assessment by cardiopulmonary exercise testing. Crit Care Resusc 2:198–208

Roviello F, Pedrazzani C, Marrelli D et al (2010) Super-extended (D3) lymphadenectomy in advanced gastric cancer. Eur J Surg Oncol 36:439–446

Sano T (2007) Tailoring treatments for curable gastric cancer. Br J Surg 94:263–264

Sano T, Sasako M, Shibata S et al (2010) Randomized controlled trial to evaluate splenectomy in total gastrectomy for proximal gastric carcinoma (JCOG 0110): analyzes of operative morbidity, operation time, and blood loss. J Clin Oncol 28:15s. Abstract 4020

Sasako M, Sano T, Yamamoto S et al (2006) Left thoraco-abdominal approach versus abdominal transhiatal approach for gastric cancer of the cardia or subcardia: a randomised trial. Lancet Oncol 7:644–651

Sasako M, Sano T, Yamamoto S (2008) D2 lymphadenectomy alone or with para-aortic nodal dissection for gastric cancer. N Engl J Med 359:453–462

Siewert JR, Bottcher K, Roder JD et al (1993) Prognostic relevance of systematic lymph node dissection in gastric carcinoma. German gastric carcinoma study group. Br J Surg 80:1015–1018

Sobin LH, Gospodarowicz MK, Wittekind C (2009) TNM Classification of malignant tumours, 7th edn. Wiley-Blackwell, John Wiley & Sons, Chichester

Songun I, Putter H, Kranenbarg EM et al (2010) Surgical treatment of gastric cancer: 15-year follow-up results of the randomised nationwide Dutch D1D2 trial. Lancet Oncol 11:439–449

Sue-Ling HM, Johnston D, Martin IG et al (1993) Gastric cancer: a curable disease. Br Med J 307:591–596

Tada M, Tanaka Y, Matsuo N et al (2000) Mucosectomy for gastric cancer. Current status in Japan. J Gastroenterol Hepatol 15:D98–D102

Ueda K, Iwahashi M, Nakamori M et al (2009) Analysis of the prognostic factors and evaluation of surgical treatment for synchronous liver metastases from gastric cancer. Langenbecks Arch Surg 394:647–653

Wu CW, Hsiung CA, Lo SS et al (2006) Nodal dissection for patients with gastric cancer: a randomised controlled trial. Lancet Oncol 7:309–315

Yokoyama H, Ikehara T, Kodera Y et al (2006) Biological significance of isolated tumour cells and micrometastasis in lymph nodes evaluated using a green fluorescent protein-tagged human gastric cancer cell line. Clin Cancer Res 15:361–368

Can Adjuvant Chemoradiotherapy Replace Extended Lymph Node Dissection in Gastric Cancer?

Edwin P. M. Jansen, Henk Boot, Cornelis J. H. van de Velde, Johanna van Sandick, Annemieke Cats and Marcel Verheij

Abstract

Surgical resection remains the essential part in the curative treatment of gastric cancer. However, with surgery only, long-term survival is poor (5-year survival <25 % in Europe). Randomized studies, which compared limited (D1) lymph node dissection with more extended (D2) resections in the Western world, failed to show a survival benefit for more extensive surgery. A substantial increase in survival was found with perioperative chemotherapy in the MAGIC study. In addition, the SWOG/Intergroup 0116 study showed that postoperative chemoradiotherapy (CRT) prolonged 5-year overall survival compared to surgery only. However, it has been argued that surgical undertreatment undermined survival in this trial. In a randomized Korean study, patients with

---

E. P. M. Jansen (✉) · M. Verheij
Department of Radiotherapy, Antoni van Leeuwenhoek Hospital,
The Netherlands Cancer Institute, Plesmanlaan 121,
1066 CX, Amsterdam, The Netherlands
e-mail: epm.jansen@nki.nl

H. Boot · A. Cats
Department of Gastroenterology, Antoni van Leeuwenhoek Hospital,
The Netherlands Cancer Institute, Plesmanlaan 121,
1066 CX, Amsterdam, The Netherlands

J. van Sandick
Department of Surgery, Antoni van Leeuwenhoek Hospital,
The Netherlands Cancer Institute, Plesmanlaan 121,
1066 CX, Amsterdam, The Netherlands

C. J. H. van de Velde
Department of Surgery,
Leiden University Medical Center, Leiden, The Netherlands

F. Otto and M. P. Lutz (eds.), *Early Gastrointestinal Cancers*,
Recent Results in Cancer Research 196, DOI: 10.1007/978-3-642-31629-6_16,
© Springer-Verlag Berlin Heidelberg 2012

advanced stage gastric cancer who received postoperative CRT had better outcome after a D2 dissection. At our institute phase I-II studies with adjuvant cisplatin and capecitabine-based CRT have been performed in over 120 patients with resected gastric cancer. Retrospective comparison of patients treated in these studies with those that had surgery only in the D1D2 study, demonstrated that postoperative CRT was associated with better outcome, especially after D1 or a R1 resection. For daily practice, it remains unclear whether patients after optimal (D2) gastric surgery will benefit from postoperative CRT. This is currently being tested in prospective randomized phase III trials (CRITICS; TOPGEAR).

Contents

1 Introduction.. 230
2 Surgery... 231
3 Chemotherapy... 232
4 Chemoradiotherapy.. 233
5 R1-Resection... 235
6 Conclusion 237
References... 237

1 Introduction

Surgical resection remains the essential part in the curative treatment of gastric cancer (Hartgrink et al. 2009). Because of poor long-term survival and high locoregional recurrence rates in Europe and North America, several (neo) adjuvant strategies as well as more extensive surgery have been evaluated during the last three decades. Intensification of surgery by means of extended lymph node dissection did not improve survival in non-Asian countries. On the contrary, perioperative chemotherapy and postoperative chemoradiotherapy (CRT) did result in better outcome. Since surgery is not standardized in the majority of studies, it is not clear whether (neo) adjuvant strategies have a role in optimally operated patients, or whether these strategies just compensate for suboptimal surgery. In this review, our own data and those from the literature on this issue are summarized.

2 Surgery

With surgery only, long-term survival is poor (5-year survival <25 % in Europe), especially because the majority of patients present with T_{3-4} tumors and/or tumor positive lymph nodes (Sant et al. 2009). Population-based studies in the Netherlands demonstrated decreased incidence of gastric cancer, but more importantly, also worsening of 5-year survival between 1990 and 2007 (Dassen et al. 2010). In this period, there was a shift toward more advanced stages of disease at presentation.

Randomized studies, which compared standard limited (D1) lymph node dissection with more extended (D2) resections in the Western world, failed to show a significant survival benefit for more extensive surgery, but did demonstrate more morbidity and mortality. 15-year follow-up of the Dutch D1D2 trial showed that D2 surgery was associated with lower locoregional recurrence rates and gastric cancer-related death rates than D1 surgery (Songun et al. 2010). The mean number of lymph nodes investigated was 17 with D1 and 30 with D2 surgery. Furthermore, in a Taiwanese single-institution study that randomized between D1 and D3 (D2 according to second edition of Japanese classification of gastric cancer) nodal dissection, overall survival was increased with more extensive surgery (Wu et al. 2006). After these studies, a spleen- and pancreatic tail preserving D2 resection with at least 15 nodes, preferably in a high-volume center is recommended as the surgical procedure for patients with resectable gastric cancer. In a Cochrane Review D2 dissections increased mortality, which was associated with spleen and pancreas resection and probably with low volume centers and inexperience (McCulloch et al. 2004). More aggressive surgery in Asian countries with D3 surgery or with the addition of para-aortic nodal dissection led to conflicting results in randomized studies (Sasako et al. 2008; Wu et al. 2006). However, these strategies were not adopted in Western countries. A European comparison of 10 population-based cancer registries showed substantial differences in 30-day mortality in gastric cancer surgery (mean 8.9 %; range 5.2–16 %) (Lepage et al. 2010). It is logical to assume that concentrating the diagnosis and treatment of gastric cancer in high-volume centers would benefit the outcome of all patients. Centralization of gastric cancer surgery in Denmark led to a decrease in 30-day mortality of 8.2 % before centralization to 2.4 % afterwards. The oncological quality of surgery also improved with an increase in the percentage of patients with at least 15 lymph nodes removed increasing from 19 to 76 (Jensen et al. 2010). In the trade-off between optimal oncological surgery and decreasing postoperative death and morbidity in the Western world, laparoscopic D2 dissection in a small study from Toronto demonstrated to be promising with a 100 % R0 resection rate and mean number of lymph nodes retrieved of 32 (Bischof et al. 2012).

3   Chemotherapy

Preoperative or neo-adjuvant chemotherapy could potentially downstage (advanced) gastric cancer and improve resectability and survival. Additionally, it is generally known that patients tolerate preoperative courses better than postoperative chemotherapy, due to surgical complications and suboptimal caloric intake. Phase II studies, indeed, showed promising results (Ajani et al. 1991; Ott et al. 2003). In a randomized study of only 59 patients, by the Dutch gastric cancer group (DGCG), however, no benefit from neo-adjuvant chemotherapy with FAMTX (5-FU, adriamycin and methotrexate) chemotherapy was found (Hartgrink et al. 2004).

Many studies have been performed testing the effect of postoperative chemotherapy. These studies have been included in several meta-analyses which demonstrated no or at the most a modest survival benefit for adjuvant chemotherapy (Earle and Maroun 1999; Gianni et al. 2001; Hermans et al. 1993; Mari et al. 2000; Hu et al. 2002; Sun et al. 2009a). The majority of chemotherapy regimens that were explored in these studies demonstrate low response rates and are viewed as old fashioned nowadays. Strikingly, in the most recent meta-analysis by the GASTRIC (Global Advanced/Adjuvant Stomach Tumor Research International Collaboration) group with 3,838 patients in 17 trials did demonstrate an overall survival benefit of 18 % reduction of the hazard of death with chemotherapy, translating in an absolute improvement of survival of 6 % at 5 years (Paoletti et al. 2010). In Asian countries, where D2 dissection is standard, adjuvant chemotherapy has a prominent role, especially after the publication of the ACTS-GC (adjuvant chemotherapy trial of TS-1 for gastric cancer) trial. This Japanese phase III study randomized 530 patients to surgery only and 529 to surgery with 1 year of adjuvant S-1, which is an oral fluoropyrimidine (Sakuramoto et al. 2007). Patients with stage II or III disease underwent gastrectomy with D2 lymph node dissection. After median follow-up of 2.9 years, overall survival was 80.1 % in the S-1 group versus 70.1 % surgery only group ($p = 0.002$); relapse-free survival was 72.2 and 59.6 % ($p < 0.001$), respectively. At a follow-up of 5 years these results were unchanged (Sasako et al. 2011). Very recently, these results were confirmed in the Capecitabine and Oxaliplatin Adjuvant Study in Stomach Cancer (CLASSIC) study from South Korea, China, and Taiwan (Bang et al. 2012). In this study 1,035 patients with stage II-IIIb gastric cancer were randomized between D2 surgery and surgery followed by eight courses of oral capecitabine and intravenous oxaliplatin. After a median follow-up of 34 months, 3-year disease free survival (DFS) was 74 % in the chemotherapy group and 59 % with surgery only. The surgical quality was very high, with 100 % R0 resections and mean number of lymph nodes examined of 44. So, at least for Asian patients postoperative chemotherapy seems a reasonable treatment option after a D2 dissection. Furthermore, it seems that at least for a subset of patients, the inclusion of targeted drugs like trastuzumab can further improve the outcome (Bang et al. 2010).

In non-Asian parts of the world, obtaining an R0 dissection seems to be a challenge. Therefore, a shift in treatment philosophy was made by introducing pre- and postoperative chemotherapy (i.e., peri-operative chemotherapy) In the United Kingdom, the Medical Research Council (MRC) randomized 503 patients with resectable gastric carcinoma between surgery only and surgery with three preoperative and three postoperative courses of ECF (epirubicin, cisplatin, and fluorouracil) in the MRC adjuvant gastric infusional chemotherapy (MAGIC) trial (Cunningham et al. 2006). After a median follow-up of 4 years, perioperative chemotherapy improved 5-year overall (36 versus 23 %) and progression-free survival, despite the fact that only 42 % of patients in the chemotherapy group completed treatment. About 40 % of patients had a D2 dissection. A French phase III trial, that randomized 224 patients between surgery and surgery with 2–3 preoperative courses of cisplatin and fluorouracil and 3–4 postoperative courses of the same regimen confirmed the improvement of DFS and OS (5-year OS 38 versus 24 %) (Ychou et al. 2011). The R0 resection rate with surgery was 74 and 84 % with the addition of perioperative chemotherapy. The median number of lymph nodes removed was 19 in both arms. In the EORTC 40954 study that examined the effect of preoperative cisplatin and fluorouracil-based chemotherapy and that was stopped early because of poor accrual, the R0 resection rate was 67 % with surgery only as compared to 82 % with neoadjuvant treatment. This did not translate in a survival benefit, notwithstanding the fact that more than 90 % of patients had a D2 dissection with a mean number of removed lymph nodes of 32 (Schuhmacher et al. 2010).

4 Chemoradiotherapy

Due to poor results of surgery in the Western part of the world with high local recurrence rates and high rate of systemic failure, the combination of radiotherapy and chemotherapy has always seemed a logical and attractive strategy. Several randomized and retrospective studies in the 1980s demonstrated a potential beneficial effect of radiotherapy in combination with 5-FU-based chemotherapy on local control and survival (GITSG 1982, 1990; Klaassen et al. 1985; Moertel et al. 1984). Based on these studies, between 1991 and 1998 the SWOG/Intergroup 0116 trial randomized 556 patients between surgery only and surgery plus postoperative CRT (Macdonald et al. 2001). The adjuvant treatment consisted of 45 Gy radiotherapy at 1.8 Gy per day, given 5 days per week for 5 weeks, with modified doses of 5-FU and leucovorin on the first four and the last 3 days of radiotherapy. Two 5-day cycles of 5-FU and leucovorin were given after CRT and one cycle was given before. Although there was significant, mainly hematological and gastrointestinal acute toxicity observed after CRT, median overall survival was 27 months after surgery only and 36 months following CRT ($p = 0.005$). Furthermore, relapse free survival was prolonged from 19 months with surgery only to 30 months with CRT. Consensus guidelines in the US nowadays recommend postoperative CRT to be considered as a treatment option, which according to surveillance, epidemiology and end results (SEER) data might be reflected by an improved survival since publication of these results (Kozak and Moody 2008; Coburn et al. 2008). However, this study has been criticized, mainly focusing on suboptimal surgery and limited interaction between radiotherapy and chemotherapy. Indeed, 54 % underwent a D0, instead of the advised D2 lymph node dissection, which could be a factor in undermining survival (Hundahl et al. 2002). However, in a Korean study with almost 1,000 patients who all underwent a D2 dissection, 544 patients received postoperative CRT accordingly to the SWOG regimen (Kim et al. 2005). Although patients were not compared in a randomized fashion, the study demonstrated a survival benefit with postoperative CRT (5 year OS 57.1 vs. 51 %, $p = 0.02$), which was consistent in all stages. The percentage of patients that had >15 lymph nodes removed was >98 % in both groups. Based on these results, a study from this group, randomized 228 patients to capecitabine/cisplatin (XP) chemotherapy and 230 patients to XP-based CRT after D2 resection (ARTIST trial; adjuvant chemoradiation therapy in stomach cancer) (Lee et al. 2012). Overall 3-year DFS was 78.2 % in the radiotherapy group versus 74.2 % in the chemotherapy only group, which was not statistically significant. This can probably explained by the fact that approximately 60 % of patients in both arms had stage IB and II disease, for whom the need for adjuvant treatment is rather unclear. However, in the subgroup with pathologic lymph nodes 3-year DFS was significantly raised from 72.3 % in the chemotherapy group to 77.5 % ($p = 0.04$) with radiotherapy. Surgical quality was very high in this trial with all patients having a R0 resection and a median number of dissected lymph nodes of 40. The follow-up trial of these investigators will compare chemotherapy versus chemotherapy with radiotherapy in patients with pathologic lymph node disease. Furthermore, two meta-analyses demonstrated pre- or postoperative (chemo) radiotherapy to be associated with improved survival (Fiorica et al. 2007; Valentini et al. 2009).

Late toxicity data of combined treatment are scarce. Progressive renal toxicity after CRT for gastric cancer with the use of common 2D or 3D radiation techniques has been described (Jansen et al. 2007c). Radiotherapy dose planning studies demonstrated that modern, intensity modulated radio therapy (IMRT) techniques are able to spare kidneys and other critical organs (Ringash et al. 2005; Wieland et al. 2004).

At the Netherlands cancer institute, phase I-II studies with daily or weekly adjuvant cisplatin and capecitabine-based CRT have been performed in over 120 patients with resected gastric cancer. These studies demonstrated that intensive postoperative concurrent CRT has manageable toxicity (Jansen et al. 2007a, b, 2010). Retrospective comparison of patients treated in these studies with those that had surgery only in the Dutch D1D2 study, demonstrated that postoperative CRT was associated with better outcome, especially after D1 or a R1 (microscopically irradical) resection (Dikken et al. 2010).

For daily practice, it remains unclear whether patients with operable gastric cancer should have pre- (and post-) operative chemotherapy or postoperative CRT. To resolve this dilemma the CRITICS (ChemoRadiotherapy after Induction chemotherapy In Cancer of the Stomach) study was developed. The CRITICS study is a randomized phase III trial (clinicaltrials.gov NCT 00407186) in which all patients receive three courses of ECC (epirubicin, cisplatin, and capecitabine) chemotherapy and then have a D2/D1+ gastric resection (Fig. 1). After surgery patients receive either another three courses of ECC chemotherapy or CRT (45 Gy in 25 fractions, with weekly cisplatin and daily capecitabine). Currently, over 400 patients have been entered in the study. In Australia, at this moment, the TOP-GEAR study is also accruing patients (TROG 08.08). In this study the balance is shifted to preoperative treatment: in one arm patients receive three courses of ECF, then at least D1 surgery followed by again three courses of ECF; in the second arm the third preoperative course of ECF is replaced by CRT (45 Gy with continuous infusion of 5 FU).

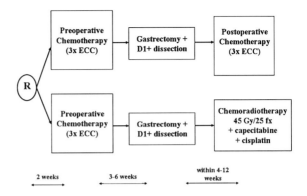

Fig. 1 Randomisation scheme of the CRITICS study. *ECC* epirubicin, cisplatin and capecitabine

At this moment, all evidence suggests that postoperative CRT is most beneficial in patients that have had adequate (D2) surgery. So, the answer in the title of this contribution should be that CRT has additive value after optimal surgery, instead of extended lymph node dissection having the ability to replace CRT.

5 R1-Resection

Another area where CRT could be of benefit is after a microscopically irradical resection (R1). Currently, there is no consensus, both in Western and Asian countries, what to do in this situation. Proposed strategies are re-resection of the anastomotic region, CRT, or just follow up. The percentage of R1 resections after curative gastric surgery varies in current series between 5.7 and 29 % (Cascinu et al. 1999; Cunningham et al. 2005; de Gara et al. 2003; Hallissey et al. 1993; Jahne et al. 2001; Morgagni et al. 2008; Siewert et al. 1998; Songun et al. 1996; Sun et al. 2009b; Yu et al. 1995). These percentages are reported from single institutions as well as from multicenter studies and from North-American, European, and Asian parts of the world. A positive surgical margin status has a strong negative prognostic impact on survival: in an American series of 18,365 patients 5-year survival was 28 % after an R0 resection and 8 % after an R1 resection; in a Taiwanese study of 1,565 patients 5-year survival was 60 % with tumor negative margins and 13.4 % with tumor positive margins (Kim et al. 1999; Shiu et al. 1987; Wanebo et al. 1993; Wang et al. 2009). In many studies, tumor positive surgical margins are associated with advanced tumor and lymph node stages, implicating that a positive margin is a sign of aggressive disease. Nevertheless, R1 status is frequently observed as an independent predictor of poor outcome. Some authors have propagated re-excision of the anastomotic line only if there are limited lymph node metastases (Kim et al. 1999). Due to a high risk on peritoneal or distant recurrence patients with pT3-4, pN2-3 disease seem not to have benefit from re-excision of a tumor positive resection line (Sun et al. 2009b; Cascinu et al. 1999). In a retrospective comparison of our postoperative CRT cohort with patients that only had surgery in the Dutch D1 versus D2 study, we have found a

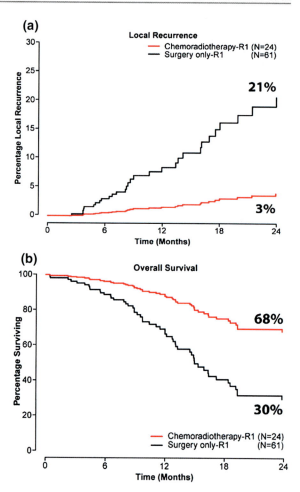

Fig. 2 Multivariate analysis of **a** local control after surgery (*black line*) versus surgery followed by chemoradiotherapy (*red line*) HR = 5.72; **b** overall survival after surgery (*black line*) versus surgery followed by chemoradiotherapy (*red line*) HR = 3.16

beneficial effect of CRT on local recurrence as well as survival after an R1 resection (Figs. 2a and b) (Dikken et al. 2010).

Therefore, we agree with Sun et al. that in patients with advanced gastric cancer and involved resection margins there is no firm indication of extensive surgical (re)treatment. Because the prognosis of these patients is mainly determined by locoregional disease extension, CRT could have a favorable role after an R1 resection.

6 Conclusion

In conclusion, at the moment there is no evidence that CRT can replace D2 dissection. More importantly, it seems that CRT will have an optimal effect after optimal surgical (D2 or D1+) dissection. After an R1 resection, CRT probably has a better trade-off between effect on disease control and toxicity than extensive reoperation.

Of course, questions regarding optimal patient care should be answered by randomized phase III trials, but these are demanding in the multimodal approach of gastric cancer. For the time being, decision making in clinical patient management could be helped by predictive tools such as the Maruyama Index of Unresected Disease or the Memorial Sloan-Kettering Cancer Center nomogram for disease-specific survival after resection for gastric cancer (Hundahl et al. 2002; Kattan et al. 2003). In the future, genetic characteristics of tissue samples that are currently collected in phase III trials will guide clinicians in what strategy to pursue in each individual patient.

References

Ajani JA, Ota DM, Jessup JM, Ames FC, McBride C, Boddie A, Levin B, Jackson DE, Roh M, Hohn D (1991) Resectable gastric carcinoma. An evaluation of preoperative and postoperative chemotherapy. Cancer 68:1501–1506

Bang YJ, Van Cutsem E, Feyereislova A, Chung HC, Shen L, Sawaki A, Lordick F, Ohtsu A, Omuro Y, Satoh T, Aprile G, Kulikov E, Hill J, Lehle M, Ruschoff J, Kang YK (2010) Trastuzumab in combination with chemotherapy versus chemotherapy alone for treatment of HER2-positive advanced gastric or gastro-oesophageal junction cancer (ToGA): a phase 3, open-label, randomised controlled trial. Lancet 376:687–697

Bang YJ, Kim YW, Yang HK, Chung HC, Park YK, Lee KH, Lee KW, Kim YH, Noh SI, Cho JY, Mok YJ, Kim YH, Ji J, Yeh TS, Button P, Sirzen F, Noh SH (2012) Adjuvant capecitabine and oxaliplatin for gastric cancer after D2 gastrectomy (CLASSIC): a phase 3 open-label, randomised controlled trial. Lancet 379:315–321

Bischof D, Swallow C, Stotland P, Hagen J, Klein L (2012) Incorporation of laparoscopic D2 dissection into the management of gastric adenocarcinoma (GCa) in a community-based setting. J Clin Oncol 30:(suppl 4; abstract 117)

Cascinu S, Giordani P, Catalano V, Agostinelli R, Catalano G (1999) Resection-line involvement in gastric cancer patients undergoing curative resections: implications for clinical management. Jpn J Clin Oncol 29:291–293

Coburn NG, Guller U, Baxter NN, Kiss A, Ringash J, Swallow CJ, Law CH (2008) Adjuvant therapy for resected gastric cancer-rapid, yet incomplete adoption following results of intergroup 0116 trial. Int J Radiat Oncol Biol Phys 70:1073–1080

Cunningham D, Allum WH, Stenning SP, Thompson JN, van de Velde CJ, Nicolson M, Scarffe JH, Lofts FJ, Falk SJ, Iveson TJ, Smith DB, Langley RE, Verma M, Weeden S, Chua YJ, MAGIC Trial P (2006) Perioperative chemotherapy versus surgery alone for resectable gastroesophageal cancer. N Engl J Med 355:11–20

Cunningham SC, Kamangar F, Kim MP, Hammoud S, Haque R, Maitra A, Montgomery E, Heitmiller RE, Choti MA, Lillemoe KD, Cameron JL, Yeo CJ, Schulick RD (2005) Survival after gastric adenocarcinoma resection: eighteen-year experience at a single institution. J Gastrointest Surg 9:718–725

Dassen AE, Lemmens VE, van de Poll-Franse LV, Creemers GJ, Brenninkmeijer SJ, Lips DJ, Vd Wurff AA, Bosscha K, Coebergh JW (2010) Trends in incidence, treatment and survival of gastric adenocarcinoma between 1990 and 2007: a population-based study in the Netherlands. Eur J Cancer 46:1101–1110

de Gara CJ, Hanson J, Hamilton S (2003) A population-based study of tumor-node relationship, resection margins, and surgeon volume on gastric cancer survival. Am J Surg 186:23–27

Dikken JL, Jansen EP, Cats A, Bakker B, Hartgrink HH, Kranenbarg EM, Boot H, Putter H, Peeters KC, van de Velde CJ, Verheij M (2010) Impact of the extent of surgery and postoperative chemoradiotherapy on recurrence patterns in gastric cancer. J Clin Oncol 28:2430–2436

Earle CC, Maroun JA (1999) Adjuvant chemotherapy after curative resection for gastric cancer in non-Asian patients: revisiting a meta-analysis of randomised trials. Eur J Cancer 35:1059–1064

Fiorica F, Cartei F, Enea M, Licata A, Cabibbo G, Carau B, Liboni A, Ursino S, Camma C (2007) The impact of radiotherapy on survival in resectable gastric carcinoma: a meta-analysis of literature data. Cancer Treat Rev 33:729–740

Gianni L, Panzini I, Tassinari D, Mianulli AM, Desiderio F, Ravaioli A (2001) Meta-analyses of randomized trials of adjuvant chemotherapy in gastric cancer. Ann Oncol 12:1178–1180

GITSG (1982) A comparison of combination chemotherapy and combined modality therapy for locally advanced gastric carcinoma. Gastrointestinal tumor study group. Cancer 49:1771–1777

GITSG (1990) The concept of locally advanced gastric cancer. Effect of treatment on outcome. Gastrointest tumor study group. Cancer 66:2324–2330

Hallissey MT, Jewkes AJ, Dunn JA, Ward L, Fielding JW (1993) Resection-line involvement in gastric cancer: a continuing problem. Br J Surg 80:1418–1420

Hartgrink HH, Jansen EP, van Grieken NC, van de Velde CJ (2009) Gastric cancer. Lancet 374:477–490

Hartgrink HH, van de Velde CJ, Putter H, Songun I, Tesselaar ME, Kranenbarg EK, de Vries JE, Wils JA, van der Bijl J, van Krieken JH (2004) Neo-adjuvant chemotherapy for operable gastric cancer: long term results of the Dutch randomised FAMTX trial. Eur J Surg Oncol 30:643–649

Hermans J, Bonenkamp JJ, Boon MC, Bunt AM, Ohyama S, Sasako M, van de Velde CJ (1993) Adjuvant therapy after curative resection for gastric cancer: meta-analysis of randomized trials. J Clin Oncol 11:1441–1447

Hu JK, Chen ZX, Zhou ZG, Zhang B, Tian J, Chen JP, Wang L, Wang CH, Chen IIY, Li YP (2002) Intravenous chemotherapy for resected gastric cancer: meta-analysis of randomized controlled trials. World J Gastroenterol 8:1023–1028

Hundahl SA, Macdonald JS, Benedetti J, Fitzsimmons T (2002) Surgical treatment variation in a prospective, randomized trial of chemoradiotherapy in gastric cancer: the effect of undertreatment. Ann Surg Oncol 9:278–286

Jahne J, Piso P, Meyer HJ (2001) 1114 total gastrectomies in the surgical treatment of primary gastric adenocarcinoma–a 30-year single institution experience. Hepatogastroenterology 48:1222–1226

Jansen EP, Boot H, Dubbelman R, Bartelink H, Cats A, Verheij M (2007a) Postoperative chemoradiotherapy in gastric cancer—a Phase I/II dose-finding study of radiotherapy with dose escalation of cisplatin and capecitabine chemotherapy. Br J Cancer 97:712–716

Jansen EP, Boot H, Dubbelman R, Verheij M, Cats A (2010) Postoperative chemoradiotherapy in gastric cancer–a phase I-II study of radiotherapy with dose escalation of weekly cisplatin and daily capecitabine chemotherapy. Ann Oncol 21:530–534

Jansen EP, Boot H, Saunders MP, Crosby TD, Dubbelman R, Bartelink H, Verheij M, Cats A (2007b) A Phase I-II Study of postoperative capecitabine-based chemoradiotherapy in gastric cancer. Int J Radiat Oncol Biol Phys 69:1424–1428

Jansen EP, Saunders MP, Boot H, Oppedijk V, Dubbelman R, Porritt B, Cats A, Stroom J, Valdes Olmos R, Bartelink H, Verheij M (2007c) Prospective study on late renal toxicity following postoperative chemoradiotherapy in gastric cancer. Int J Radiat Oncol Biol Phys 67:781–785

Jensen LS, Nielsen H, Mortensen PB, Pilegaard HK, Johnsen SP (2010) Enforcing centralization for gastric cancer in Denmark. Eur J Surg Oncol 36 Suppl 1:S50–S54

Kattan MW, Karpeh MS, Mazumdar M, Brennan MF (2003) Postoperative nomogram for disease-specific survival after an R0 resection for gastric carcinoma. J Clin Oncol 21:3647–3650

Kim S, Lim do H, Lee J, Kang WK, Macdonald JS, Park CH, Park SH, Lee SH, Kim K, Park JO, Kim WS, Jung CW, Park YS, Im YH, Sohn TS, Noh JH, Heo JS, Kim YI, Park CK, Park K (2005) An observational study suggesting clinical benefit for adjuvant postoperative chemoradiation in a population of over 500 cases after gastric resection with D2 nodal dissection for adenocarcinoma of the stomach. Int J Radiat Oncol Biol Phys 63:1279–1285

Kim SH, Karpeh MS, Klimstra DS, Leung D, Brennan MF (1999) Effect of microscopic resection line disease on gastric cancer survival. J Gastrointest Surg 3:24–33

Klaassen DJ, MacIntyre JM, Catton GE, Engstrom PF, Moertel CG (1985) Treatment of locally unresectable cancer of the stomach and pancreas: a randomized comparison of 5-fluorouracil alone with radiation plus concurrent and maintenance 5-fluorouracil–an eastern cooperative oncology group study. J Clin Oncol 3:373–378

Kozak KR, Moody JS (2008) The survival impact of the intergroup 0116 trial on patients with gastric cancer. Int J Radiat Oncol Biol Phys 72:517–521

Lee J, Lim do H, Kim S, Park SH, Park JO, Park YS, Lim HY, Choi MG, Sohn TS, Noh JH, Bae JM, Ahn YC, Sohn I, Jung SH, Park CK, Kim KM, Kang WK (2012) Phase III trial comparing capecitabine plus cisplatin versus capecitabine plus cisplatin with concurrent capecitabine radiotherapy in completely resected gastric cancer with D2 lymph node dissection: the ARTIST trial. J Clin Oncol 30:268–273

Lepage C, Sant M, Verdecchia A, Forman D, Esteve J, Faivre J (2010) Operative mortality after gastric cancer resection and long-term survival differences across Europe. Br J Surg 97:235–239

Macdonald JS, Smalley SR, Benedetti J, Hundahl SA, Estes NC, Stemmermann GN, Haller DG, Ajani JA, Gunderson LL, Jessup JM, Martenson JA (2001) Chemoradiotherapy after surgery compared with surgery alone for adenocarcinoma of the stomach or gastroesophageal junction. N Engl J Med 345:725–730

Mari E, Floriani I, Tinazzi A, Buda A, Belfiglio M, Valentini M, Cascinu S, Barni S, Labianca R, Torri V (2000) Efficacy of adjuvant chemotherapy after curative resection for gastric cancer: a meta-analysis of published randomised trials. A study of the GISCAD (Gruppo Italiano per lo studio dei carcinomi dell'apparato digerente). Ann Oncol 11:837–843

McCulloch P, Nita ME, Kazi H, Gama-Rodrigues J (2004) Extended versus limited lymph nodes dissection technique for adenocarcinoma of the stomach. Cochrane Database Syst Rev 4:CD001964

Moertel CG, Childs DS, O'Fallon JR, Holbrook MA, Schutt AJ, Reitemeier RJ (1984) Combined 5-fluorouracil and radiation therapy as a surgical adjuvant for poor prognosis gastric carcinoma. J Clin Oncol 2:1249–1254

Morgagni P, Garcea D, Marrelli D, de Manzoni G, Natalini G, Kurihara H, Marchet A, Saragoni L, Scarpi E, Pedrazzani C, Di Leo A, De Santis F, Panizzo V, Nitti D, Roviello F (2008) Resection line involvement after gastric cancer surgery: clinical outcome in nonsurgically retreated patients. World J Surg 32:2661–2667

Ott K, Sendler A, Becker K, Dittler HJ, Helmberger H, Busch R, Kollmannsberger C, Siewert JR, Fink U (2003) Neoadjuvant chemotherapy with cisplatin, 5-FU, and leucovorin (PLF) in locally advanced gastric cancer: a prospective phase II study. Gastric Cancer 6:159–167

Paoletti X, Oba K, Burzykowski T, Michiels S, Ohashi Y, Pignon JP, Rougier P, Sakamoto J, Sargent D, Sasako M, Van Cutsem E, Buyse M (2010) Benefit of adjuvant chemotherapy for resectable gastric cancer: a meta-analysis. JAMA 303:1729–1737

Ringash J, Perkins G, Brierley J, Lockwood G, Islam M, Catton P, Cummings B, Kim J, Wong R, Dawson L (2005) IMRT for adjuvant radiation in gastric cancer: a preferred plan? Int J Radiat Oncol Biol Phys 63:732–738

Sakuramoto S, Sasako M, Yamaguchi T, Kinoshita T, Fujii M, Nashimoto A, Furukawa H, Nakajima T, Ohashi Y, Imamura H, Higashino M, Yamamura Y, Kurita A, Arai K (2007) Adjuvant chemotherapy for gastric cancer with S-1, an oral fluoropyrimidine. N Engl J Med 357:1810–1820

Sant M, Allemani C, Santaquilani M, Knijn A, Marchesi F, Capocaccia R (2009) EUROCARE-4. Survival of cancer patients diagnosed in 1995–1999. Results and commentary. Eur J Cancer 45:931–991

Sasako M, Sakuramoto S, Katai H, Kinoshita T, Furukawa H, Yamaguchi T, Nashimoto A, Fujii M, Nakajima T, Ohashi Y (2011) Five-year outcomes of a randomized phase III trial comparing adjuvant chemotherapy with S-1 versus surgery alone in stage II or III gastric cancer. J Clin Oncol 29:4387–4393

Sasako M, Sano T, Yamamoto S, Kurokawa Y, Nashimoto A, Kurita A, Hiratsuka M, Tsujinaka T, Kinoshita T, Arai K, Yamamura Y, Okajima K (2008) D2 lymphadenectomy alone or with para-aortic nodal dissection for gastric cancer. N Engl J Med 359:453–462

Schuhmacher C, Gretschel S, Lordick F, Reichardt P, Hohenberger W, Eisenberger CF, Haag C, Mauer ME, Hasan B, Welch J, Ott K, Hoelscher A, Schneider PM, Bechstein W, Wilke H, Lutz MP, Nordlinger B, Cutsem EV, Siewert JR, Schlag PM (2010) neoadjuvant chemotherapy compared with surgery alone for locally advanced cancer of the stomach and cardia: european organisation for research and treatment of cancer randomized trial 40954. J Clin Oncol 28:5210–5218

Shiu MH, Moore E, Sanders M, Huvos A, Freedman B, Goodbold J, Chaiyaphruk S, Wesdorp R, Brennan MF (1987) Influence of the extent of resection on survival after curative treatment of gastric carcinoma. A retrospective multivariate analysis. Arch Surg 122:1347–1351

Siewert JR, Bottcher K, Stein HJ, Roder JD (1998) Relevant prognostic factors in gastric cancer: ten-year results of the German gastric cancer study. Ann Surg 228:449–461

Songun I, Bonenkamp JJ, Hermans J, van Krieken JH, van de Velde CJ (1996) Prognostic value of resection-line involvement in patients undergoing curative resections for gastric cancer. Eur J Cancer 32A:433–437

Songun I, Putter H, Kranenbarg EM, Sasako M, van de Velde CJ (2010) Surgical treatment of gastric cancer: 15-year follow-up results of the randomised nationwide Dutch D1D2 trial. Lancet Oncol 11:439–449

Sun P, Xiang JB, Chen ZY (2009a) Meta-analysis of adjuvant chemotherapy after radical surgery for advanced gastric cancer. Br J Surg 96:26–33

Sun Z, Li DM, Wang ZN, Huang BJ, Xu Y, Li K, Xu HM (2009b) Prognostic significance of microscopic positive margins for gastric cancer patients with potentially curative resection. Ann Surg Oncol 16:3028–3037

Valentini V, Cellini F, Minsky BD, Mattiucci GC, Balducci M, D'Agostino G, D'Angelo E, Dinapoli N, Nicolotti N, Valentini C, La Torre G (2009) Survival after radiotherapy in gastric cancer: systematic review and meta-analysis. Radiother Oncol 92:176–183

Wanebo HJ, Kennedy BJ, Chmiel J, Steele G, Jr., Winchester D, Osteen R (1993) Cancer of the stomach. A patient care study by the American college of surgeons. Ann Surg 218:583–592

Wang SY, Yeh CN, Lee HL, Liu YY, Chao TC, Hwang TL, Jan YY, Chen MF (2009) Clinical impact of positive surgical margin status on gastric cancer patients undergoing gastrectomy. Ann Surg Oncol 16:2738–2743

Wieland P, Dobler B, Mai S, Hermann B, Tiefenbacher U, Steil V, Wenz F, Lohr F (2004) IMRT for postoperative treatment of gastric cancer: covering large target volumes in the upper abdomen: a comparison of a step-and-shoot and an arc therapy approach. Int J Radiat Oncol Biol Phys 59:1236–1244

Wu CW, Hsiung CA, Lo SS, Hsieh MC, Chen JH, Li AF, Lui WY, Whang-Peng J (2006) Nodal dissection for patients with gastric cancer: a randomised controlled trial. Lancet Oncol 7:309–315

Ychou M, Boige V, Pignon JP, Conroy T, Bouche O, Lebreton G, Ducourtieux M, Bedenne L, Fabre JM, Saint-Aubert B, Geneve J, Lasser P, Rougier P (2011) Perioperative chemotherapy compared with surgery alone for resectable gastroesophageal adenocarcinoma: an FNCLCC and FFCD multicenter phase III trial. J Clin Oncol 29:1715–1721

Yu CC, Levison DA, Dunn JA, Ward LC, Demonakou M, Allum WH, Hallisey MT (1995) Pathological prognostic factors in the second British stomach cancer group trial of adjuvant therapy in resectable gastric cancer. Br J Cancer 71:1106–1110

Predicting the Response to Chemotherapy in Gastric Adenocarcinoma: Who Benefits from Neoadjuvant Chemotherapy?

William B. Robb and Christophe Mariette

Abstract

Despite a decline in the overall incidence, gastric adenocarcinoma remains the second most common cause of cancer death worldwide and thus a significant global health problem. Even in early-stage locoregional confined disease the 5-year survival rarely exceeds 25–35 %. Randomized trials have demonstrated a benefit from neoadjuvant and perioperative chemotherapy. However the optimal approach in individual patients is not clear and remains controversial. A consistent finding is that patients who have a histopathological response to neoadjuvant therapy are more likely to receive a survival benefit. These clinical data provide a strong argument for the urgent development of methods to predict histopathological response to neoadjuvant therapies for gastric adenocarcinomas. Published data demonstrate that clinico-pathological features (tumour histology and location), imaging through metabolic response by FDG-PET and tissue/molecular biomarkers may all have a predictive value for neoadjuvant therapies. However it is still uncertain from published data whether or not they will be useful for clinical decision making in individual patients. Existing candidate biomarkers need to be properly qualified and validated and

---

W. B. Robb · C. Mariette
Department of Digestive and Oncological Surgery, University Hospital Claude
Huriez Regional University Hospital Center, Place de Verdun, 59037 Lille Cedex, France

C. Mariette (✉)
University of Lille 2, Lille, France
e-mail: christophe.mariette@chru-lille.fr

C. Mariette
Inserm, UMR837, Team 5 "Mucins epithelial differentiation and carcinogenesis", JPARC,
Rue Michel Polonovski, 59045 Lille cedex, France

F. Otto and M. P. Lutz (eds.), *Early Gastrointestinal Cancers*,
Recent Results in Cancer Research 196, DOI: 10.1007/978-3-642-31629-6_17,
© Springer-Verlag Berlin Heidelberg 2012

Contents

1 Introduction.. 244
2 Histological Response Evaluation 245
3 Histological Tumour Characteristics as a Predictive Marker
  of Chemotherapy Response.. 245
  3.1 Efficacy of Neoadjuvant Treatment in SRC Gastric Cancer.................... 246
  3.2 Chemoresistance SRC Gastric Cancer: Postulated Mechanisms.............. 247
4 Imaging as a Predictive Biomarker of Chemotherapy Response 247
  4.1 Response Evaluation: EUS and CT.. 248
  4.2 18-F-Fluoro-2-deoxyglucose Positron EmissionTomography: FDG-PET.............. 248
  4.3 Is Response Prediction Improved with Other Radiotracers? FLT-PET 251
5 Molecular Markers: Predicting Response to Chemotherapy and Targeting Treatment ... 252
  5.1 Thymidylate Synthase 252
  5.2 Thymidine Phosphorylase and Dihydropyrimidine Dehydrogenase........................ 254
  5.3 Glutathione S-Transferase 255
  5.4 p53.. 257
  5.5 Bcl-2... 257
  5.6 Survivin... 257
  5.7 Microsatellite Instability... 259
  5.8 Inhibition of Angiogenesis: Vascular Endothelial Derived Growth Factor............ 260
6 Targeted Therapies in Gastric Cancer: Signs of Future Promise...................... 260
  6.1 Tyrosine Kinase Inhibitors... 260
  6.2 Monoclonal Antibodies Against VEGF.. 261
  6.3 HER Family... 262
7 Conclusions and Future Directions.. 263
References.. 264

1 Introduction

Despite a decline in overall incidence, gastric cancer (GC) remains the second most common cause of cancer death worldwide and continues to pose a significant global health problem. Even when diagnosed with early stage loco regional disease 5 year survival rarely exceeds 25–35 %. The pattern of disease is changing with the increase in the proportion of GC arising from the oesophagogastric junction (OGJ) being most marked in the developed world (Kamangar et al. 2006). Geographical variation in disease presentation is matched by geographical variation in treatment. In Japan, D2 resection and adjuvant oral fluoropyrimidine monotherapy has resulted in unprecedented survival rates (Sakuramoto et al. 2007). Practice in North America is influenced by the findings of MacDonald et al. (2001) and patients are more often referred for adjuvant chemoradiation after resection, while in Europe most commonly practice involves perioperative chemotherapy (PCT) combined with D2 resection (Cunningham et al. 2006; Ychou et al. 2011).

Consistently, patients who exhibit a histopathological response to PCT are more likely to have a survival benefit, and patients who do not respond to neoadjuvant treatment have survival rates not significantly different to patients treated with surgery alone (Berger et al. 2005, 2006, 2009; Kelsen et al. 2007). Those patients whose tumours are not responsive to neoadjuvant therapy are subjected to the toxicity of an ineffective treatment and also a delay in surgical resection which may allow tumour progression.

Despite the advances in perioperative therapy (Cunningham et al. 2006; Ychou et al. 2011), treatment is still largely administered as a "one size fits all" strategy. The optimal approach for each individual patient remains unclear. This scenario provides a clear impetus to develop methods of predicting which patients will have a histopathological response to neoadjuvant therapy. Reliable predictive markers of response would be invaluable to discriminate patients likely to benefit from treatment from those who are not. Tumour characteristics, modern modality imaging and identification of molecular biomarkers predicting responsiveness to neoadjuvant treatment have all shown some promise in this regard.

2 Histological Response Evaluation

Currently, histopathological response is ultimately determined upon examination of the surgical specimen. Limiting the assessment of response rates to only those patients who proceed to resection introduces a significant bias. Evaluation of rates of pathological response must include patients whose disease has progressed during chemotherapy. Mandard et al. (1994) first described a histological regression score for oesophageal cancer after chemotherapy and this has been modified by Becker et al. (2003) for GC. No matter which type of response evaluation is used, increased response correlates highly with improved prognosis. If future studies of response to induction chemotherapy are to be more easily comparable it is desirable that a unifying method of response evaluation and reporting is utilised.

3 Histological Tumour Characteristics as a Predictive Marker of Chemotherapy Response

The Lauren classification is commonly used to histologically classify gastric adenocarcinomas (ADC). It primarily differentiates between "intestinal" and "diffuse" types. The intestinal type corresponds to tubular or villous well-differentiated ADC whereas the diffuse type corresponds to the less differentiated and more infiltrative ADC and includes signet-ring cell carcinomas (SRC). GC shows much heterogeneity in histological pattern, and SRC has been further classified by the World Health Organisation as an ADC in which the predominant component (more than 50 % of the tumour) consists of isolated or small groups of malignant cells containing intracytoplasmic mucins (Watanabe and Sobin 1990). The incidence of diffuse type GC, particularly SRC type has been increasing and composes 28 to 70 % of gastric

ADC in western studies (Cunningham et al. 2005; Henson et al. 2004; Novotny et al. 2006). Tumours of SRC histology have several characteristics which differentiate them from other tumour types. They appear to affect patients at an earlier age (Smith and Stabile 2009), typically present with a more advanced tumour stage at diagnosis and carry a worse prognosis (Piessen et al. 2009).

3.1 Efficacy of Neoadjuvant Treatment in SRC Gastric Cancer

Two European studies have established a 5 year survival benefit for patients treated perioperatively with either epirubicin/cisplatin/5-fluorouracil (ECF) (Cunningham et al. 2006) or cisplatin/5-fluorouracil (CF) (Ychou et al. 2011) chemotherapy. However, in neither study was subgroup analysis performed for patients with SRC-type tumours or diffuse-type histology. Few conclusions can be made regarding the efficacy of other standard GC treatments on SRC, such as adjuvant chemoradiotherapy in the USA, or adjuvant oral S1-based chemotherapy in Asia, because of the absence of SRC subtype analyses in both pivotal trials (Macdonald et al. 2001; Sakuramoto et al. 2007). It is certainly noteworthy that the 10 year follow-up of the INT0116 trial suggests that the diffuse histology subgroup does not benefit from adjuvant chemoradiation (Macdonald 2009).

Recently Messager et al. (2011) have published the results of a large multicentre comparative cohort study investigating the impact of PCT on survival in patients with SRC gastric ADC. It represents the largest study conducted on this histological subtype and involved analysis of 1,050 patients diagnosed with SRC gastric tumours. When PCT was given ($n = 171$, 18.5 %), the regimen was based mainly on a fluorouracil-platinum therapy, with doublet (39.2 %) or triplet therapy (42.3 %) in association with epirubicin, being used. Other combinations included fluorouracil-irinotecan (8.8 %) and combinations in doublet or triplet forms with docetaxel (8.8 %). No survival benefit was demonstrated for patients with SRC histology receiving PCT. Nor did neoadjuvant therapy result in tumour down-staging, down-staging of nodal disease or decrease the risk of disease recurrence. Indeed the authors found some evidence that disease progression during neoadjuvant treatment may have occurred in this subgroup of patients. Supporting this assertion, extended resections were more commonly required and a longer median survival for patients treated with surgery alone were found in the first period of study—prior to the incorporation of PCT into the French guidelines for GC in 2006.

If patients with tumours of SRC histology are not to be given preoperative chemotherapy it is vital that the diagnostic biopsy is both highly sensitive and specific in making the diagnosis of this tumour subtype. Piessen et al. (2012) have documented pre-treatment biopsies to have a sensitivity of 88.1 % and specificity of 95.6 % for SRC tumours. The specific therapeutic strategy can consequently be considered from the initial diagnosis.

3.2 Chemoresistance SRC Gastric Cancer: Postulated Mechanisms

Precise mechanisms responsible for SRC chemoresistance are unknown. However some hypotheses can be drawn. First, systemic chemotherapy is known to have little effect on peritoneal tumour invasion, whereas such tropism is a feature of SRC histology. Second, the patients' performance status deterioration during chemotherapy leads to relative immunodeficiencies as a result of chemotherapeutic toxicities. Usually, the possibility of serious drug adverse events on the patient's general status is counterbalanced by a clear survival benefit of PCT. In the absence of an improvement in survival, chemotherapy toxicities may negatively impact the general status of the patient and may contribute to tumour progression, earlier relapse and death. Third, it has been suggested that the massive intracytoplasmic vacuole of mucinous content (which defines the histological features of SRC) could play an important role by competing with drug—cell interactions within the tumour (Jonckheere and Seuningen 2010). Hypothetically, specific patterns of the secretion and membranous expression of mucins could play a crucial role in drug—cell interactions, leading to chemoresistance (Jonckheere and Seuningen 2008).

To summarise, whatever the mechanisms involved, the best analysis of current data suggests that PCT in its current form does not provide a survival advantage in SRC gastric tumours. This group of tumours provides an example of where treatment of all GC in the same manner seems increasingly inappropriate. Therapeutic strategies for SRC urgently need to be tested in randomised trials dedicated to SRC histology, or future trials need to include histological subtype analysis of benefit. One phase II/III trial just funded will begin in the near future to test the impact of primary chemotherapy versus primary surgery in a population of SRC gastric ADC (PI C Mariette, France). Some other trials will evaluate the role of adjuvant intraperitoneal chemotherapy in such situation (PI O Glehen, France) or the impact of adjuvant catumaxomab in patients already with peritoneal disease (PI D Elias, France). Further studies are required to delineate tumour biology, characterise mechanisms of chemoresistance and identify signalling pathways which may be exploited for therapeutic advantage. Individually tailored therapy is the long-term goal.

4 Imaging as a Predictive Biomarker of Chemotherapy Response

The standard imaging tools for gastric cancer are computed tomography (CT), endoscopic ultrasound (EUS) and selective staging laparoscopy. These imaging techniques only have a moderate degree of sensitivity and specificity in staging the primary tumour and in detecting lymph node metastases (Bentrem et al. 2007; Burke et al. 1997; Yun et al. 2005a). CT's limited sensitivity in detecting lymph node metastases is derived from its anatomical nature and due to non-enlarged lymph nodes harbouring tumour cells. In addition, enlarged inflammatory nodes limit this modality's specificity. Indeed, over 20 % of patients who are staged clinically and on CT scanning as being free of distant metastases have distant abdominal metastases on surgical exploration (Sarela et al. 2006). Evidently better non-invasive staging modalities are necessitated.

4.1 Response Evaluation: EUS and CT

Despite being well established that patients who respond to induction chemotherapy have a significantly improved survival compared to non-responders (Lowy et al. 1999), to date, no standard method of preoperative response evaluation has been validated. Morphological imaging techniques have specific limitations in evaluating clinical response of gastric cancers to preoperative treatment. The criteria from the RECIST (Response Evaluation Criteria in Solid Tumours) Group are in principle applicable, however, the measurement of gastric wall thickness is critically dependent on appropriate gastric distension during CT scanning (Therasse et al. 2000). In experienced tertiary centres a combination of endoscopy, EUS and CT scanning in re-staging patients after one cycle of chemotherapy or preoperatively may be predictive of histological response and prognosis (Lowy et al. 1999; Ott et al. 2003a, 2006a; Weber et al. 2001).

4.2 18-F-Fluoro-2-deoxyglucose Positron Emission Tomography: FDG-PET

The advent of FDG-PET scanning has added greatly to the preoperative staging of oesophageal cancers. The MUNICON study confirmed prospectively the usefulness of early metabolic response evaluation and demonstrated the feasibility of a PET-guided treatment algorithm, an important step in tailoring multimodality treatment in accordance with tumour biology (Lordick et al. 2007). Results of studies, relating to FDG-PET's ability to predict histological response in the setting of OGJ carcinomas are more robust than in the setting of gastric ADC - Table 1 (Lordick et al. 2007; Ott et al. 2006b; Weber et al. 2001; Wieder et al. 2007). The promising results of FDG-PET being a predictive biomarker of response has lead to investigation of its role in both preoperative staging of GC and whether metabolic response to neoadjuvant treatment is a reliable predictive marker of histopathological response.

4.2.1 Limitations of FDG-PET in the Setting of Gastric Cancer

FDG-PET is not an accurate diagnostic imaging technique for GC since approximately 30 % of GC, even those patients with locally advanced tumours, exhibit insufficient FDG uptake for quantification (Ott et al. 2008c). High physiological uptake in normal gastric mucosa due to its rich blood supply and variable, but

Table 1 FDG-PET response as a biomarker for histopathological response to neoadjuvant treatment in adenocarcinomas of the gastro-oesophageal junction

Study	n	Tumour site	Neoadjuvant CTx	Repeat FDG-PET	FDG-PET response definition	MHR Rate for metabolic responders and non-responders Metabolic response—sensitive and specific for MHR	Survival
Weber (2001)	40	Siewert type I and II	Cisplatin Leucovorin 5-FU	Day 14	>35 % Reduction in SUV	Responders—8/15—PPV 53 % Non-responders—1/22—NPV 95 % Sensitivity—89 % Specificity—75 %	2 year survival Responders—60 % Non-responders—37 % ($p = 0.04$)
Ott (2006)	65	Siewert type I and II	Cisplatin Leucovorin 5-FU	Day 14	>35 % Reduction in SUV	Responders—8/18—PPV 44 % Non-Responders—2/38—NPV 95 % Sensitivity—80 % Specificity—78 %	3 year survival Responders—70 % Non-Responders—35 % ($p = 0.01$)
Wieder (2007)	24	Siewert type I and II	Cisplatin Leucovorin 5-FU	Day 14 and post treatment	Day 14—>35 % reduction in SUV Post-Tx—≥ 63 % reduction in SUV	*Day 14* Responders—7/12—PPV 58 % Non-Responders—1/12—NPV 92 % Sensitivity—88 % Specificity—69 %	3 year survival *Day 14 data* Responders—83 % Non-Responders—33 % ($p = 0.03$) Responders—73 % Non-Responders—46 % ($p = 0.09$)
Lordick (2007)	110	Siewert type I and II	Cisplatin/5-FU (44 %) Cisplatin/Oxaliplatin (15 %) Cisplatin/5-FU/ Paclitaxel (41 %)	Day 14	≥35 % Reduction in SUV	Responders—29/50—PPV 58 % Non-Responders—0/54—NPV 100 % Sensitivity—100 % Specificity—72 %	Median survival Responders—not reached Non-Responders—25.8 months ($p = 0.015$)

N number of patients; *CTx* chemotherapy; *5-FU* 5-fluorouracil; *FDG-PET* Fluoro-2-deoxyglucose positron emission tomography; *SUV* specific uptake variable; *Resp* responder; *Non-Resp* non-responder; *PPV* positive predictive value; *NPV* negative predictive value

sometimes intense, background activity noted in the normal gastric wall, mean false positive rates are high. Sensitivity rates, for detecting the primary tumour, vary from 58 to 94 % (Dassen et al. 2009). During imaging, gastric distension with water may serve to improve specificity (Yun et al. 2005b). Proximal tumours appear to be diagnosed with more accuracy than distal tumours (Koga et al. 2003) and the sensitivity of FDG-PET increases with increasing tumour size and T stage, meaning it is not a useful tool for either screening or primary tumour detection (Shoda et al. 2007). Poor uptake of FDG is also associated with diffuse-type GC with signet ring cells and mucinous content. In summary, FDG non-avid tumours are likely to be small, well differentiated, diffuse type with mucinous content and found in the distal stomach (Ott et al. 2008c).

4.2.2 FDG-PET: Promise as a Biomarker of Response in Gastric Cancer?

Despite the numerous limitations of this metabolic imaging technique in GC, its ability to predict histopathological response in patients with FDG avid tumours has been a subject of interest. In particular, if failure to exhibit a metabolic response to treatment identifies patients whose tumours are unresponsive to chemotherapy and whose disease may progress during treatment, then these patients could be appropriately changed to alternative chemotherapy regimens or proceed directly to surgery. This would be of significant clinical advantage.

Ott et al. (2003b) reported that 14 days after the commencement of cisplatin-based neoadjuvant chemotherapy, a decrease of more than 35 % of the baseline metabolic uptake allowed for accurate prediction of response in metabolically avid tumours. Metabolic response showed a correlation with both histological and clinical response. Their subsequent report on a larger cohort of patients aimed to identify subgroups of patients with locally advanced GC with differing tumour biology, based on their metabolic baseline uptake and metabolic response to treatment (Ott et al. 2008a). Three groups of patients were identified: metabolic responders, metabolic non-responders and patients with FDG non-avid tumours. A major histological response (<10 % residual tumour cells) was seen in 69 % of metabolical responders and only 17 % of non-responders. The histopathological response rate (24 %) for patients with FDG-PET non-avid tumours did not differ significantly from non-responders ($p = 0.72$), nor did survival ($p = 0.46$). In FDG non-avid tumours, the histopathological response rate (5/21 resected patients) was significantly different from the histopathological response rate of metabolic responders (11/16 resected patients). Different from ADC of the OGJ, the study confirmed that, about one-third of gastric tumours do not uptake FDG sufficiently for quantification. The proportion of FDG non-avid tumours was significantly higher in the distal stomach ($p = 0.029$) and contained significantly more signet ring cells ($p = 0.013$). This single centre study with 70 % of tumours being localised in the proximal third of the stomach remains the sole published study documenting early FDG-PET response as being predictive of histological response and prognosis in GC.

A decrease of greater than 45 % of the initial specific uptake variable (SUV) after 35 days was investigated retrospectively by Shah et al. (2007) as the best criterion for prediction of tumour response and prognosis. Using these parameters a decrease of more than 45 % in initial SUV was correlated with both histological response ($p = 0.007$) and disease-free survival ($p = 0.01$). When the FDG-PET scan was repeated at day 15, it was not significantly correlated with a histological response, or with disease-free survival. Vallbohmer et al. (2010) have recently published their series of 42 patients recruited from a prospective observation trial. FDG-PET was performed before and 2 weeks after finishing neoadjuvant treatment. No significant correlations were documented in this study between baseline, interval or percentage change in SUV and histopathological response or prognosis. They conclude that FDG-PET does not appear to hold promise as an imaging modality to effectively characterise response and survival in patients undergoing neoadjuvant treatment. These results are summarised in Table 2.

4.3 Is Response Prediction Improved with Other Radiotracers? FLT-PET

At present, the radiotracer most extensively investigated in association with positron emission tomography is 18F-FDG. Recent study has also looked at 18F-fluorothymidine (FLT) (Ott et al. 2011). FLT represents the activity of thymidine kinase a key enzyme in the salvage pathway for the production of thymidine monophosphate, and has been used successfully for imaging drug-related inhibition of thymidylate synthase (TS) (Weber et al. 1991; Wells et al. 2003). FLT has been shown to have a higher sensitivity in the detection of primary GC, including those of SRC histology (Kameyama et al. 2009). Remembering that thymidylate synthase is a target enzyme for 5-fluorouracil, such higher sensitivity and the ability to image thymidylate synthase inhibition is of evident interest for in vivo testing of GC sensitivity to neoadjuvant chemotherapy.

A recent German study of 45 patients with GC undergoing both FDG and FLT-PET before and after 2 weeks the start of neoadjuvant therapy found no significant association of histological response with any of the analysed metabolic parameters (Ott et al. 2011). Multivariate analysis revealed only Lauren's classification and FLT SUV day 14 as the sole significant prognostic factors ($p = 0.006$ and $p = 0.002$, respectively). This contrasts to the same groups previously published data of FDG uptake predicting both response and prognosis (Ott et al. 2008a). The authors argue that small sample size, the high rate of poorly differentiated tumours, poor response rate and overall poor survival rate (median survival of 20 months) may explain why FDG decrease was not confirmed as being of predictive value. The results, however, corroborate the findings of others, that at present, FDG-PET is of limited value in the prediction of histological response and prognosis in GC Vallbohmer (2010).

To summarise, the difficulties of incorporating FDG-PET into current treatment algorithms are demonstrated by the evident heterogeneity of uptake, response and biology of GC. Before metabolic PET findings can have clinical applicability, thresholds of both what defines metabolic response and histopathological response need to be harmonised and further tested in a multicentre setting. Currently, it cannot be used to individualise patient treatment or for decision making in the preoperative patient care algorithm. As knowledge of the capabilities of different radiotracers becomes known, metabolic-based imaging may hold future promise in selecting the patients who gain benefit from neoadjuvant therapy.

5 Molecular Markers: Predicting Response to Chemotherapy and Targeting Treatment

Molecular predictive biomarkers can be divided into two groups. Those which predict tumour chemosensitivity and the likelihood of histopathological response, and molecular markers which may be used for individualised targeted therapies. The recognition of the heterogeneity of gastric cancer may be of less relevance for treatment with cytotoxic drugs, but the evidence summarised in this review suggests there may be a differential response to the emerging targeted therapies for the differing histological and molecular tumour subtypes. Individualised treatment may become more feasible as molecular biomarkers increasingly predict the efficacy of a particular chemotherapeutic strategy for each individual tumour. The subsequent discussion relates to molecular biomarkers which have shown some promise in histopathological response prediction or as future therapeutic targets.

5.1 Thymidylate Synthase

5.1.1 Role of TS

The current neoadjuvant regimes in gastric cancer commonly employ combination chemotherapy based on treatment with 5-fluorouracil (5-FU). 5-FU is an antimetabolite which inhibits the conversion of uracil in thymidine and so blocks DNA synthesis. TS catalyses the conversion of fluorodeoxyuridine monophosphate (dUMP) to deoxythymidine monophosphate (dTMP), and is the target enzyme for 5-FU. Thymidine phosphorylase (TP) converts 5-FU to its active metabolite, fluorouridine monophosphate (FdUMP), which blocks DNA replication by inhibiting the synthesis of thymidine. In a study of 65 patients with gastric cancer and undergoing 5-FU and cisplatin neoadjuvant treatment, Lenz et al. (1996) found TS expression to be correlated with response to chemotherapy. Patients overexpressing TS mRNA exhibited lower tumoural response rates to treatment. Overexpression of TS and poor clinical outcome was subsequently confirmed in other studies measuring TS levels by either immunohistochemistry or mRNA expression (Boku et al. 1998; Yeh et al. 1998), while others have failed to confirm

Predicting the Response to Chemotherapy

Table 2 Studies evaluating FDG-PET metabolic response, histopathological response and survival in patients undergoing neoadjuvant treatment with chemotherapy for gastric cancer

Variables	Shah et al. (2007)	Ott et al. (2008)	Valbohmer et al. (2010)
Total no. of patients	42	71	42
Definition of metabolic PET response	>45 %	>35 %	% change in SUV
Definition of histological response(%) residual tumour cells	<10 %	<10 %	<10 %
Number of patients with major histopathological response (%)	NS	21 (30 %)	6 (15 %)
Chemotherapy regime	CPT CIS	Cisplatin, Leucovorin, 5-Fluorouracil	Cisplatin, Leucovorin, 5-Fluorouracil
Time of follow-up PET scan	Day 15, and then at Day 35	14 days after *start* of chemotherapy	14 days after *completion* of chemotherapy
Tumour stages included	cT2,N + ,M0, or cT3–4,N0-3,M0	cT3-4, cN0-3, cM0	cT3-4, cN0-3, cM0
Metabolically avid tumours (% of total)	31 (73.8 %)	49 (69.0 %)	42 (100 %)
Tumour localisation	Gastric: 31, OGJ: 11		
Proximal: Middle and distal	As above	50:21	26:14
Metabolic activity significantly higher in proximal tumours	NS	Yes, $p = 0.029$	Yes, $p = 0.041$
Tumour Histology—Lauren Classification Intestinal: Diffuse Less metabolic activity in diffuse histology—yes/no (p value)	NS	33:38 Yes ($p = 0.013$)	16:24 Yes ($p = 0.023$)
Correlation between metabolic responders and histological response	Day 15—No Day 35—Yes ($p = 0.007$)	11 of 16 (69 %)	None
Correlation between metabolic response and improved survival	Day 15—No Day 35—Yes ($p = 0.01$)	Yes	None

PET positron emission tomography; *SUV* specific uptake variable; *CPT* irinotecan; *CIS* cisplatin; *OGJ* oesophago-gastric junction; *NS* not stated

such a predictive value for TS activity (Terashima et al. 2003). Most recently, in a study of 64 patients with advanced GC treated preoperatively with 5-FU, leucovorin and oxaliplatin, Kwon et al. (2007) have found no significant relationship between tumour response and TS protein expression—Table 3. Inconsistency in results may be a reflection of the molecular diversity of this tumour group.

5.1.2 TS Polymorphism

The therapeutic efficacy of 5-FU chemotherapy may be altered by genetic polymorphisms which alter the activity of TS. An improved survival (10.2 vs. 6 months) was reported by Goekkurt et al. (2006) for patients with advanced GC having specific TS genotypes. Further, Lu et al. (2006) analysed DNA from peripheral blood leucocytes in 106 patients with GC and classified polymorphisms in the 3'-untranslated region (3'-UTR) into 3 groups depending on the presence of a 6 bp nucleotide fragment. Histological response rates in the $-6/-6$ bp and $-6/+6$ bp groups were significantly higher than that in the $+6/+6$ bp group ($p = 0.045$). These findings have recently been substantiated by Kearn et al. (2008) who found, in a study of 73 patients with GC treated with preoperative 5-FU and oxaliplatin, homozygote deletion of 6 bp in the 3'-UTR of TS correlated with a significantly higher histopathological response rate ($p = 0.03$) and overall survival. DNA polymorphisms in TS and 5,10-methylene-tetrahydrofolate reductase (MTHFR) genes were analysed in 238 patients with locally advanced GC by the Munich group (Ott et al. 2006a). In 105 patients who received 5-FU based chemotherapy, genotyping, of the tandem repeat and the G/C polymorphism in the triple repeat, in the promoter region of the TS gene was performed. Upon analysis of patients undergoing R0 resection with or without preoperative treatment, a significant survival benefit was noted for those patients receiving neoadjuvant treatment and being homozygote for the double repeat polymorphism ($p = 0.002$), or heterozygote for the double repeat/triple repeat polymorphism ($p = 0.004$). Chemotherapy did not improve survival for patients with the homozygote triple repeat genotype ($p = 0.93$), suggesting that this group of patients may either require a different therapeutic strategy or should proceed straight to surgery. The authors suggest that the association in the neoadjuvant treated group, between the TS tandem repeat polymorphism and survival, but not histological response, may point to a cellular response mechanism which is not measurable by current standard response evaluation methods—tumour shrinkage.

5.2 Thymidine Phosphorylase and Dihydropyrimidine Dehydrogenase

Thymidine phosphorylase may have a prominent role in the efficacy of 5-FU based chemotherapy. Enzymatic conversion of 5'-deoxy-5-fluorouridine to the biologically active 5-FU occurs in tumour tissues rich in TP (Kono et al. 1983). Studies examining TP expression in GC and its relationship to tumour response and survival have yielded mixed results. While Koizumi et al. (1999) have reported response rates among TP positive tumours to be higher (82.4 %) than TP weakly positive or negative tumours (29.2 %), other authors have failed to show any

Predicting the Response to Chemotherapy 253

association between TP expression and histological response (Napieralski et al. 2005; Terashima et al. 2002, 2003). It may be that TP expression in combination with other markers may be more predictive of chemotherapeutic response.

Dihydropyrimidine dehydrogenase (DPD) in the liver is responsible for the breakdown of 80–90 % of 5-FU to its inactive metabolite 5,6-dihydro-5-FU (Diasio and Harris 1989). Nishina et al. (2004) demonstrated that while TP alone was not predictive of response to neoadjuvant treatment, in metastatic cancer a high TP: DPD ratio was predictive of significantly better chemotherapeutic response and survival. Similar results were reported by Napieralski et al., who studied the expressions of the 5-FU related genes TS, TP and DPD as well as the cisplatin-related genes ERCC1, ERCC4, KU80 and GADD45A in a cohort of 61 patients with advanced gastric cancer treated with 5-FU/cisplatin neoadjuvant chemotherapy (Napieralski et al. 2005). Low expression levels of GADD45A were predictive of improved survival and good response to chemotherapy, especially if found in association with low levels of TP. Conversely, high dual expression of TP and/or GADD45 were exclusively found in non-responding patients ($p = 0.002$) and were associated with a significantly poorer survival ($p = 0.04$).

Taken together, studies of the role of TP as a predictor of response to treatment in GC have reported conflicting results. Used in isolation it appears to have limited suitability as a predictive biomarker. In association with other variables such as GADD45 or DPD, the expression of TP may give some additional information on the likelihood of tumoural response to treatment with fluoropyrimidines (Table 4).

5.3 Glutathione S-Transferase

Glutathione-*S*-transferase (GST) conjugates glutathione to diverse electrophiles and plays a major role in the detoxification of alkylating and platinating agents. The cytotoxicity of platinating agents including cisplatin, carboplatin and oxaliplatin, is due to their ability to bind to DNA and produce crosslinks. Treatment with these agents may be characterised by resistance, both acquired and intrinsic. Such resistance can be caused by a number of cellular adaptations including reduced uptake, inactivation by glutathione or other antioxidants and increased levels of DNA repair or DNA tolerance. The isoenzyme glutathione-s-transferase pi 1 (GSTP1) and its polymorphisms have been most extensively studied in colorectal and gastric cancers. Analysis of GSTP-105 polymorphisms, which may alter GSTP1functional capacity, was studied in 52 patients with advanced GC, treated with neoadjuvant 5-FU/cisplatin (Goekkurt et al. 2006). The GSTP-105 Val/Val genotype showed a significantly superior response rate to treatment (67 %) compared to only 21 % of patients with at least one 105Ile allele. Ott et al. (2008b) isolated DNA from 139 patients with locally advanced GC before chemotherapy, but found that none of the common GST polymorphisms predicted response to cisplatin based neoadjuvant chemotherapy. The GSTM1+ genotype was associated with a better prognosis in completely resected patients.

Table 3 Biomarkers relating to metabolism of 5-FU and response to chemotherapy in gastric cancer

Study	n	Chemotx.	Biomarker	Result summary
Lenz et al. (1996)	65	5-FU, Leucovorin, Cisplatin	TS (mRNA)	Mean TS mRNA in responding an resistant patients statistically different ($p < 0.001$) ↓ TS associated with ↑ survival
Metzger et al. (1998)	38	5-FU, Cisplatin	TS (mRNA)	TS mRNA > median—20 % histological response TS mRNA < median—85 % histological response ↓ TS associated with ↑ tumoural response
Yeh et al. (1998)	30		TS (protein)	↓ TS associated with ↑ tumoural response and ↑ survival
Boku et al. (1998)	39	5-FU, Cisplatin	TS (protein)	↓ TS associated with ↑ tumoural response
Ishikawa et al. (2000)	41	5-FU	TS and DPD (mRNA)	↑ DPD activity associated with ↓ 5-FU sensitivity No correlation between TS expression and 5-FU sensitivity
Kikuyama et al. (2001)	28	5-FU, Cisplatin, Pirarubicin	TP (protein)	↑ TP expression associated ↑ response to chemotherapy
Napieralski (2005)	61	5-FU, Cisplatin	TS, TP and DPD (mRNA)	↑ DPD activity ↓ response/survival TS not associated with tumoural response ↑ TP ± GADD45A exclusively found in non-responding patients ($p = 0.002$)
Ott et al. (2006)	238	5-FU, Leucovorin, Cisplatin	TS promoter region polymorphism, MTHFR C677T polymorphism	No association with histopathological response Chemotherapy did not improve survival in patients with the homozygote triple repeat TS genotype.
Lu et al. (2006)	106	5-FU	TS polymorphism in 3'-UTR	↓ histological response rates with homozygote +6/+ 6 bp polymorphism in the 3'-UTR
Fukuda et al. (2006)	62	5-FU, Cisplatin	TS and DPD protein	↓ TS and ↓ DPD expression both associated with ↑ tumoural response
Kwon et al. (2007)	64	5-FU, Leucovorin, Oxaliplatin	TS (IHC)	No significant association of response or survival and TS expression ($p = 0.813$ and 0.4578, respectively)

(continued)

Predicting the Response to Chemotherapy 255

Table 3 (continued)

Study	n	Chemotx.	Biomarker	Result summary
Kearn et al. (2008)	73	5-FU, Oxaliplatin	TS polymorphism in 3'-UTR	TS homozygote deletion of 6 bp in the 3'-UTR—↑ histopathological response rate ($p = 0.03$)

5-FU 5-Fluorouraci; *TS* thymidylate synthase; *DPD* Dihydropyrimidine Dehydrogenase; *TP* Thymidine Phosphorylase; *MTHFR* 5,10-methylenetetrahydrofolate reductase; *3'-UTR* 3'-untranslated region; *IHC* immunohistochemistry

5.4 p53

Inactivation of tumor-suppressor genes is one of the key hallmarks of a tumour. Unlike other tumor-suppressor genes, p53 is inactivated by missense mutations in half of all human cancers. It is increasingly clear that the resulting mutant p53 proteins do not represent only the loss of wild-type p53 tumor-suppressor activity, but also the gain of new oncogenic properties favouring maintenance, spreading and chemoresistance of malignant tumours. As mutant p53 tends to be resistant to breakdown, the presence of p53 in tumours is taken as a marker for p53 mutation. In GC, several studies have documented p53 negativity with good response to treatment (Boku et al. 1998; Nagashima et al. 2005; Nakata et al. 1998). These consistent findings conflict with the findings of Bataille et al. (2003) who found that overexpression of p53 and the presence of p53 mutations in pre-treatment biopsies was associated with improved survival as well as tumour histological response. Similarly, conflicting results have been observed in oesophageal cancer (Fareed et al. 2009), making the predictive role of p53 expression unclear.

5.5 Bcl-2

Apoptosis induced by p53 may be induced by the bcl-2 family of proteins which are involved in regulation of the cell cycle. Bcl-2 proteins include both anti-apoptotic and pro-apoptotic members and have been investigated in the setting of GC as possible predictors of the chemotherapeutic response. In a study of 39 unresectable GC patients treated with 5-FU and cisplatin, Boku et al. (1998) examined a range of markers to predict chemotherapy response and survival. Bcl-2 negativity was not independently predictive of response. When combined with the expression of favourable phenotypes of 4 other markers, it was found that in 10 cases expressing either 4 or 5 favourable phenotypes the chemotherapy response rate was 70 %, with significantly prolonged median survival ($p = 0.0069$). In a similar study, Nagashima et al. (2005) found favorable phenotypes for chemotherapy response to be p53-ve, bcl-2-ve, and vascular endothelial derived growth factor (VEGF) +ve tumours, with the response rate being significantly correlated to the number of these favorable phenotypes expressed ($p = 0.043$). This provides some evidence that a panel of biomarkers may add to the ability to predict histological response to current chemotherapy.

Table 4 Biomarkers relating to transcription factor p53, angiogenesis and other pathways and response to chemotherapy in gastric cancer

Study	n	Chemotx.	Biomarker	Result summary
Transcription factor, p53				
Nakata et al. (1998)	23	5-FU, Cisplatin	P53 protein (IHC)	↑ response in p53 −ve tumours
				p53 useful predictor of chemotherapy outcome
Boku et al. (1998)	39	5-FU, Cisplatin	P53 protein (IHC)	↑ response in p53 −ve tumours
				Expression of p53, bcl-2, TS, GST, VEGF—patients with 4 or 5 favourable phenotypes survived longer ($p = 0.0069$)
Kikuyama et al. (2001)	67	5-FU, Pirarubicin Cisplatin	P53 protein (IHC)	↑survival in p53 −ve tumours—no correlation with tumour response
Ott et al. (2003)	53	Cisplatin based therapy	DNA analysis: MSI/ LOH/p53 mutation analysis	p53 protein expression not associated with tumour response
				↑ chromosomal instability (high FAL), ↑benefit from neoadjuvant therapy
Nagashima et al. (2005)	55	Cisplatin, Irinotecan	P53 protein (IHC)	↑ response in p53 −ve tumours
Angiogenesis				
Nagashima et al. (2005)	55	Cisplatin, Irinotecan	VEGF protein (IHC)	VEGF +ve tumours, favourable phenotype for chemotherapy response
Fukuda et al. (2006)	62	5-FU, Cisplatin	VEGF protein (IHC)	VEGF expression—No association with histological response
Other Pathways				
Metzger et al. (1998)	38	5-FU, Cisplatin	(ERCC1) mRNA levels	↓ ERCC1 mRNA—↑ response and ↑ median survival
Boku et al. (1998)	39	5-FU, Cisplatin	GST-π protein (IHC)	GST-π −ve tumours—↑ tumoural chemotherapy response
Kikuyama et al. (2001)	67	5-FU, Pirarubicin Cisplatin	bcl-2 protein (IHC)	bcl-2 negative tumours showed improved survival
Nagashima et al. (2005)	55	Cisplatin, Irinotecan	bcl-2 protein (IHC)	bcl-2 negative tumours favourable phenotype for chemotherapy response
Napieralski et al. (2005)	61	5-FU, Cisplatin	GADD45A mRNA	↑ TP ± GADD45A—predicted non-responsive tumours ($p = 0.002$) and ↓ survival ($p = 0.04$)
Kwon et al. (2007)	64	5-FU, Leucovorin, Oxaliplatin	ERCC1 protein (IHC)	↓ ERCC1 expression ↑chemotherapy response ($p = 0.045$)

IHC immunohistochemistry; *TS* thymidylate synthase; *GST* Glutathione S-transferase; *VEGF* Vascular Endothelial Derived Growth Factor; *MSI* microsatellite instability; *LOH* loss of heterozygosity; *ERCC* excision repair cross complement gene

5.6 Survivin

Survivin is a member of the inhibitor of apoptosis gene family and has an important role in cell division and the upstream initiation of mitochondrial-dependent apoptosis (Vallbohmer et al. 2009). Molecular biological studies in gastric cancer have suggested that survivin expression is associated with poor prognosis, leading to the development of survivin-inhibitors to suppress tumour growth by increasing apoptotic activity (Wang et al. 2007). Subsequent studies have questioned the association between high expression of survivin and poor prognosis and have suggested that it may in fact be associated with a favourable prognosis (Okada et al. 2001; Warnecke-Eberz et al. 2005). Most recently, Vallbohmer et al. (2009) studied 40 patients with gastric cancer receiving neoadjuvant cisplatin, leucovorin and 5-FU and found no correlation between pre-and post-therapeutic survivin protein expression and histopathological response rates. Patients with a higher pre-therapeutic survivin expression did have a significant survival benefit, indicating it to be an independent prognostic marker in the multimodality treatment of advanced GC but not a marker predictive of a therapeutic response.

5.7 Microsatellite Instability

Gastric tumours show one of the highest prevalences of MSI, with up to 33 % of tumours having been documented to have this abnormality (Milano et al. 1999). Cell lines defective in mismatch repair and which exhibit MSI show resistance to treatment with cisplatin (Fink et al. 1996). These observations lead to suggestion that chemoresistance in vivo to cisplatin based therapy may be associated with MSI.

A study examining whether loss of heterozygosity (LOH) and MSI were predictive markers of clinical response to neoadjuvant treatment in gastric carcinoma, at 11 microsatellite locations of chromosomal sites known to be involved in gastric carcinogenesis, found that responding tumours had significantly higher rates of LOH (Grundei et al. 2000). Expressing the level of LOH per tumour as fractional allelic loss (FAL), high FAL values were found to correlate with tumours that responded well. A high FAL can be interpreted as an indication of a high level of chromosomal aberrations and good clinical response was associated with both Lauren's intestinal type histology and a high rate of FAL. The authors recognise the limitations of assessing clinical response by CT scan, endoscopy and EUS. The same group analysed 53 patients with GC treated with cisplatin based neoadjuvant treatment to evaluate MSI, LOH and mutation in the p53 gene in relation to patient response to therapy and survival (Ott et al. 2003b). There was no significant response benefit related to p53 mutation, p53 protein expression or MSI of either high or low grade. LOH at chromosome 17p13 (the chromosomal region of the p53 gene) did show a significant association with therapy response ($p = 0.022$) but not with survival. A high FAL, reflecting chromosomal instability, was related to improved response to therapy and may define a subset of patients who are more likely to benefit from a cisplatin based neoadjuvant regime because of a reduction in the capacity for cellular DNA repair.

5.8 Inhibition of Angiogenesis: Vascular Endothelial Derived Growth Factor

The ability of a tumour to propagate and progress is critically dependent upon the induction of a tumour vasculature. Hypoxia in tumours sets in early as the rapidly expanding tumour mass outgrows the host vasculature. Hypoxic clones may survive after initiating an angiogenic pathway. The hypoxia-inducible transcription factor-1 (HIF-1)-mediated pathway is critical for tumour angiogenesis and activates the expression of VEGF. As with many putative biomarkers of response to therapy, analysis of VEGF expression has shown mixed results with some study showing no relationship between VEGF expression and histopathological response (Fukuda et al. 2006) and others finding that VEGF positive tumours had a favourable phenotype for response, with the response rate being significantly correlated with the total number of favourable phenotypes expressed (p53 negative, bcl-2 negative, VEGF positive tumours) (Nagashima et al. 2005). Recognition of VEGF as a key pathway in angiogenesis has led to agents being developed that are either antibodies to VEGR or the VEGF receptor (VEGFR) as well as TKIs targeting the VEGFR.

6 Targeted Therapies in Gastric Cancer: Signs of Future Promise

6.1 Tyrosine Kinase Inhibitors

The TKI sunitinib is currently approved for the first line treatment of renal cell cancers and is also used in the second line therapy of gastrointestinal stromal cell tumours. Two non-randomised phase II studies have evaluated sunitinib's role in advanced GC (Bang et al. 2011; Moehler et al. 2011). The European-based trial has shown results of some promise for improved survival, suggesting the inclusion of sunitinib in a randomised trial would be of value (Moehler et al. 2011). Sorafenib is a further inhibitor of several tyrosine kinase receptors involved in the progression of GC. A phase II study of 44 patients, with either locally advanced (20 %) or metastatic (80 %) gastric or OGJ tumours, treated patients with sorafenib in combination with docetaxel and cisplatin. Eighteen of the 44 eligible and treated patients showed partial responses with tolerable toxicity, suggesting additional studies of sorafenib with chemotherapy are warranted (Sun 2010).

6.2 Monoclonal Antibodies Against VEGF

Prolonged survival in patients with metastatic colorectal cancer has been established in a phase III trial of the addition of bevacizumab, a humanised mAb against VEGFA, to chemotherapy with irinotecan, 5-FU and leucovorin (Hurwitz et al. 2004). Available clinical evidence of angiogenesis inhibitors in patients with advanced GC tumours is limited to some phase II and one phase III trials. A pivotal phase II trial of bevacizumab combined with irinotecan and cisplatin in 47 patients with advanced disease (51 % gastric and 49 % OGJ adenocarcinomas), observed an objective response rate of 65 % and a median survival of 12.3 months (Shah et al. 2006). Bevacizumab toxicity countered its evident efficacy, with a 6 % perforation rate and 25 % of patients suffering grade III and IV thromboembolic events. In a further phase II trial (Shah et al. 2011), of a modified docetaxel, cisplatin and fluorouracil (DCF) regime combined with bevacizumab, in the first line treatment of patients with metastatic gastric and OGJ ADC, a response rate of 64 % was noted with a further 9 % of patients showing stable disease. Grade III and IV venous thromboembolism occurred in 29 %, of whom 93 % were asymptomatic but diagnosed on per protocol scanning. This trial does confirm venous thromboembolism in more than one quarter of patients treated which compares less favourably to the traditional cisplatin based regimes. In the phase III AVAGAST study (Ohtsu et al. 2011), 774 patients with inoperable, locally advanced or metastatic stomach/OGJ ADC, were randomised to capecitabine plus cisplatin and either bevacizumab or placebo. While the primary endpoint, improvement in overall survival, was not met, there was a significant improvement in progression-free survival and overall response rate, especially in European patients with an acceptable safety profile. The majority of the data accumulated on targeted therapy comes from trials in the setting of advanced disease. Little information is available for the efficacy of such targeted treatment in resectable patients in combination with perioperative chemotherapeutic regimes. The ongoing MRC-STO3 study,[1] a phase II/III trial adding bevacizumab to perioperative epirubicin, cisplatin and xeloda, will hopefully confirm the promise of this targeted therapy in the clinical setting of resectable disease. If positive this trial will mark the exciting opening of a new avenue in the expanding network of targeted therapy.

6.3 HER Family

One of the targeted pathways through which TKIs and mAbs act is via the human epidermal growth factor receptor (EGFR or HER) pathway. HER is a proto-oncogene which encodes for a tyrosine kinase growth factor receptor that plays a

---

[1] http://clinicaltrials.gov Combination chemotherapy with or without bevacizumab in treating patients with previously untreated stomach cancer, gastroesophageal junction cancer or lower oesophageal cancer that can be removed by surgery (ST03).

key role in tumourigenesis and tumour progression. The HER family consists of a transmembrane tyrosine kinase receptor, overexpression of which is associated with adverse outcomes for solid tumours. The four receptors comprising the HER family are HER1 (EGFR), HER2, HER3 and HER4 (Kaur and Dasanu 2011).

With initial recognition of the HER2/neu overexpression in breast cancer (Witton et al. 2003), studies have also shown its overexpression in gastric (Becker et al. 2006; Ghaderi et al. 2002) and oesophageal tumours (Kawaguchi et al. 2007). In gastric cancer, the anatomical location of the tumour is associated with variable HER2 expression, a finding recently confirmed in the ToGA trial, with HER2 positivity was noted in 32 and 19 % of OGJ and gastric tumours, respectively (Bang et al. 2010). Trastuzumab is a monoclonal antibody that targets HER2, induces antibody-dependent cellular cytotoxicity, inhibits HER2-mediated signalling, and prevents cleavage of the extracellular domain of HER2 (Hudis 2007). In view of the good tolerance profile of trastuzumab, a HER2 positivity rate similar to breast cancer and the evident medical need for targeted therapy in gastric cancer, its addition to traditional chemotherapy in advanced gastric cancer was investigated in the trastuzamab for gastric cancer (ToGA) trial (Bang et al. 2010). Out of more than 3800 cases screened in 24 countries, 22 % showed HER2 expression, with a good concordance rate between immunohistochemical (IHC) staining and fluorescence in situ hybridisation (FISH). 594 patients were randomly assigned to treatment (trastuzumab plus chemotherapy, $n = 298$; chemotherapy alone, $n = 296$). Median overall survival was 13·8 months (95 % CI 12–16) in those assigned to trastuzumab plus chemotherapy compared with 11·1 months (10–13) in those assigned to chemotherapy alone (hazard ratio 0.74; 95 % CI 0.60–0.91; $p = 0.0046$). Despite being statistically significant, the improvement in survival is relatively modest and treatment is expensive. The study concluded that trastuzumab in combination with chemotherapy can be considered as a new standard option for patients with HER2-positive advanced disease. This has established a new standard of care and given hope that targeted agents will play an ever increasing role in treatment.

Lapatinib is an orally effective, dual TKI of HER1 and HER2 with a proven use in trastuzumab resistant breast cancer. In preclinical trials, Lapatinib's efficacy has been reported in gastric cancer cell lines and it also has activity against selected EGFR-negative cell lines and a synergistic effect with the antitumor activity of 5-fluorouracil, cisplatin, oxaliplatin, paclitaxel, irinorectan and trastuzumab. The preliminary results of a Phase II trial conducted for lapatinib as a monotherapy for advanced gastric cancer appear to be relatively modest (Iqbal et al. 2011). The final results of this trial are awaited.

Phase II studies with cetuximab and nimotuzumab (Lordick et al. 2010; Pinto et al. 2007, 2009), both EGFR antibodies have shown some promise. The encouraging results from such phase II trials prompted the initiation of phase III trials to test their efficacy. Two large phase III studies for chemotherapy with or without an EGFR inhibitory monoclonal antibody are at present open to recruitment. The REAL-3 trial of the efficacy of epirubicin, oxaliplatin and capecitabine (EOX) with or without panitumumab in untreated advanced oesophago-gastric cancer will give data on this mAb's effect on overall survival and rates of toxicity.[2] In the EXPAND trial,[3] a multi-centre, randomised controlled study involving 185 centres in 25 countries, patients with advanced or metastatic gastric cancer are randomised to receive cisplatin/xeloda chemotherapy with or without cetuximab—an anti-EGFR mAb. Recruitment has been completed and results are awaited. Neither trial is restricted to patients with wild-type KRAS tumour status, as at present there are no data suggesting that the presence of a mutation predicts a lack of response to EGFR inhibitors in gastric cancers. The perioperative use of cetuximab combined with 5-FU and cisplatin is also under investigation in patients with resectable gastric and junctional cancers in the Federation Francophone de Cancerologie Digestive (FFCD) 0901 trial.[4]

To date, little information is available for the efficacy of targeted treatment in resectable patients in combination with perioperative chemotherapeutic regimes. Results of both the MAGIC 2 (see footnote 1) and FFCD 0901 (see footnote 4) trials are anticipated and will give helpful data.

7 Conclusions and Future Directions

The heterogeneity of gastric cancer, the distinct histological subtypes and the intrinsic molecular diversity represent a challenge and an opportunity in developing individually tailored therapy. This review clearly illustrates the need for the emergence of reliable predictive biomarkers of both histological response and clinical benefit of neoadjuvant treatment in gastric cancer. Currently, despite extensive study, neither imaging nor molecular biomarkers can provide a sufficiently sensitive test to warrant excluding a cohort of patients from the potential benefit of preoperative treatment.

Due to its inherent limitations, the promise that FDG-PET has shown as a biomarker for chemosensitivity in OGJ tumours is not transferrable to gastric cancers. As both knowledge of tumour biology and the development of metabolic tracers increase, it may be hoped that metabolic imaging will evolve to become the sensitive test of chemotherapy's efficacy for which it has held promise. The goal of imaging contributing to decision making in the patient algorithm is tangible. Despite the voluminous literature relating to the investigation of molecular markers to predict tumour chemo-responsiveness, no single marker has emerged of real clinical benefit. Increasingly tumour histology appears to be linked to

---

[2] http://clinicaltrials.gov A randomised open-labelled multicentre trial of the efficacy of epirubicin, oxaliplatin and capecitabine (EOX) with or without panitumumab in previously untreated advanced oesophago-gastric cancer.

[3] http://clinicaltrials.gov Erbitux in combination with xeloda and cisplatin in advanced esophagogastric cancer (EXPAND).

[4] http://clinicaltrials.gov Trial evaluating the efficacy and tolerance of perioperative chemotherapywith 5FU-cisplatin-cetuximab in adenocarcinomas of the stomach and gastroesophageal junction. Phase II single arm, multicenter.

histological response. SRC tumours may not benefit from conventional preoperative cytotoxic treatment. This assertion needs to be clarified, and future clinical trial design needs to take into account tumour diversity and allow for an analysis of distinct histological subtypes. Analysed together, these observations mean that a proportion of patients continue to undergo toxic neoadjuvant treatment, which is ineffective for their tumour subtype, and allows for interval disease progression, while they await definitive surgical resection.

While individualised therapy is the future aspiration, currently, changing patients from established treatment strategies and introducing targeted therapies should be limited to the setting of ongoing and future clinical trials. It is clear that trials need to take account of the diversity of tumour biology, and further research needs to elucidate the molecular pathways and mechanisms responsible for both metabolic and histological tumour response. The identification of predictive biomarkers to select those patients who do, and do not, benefit from chemotherapy and targeted therapy remains a critical but yet elusive goal.

Conflicts of Interest The authors declare that they have no competing interests.

Funding Source: none

References

Bang YJ, Van Cutsem E, Feyereislova A, Chung HC, Shen L, Sawaki A, Lordick F, Ohtsu A, Omuro Y, Satoh T, Aprile G, Kulikov E, Hill J, Lehle M, Ruschoff J, Kang YK (2010) Trastuzumab in combination with chemotherapy versus chemotherapy alone for treatment of HER2-positive advanced gastric or gastro-oesophageal junction cancer (ToGA): a phase 3, open-label, randomised controlled trial. Lancet 376:687–697

Bang YJ, Kang YK, Kang WK, Boku N, Chung HC, Chen JS, Doi T, Sun Y, Shen L, Qin S, Ng WT, Tursi JM, Lechuga MJ, Lu DR, Ruiz-Garcia A, Sobrero A (2011) Phase II study of sunitinib as second-line treatment for advanced gastric cancer. Invest New Drugs 29:1449–1458

Bataille F, Rummele P, Dietmaier W, Gaag D, Klebl F, Reichle A, Wild P, Hofstadter F, Hartmann A (2003) Alterations in p53 predict response to preoperative high dose chemotherapy in patients with gastric cancer. Mol Pathol 56:286–292

Becker K, Mueller JD, Schulmacher C, Ott K, Fink U, Busch R, Bottcher K, Siewert JR, Hofler H (2003) Histomorphology and grading of regression in gastric carcinoma treated with neoadjuvant chemotherapy. Cancer 98:1521–1530

Becker JC, Muller-Tidow C, Serve H, Domschke W, Pohle T (2006) Role of receptor tyrosine kinases in gastric cancer: new targets for a selective therapy. World J Gastroenterol 12:3297–3305

Bentrem D, Gerdes H, Tang L, Brennan M, Coit D (2007) Clinical correlation of endoscopic ultrasonography with pathologic stage and outcome in patients undergoing curative resection for gastric cancer. Ann Surg Oncol 14:1853–1859

Berger AC, Farma J, Scott WJ, Freedman G, Weiner L, Cheng JD, Wang H, Goldberg M (2005) Complete response to neoadjuvant chemoradiotherapy in esophageal carcinoma is associated with significantly improved survival. J Clin Oncol 23:4330–4337

Boku N, Chin K, Hosokawa K, Ohtsu A, Tajiri H, Yoshida S, Yamao T, Kondo H, Shirao K, Shimada Y, Saito D, Hasebe T, Mukai K, Seki S, Saito H, Johnston PG (1998) Biological markers as a predictor for response and prognosis of unresectable gastric cancer patients treated with 5-fluorouracil and cis-platinum. Clin Cancer Res 4:1469–1474

Brucher BL, Becker K, Lordick F, Fink U, Sarbia M, Stein H, Busch R, Zimmermann F, Molls M, Hofler H, Siewert JR (2006) The clinical impact of histopathologic response assessment by residual tumor cell quantification in esophageal squamous cell carcinomas. Cancer 106:2119–2127

Brucher BL, Swisher SG, Konigsrainer A, Zieker D, Hartmann J, Stein H, Kitagawa Y, Law S, Ajani JA (2009) Response to preoperative therapy in upper gastrointestinal cancers. Ann Surg Oncol 16:878–86

Burke EC, Karpeh MS, Conlon KC, Brennan MF (1997) Laparoscopy in the management of gastric adenocarcinoma. Ann Surg 225:262–267

Cunningham SC, Kamangar F, Kim MP, Hammoud S, Haque R, Maitra A, Montgomery E, Heitmiller RE, Choti MA, Lillemoe KD, Cameron JL, Yeo CJ, Schulick RD (2005) Survival after gastric adenocarcinoma resection: eighteen-year experience at a single institution. J Gastrointest Surg 9:718–725

Cunningham D, Allum WH, Stenning SP, Thompson JN, Van de Velde CJ, Nicolson M, Scarffe JH, Lofts FJ, Falk SJ, Iveson TJ, Smith DB, Langley RE, Verma M, Weeden S, Chua YJ, Participants MT (2006) Perioperative chemotherapy versus surgery alone for resectable gastroesophageal cancer. N Engl J Med 355:11–20

Dassen AE, Lips DJ, Hoekstra CJ, Pruijt JF, Bosscha K (2009) FDG-PET has no definite role in preoperative imaging in gastric cancer. Eur J Surg Oncol 35:449–455

Diasio RB, Harris BE (1989) Clinical pharmacology of 5-fluorouracil. Clin Pharmacokinet 16:215–237

Fareed KR, Kaye P, Soomro IN, Ilyas M, Martin S, Parsons SL, Madhusudan S (2009) Biomarkers of response to therapy in oesophago-gastric cancer. Gut 58:127–143

Fink D, Nebel S, Aebi S, Zheng H, Cenni B, Nehme A, Christen RD, Howell SB (1996) The role of DNA mismatch repair in platinum drug resistance. Cancer Res 56:4881–4886

Fukuda H, Takiguchi N, Koda K, Oda K, Seike K, Miyazaki M (2006) Thymidylate synthase and dihydropyrimidine dehydrogenase are related to histological effects of 5-fluorouracil and cisplatin neoadjuvant chemotherapy for primary gastric cancer patients. Cancer Invest 24:235–241

Ghaderi A, Vasei M, Maleck-Hosseini SA, Gharesi-Fard B, Khodami M, Doroudchi M, Modjtahedi H (2002) The expression of c-erbB-1 and c-erbB-2 in Iranian patients with gastric carcinoma. Pathol Oncol Res 8:252–256

Goekkurt E, Hoehn S, Wolschke C, Wittmer C, Stueber C, Hossfeld DK, Stoehlmacher J (2006) Polymorphisms of glutathione S-transferases (GST) and thymidylate synthase (TS)–novel predictors for response and survival in gastric cancer patients. Br J Cancer 94:281–286

Grundei T, Vogelsang H, Ott K, Mueller J, Scholz M, Becker K, Fink U, Siewert JR, Hofler H, Keller G (2000) Loss of heterozygosity and microsatellite instability as predictive markers for neoadjuvant treatment in gastric carcinoma. Clin Cancer Res 6:4782–4788

Henson DE, Dittus C, Younes M, Nguyen H, Albores-Saavedra J (2004) Differential trends in the intestinal and diffuse types of gastric carcinoma in the United States, 1973–2000: increase in the signet ring cell type. Arch Pathol Lab Med 128:765–770

Hudis CA (2007) Trastuzumab–mechanism of action and use in clinical practice. N Engl J Med 357:39–51

Hurwitz H, Fehrenbacher L, Novotny W, Cartwright T, Hainsworth J, Heim W, Berlin J, Baron A, Griffing S, Holmgren E, Ferrara N, Fyfe G, Rogers B, Ross R, Kabbinavar F (2004) Bevacizumab plus irinotecan, fluorouracil, and leucovorin for metastatic colorectal cancer. N Engl J Med 350:2335–2342

Iqbal S, Goldman B, Fenoglio-Preiser CM, Lenz HJ, Zhang W, Danenberg KD, Shibata SI, Blanke CD (2011) Southwest Oncology Group study S0413: a phase II trial of lapatinib (GW572016) as first-line therapy in patients with advanced or metastatic gastric cancer. Ann Oncol 22:2610–2615

Ishikawa Y, Kubota T, Otani Y, Watanabe M, Teramoto T, Kumai K, Takechi T, Okabe H, Fukushima M, Kitajima M (2000) Dihydropyrimidine dehydrogenase and messenger RNA levels in gastric cancer: possible predictor for sensitivity to 5-fluorouracil. Jpn J Cancer Res 91:105–112

Jonckheere N, Van Seuningen I (2008) The membrane-bound mucins: how large O-glycoproteins play key roles in epithelial cancers and hold promise as biological tools for gene-based and immunotherapies. Crit Rev Oncog 14:177–196

Jonckheere N, Van Seuningen I (2010) The membrane-bound mucins: From cell signalling to transcriptional regulation and expression in epithelial cancers. Biochimie 92:1–11

Kamangar F, Dores GM, Anderson WF (2006) Patterns of cancer incidence, mortality, and prevalence across five continents: defining priorities to reduce cancer disparities in different geographic regions of the world. J Clin Oncol 24:2137–2150

Kameyama R, Yamamoto Y, Izuishi K, Takebayashi R, Hagiike M, Murota M, Kaji M, Haba R, Nishiyama Y (2009) Detection of gastric cancer using 18F-FLT PET: comparison with 18F-FDG PET. Eur J Nucl Med Mol Imaging 36:382–388

Kaur A, Dasanu CA (2011) Targeting the HER2 pathway for the therapy of lower esophageal and gastric adenocarcinoma. Expert Opin Pharmacother 12:2493–2503

Kawaguchi Y, Kono K, Mimura K, Mitsui F, Sugai H, Akaike H, Fujii H (2007) Targeting EGFR and HER-2 with cetuximab- and trastuzumab-mediated immunotherapy in oesophageal squamous cell carcinoma. Br J Cancer 97:494–501

Keam B, Im SA, Han SW, Ham HS, Kim MA, Oh DY, Lee SH, Kim JH, Kim DW, Kim TY, Heo DS, Kim WH, Bang YJ (2008) Modified FOLFOX-6 chemotherapy in advanced gastric cancer: results of phase II study and comprehensive analysis of polymorphisms as a predictive and prognostic marker. BMC Cancer 8:148

Kelsen DP, Winter KA, Gunderson LL, Mortimer J, Estes NC, Haller DG, Ajani JA, Kocha W, Minsky BD, Roth JA, Willett CG (2007) Long-term results of RTOG trial 8911 (USA Intergroup 113): a random assignment trial comparison of chemotherapy followed by surgery compared with surgery alone for esophageal cancer. J Clin Oncol 25:3719–3725

Kikuyama S, Inada T, Shimizu K, Miyakita M, Ogata Y (2001) p53, bcl-2 and thymidine phosphorylase as predictive markers of chemotherapy in patients with advanced and recurrent gastric cancer. Anticancer Res 21:2149–2153

Koga H, Sasaki M, Kuwabara Y, Hiraka K, Nakagawa M, Abe K, Kaneko K, Hayashi K, Honda H (2003) An analysis of the physiological FDG uptake pattern in the stomach. Ann Nucl Med 17:733–738

Koizumi W, Saigenji K, Nakamaru N, Okayasu I, Kurihara M (1999) Prediction of response to 5′-deoxy-5-fluorouridine (5′-DFUR) in patients with inoperable advanced gastric cancer by immunostaining of thymidine phosphorylase/platelet-derived endothelial cell growth factor. Oncology 56:215–222

Kono A, Hara Y, Sugata S, Karube Y, Matsushima Y, Ishitsuka H (1983) Activation of 5′-deoxy-5-fluorouridine by thymidine phosphorylase in human tumors. Chem Pharm Bull (Tokyo) 31:175–178

Kwon HC, Roh MS, Oh SY, Kim SH, Kim MC, Kim JS, Kim HJ (2007) Prognostic value of expression of ERCC1, thymidylate synthase, and glutathione S-transferase P1 for 5-fluorouracil/oxaliplatin chemotherapy in advanced gastric cancer. Ann Oncol 18:504–509

Lenz HJ, Leichman CG, Danenberg KD, Danenberg PV, Groshen S, Cohen H, Laine L, Crookes P, Silberman H, Baranda J, Garcia Y, Li J, Leichman L (1996) Thymidylate synthase mRNA level in adenocarcinoma of the stomach: a predictor for primary tumor response and overall survival. J Clin Oncol 14:176–182

Lordick F, Ott K, Krause BJ, Weber WA, Becker K, Stein HJ, Lorenzen S, Schuster T, Wieder H, Herrmann K, Bredenkamp R, Hofler H, Fink U, Peschel C, Schwaiger M, Siewert JR (2007) PET to assess early metabolic response and to guide treatment of adenocarcinoma of the oesophagogastric junction: the MUNICON phase II trial. Lancet Oncol 8:797–805

Lordick F, Luber B, Lorenzen S, Hegewisch-Becker S, Folprecht G, Woll E, Decker T, Endlicher E, Rothling N, Schuster T, Keller G, Fend F, Peschel C (2010) Cetuximab plus oxaliplatin/leucovorin/5-fluorouracil in first-line metastatic gastric cancer: a phase II study of the Arbeitsgemeinschaft Internistische Onkologie (AIO). Br J Cancer 102:500–505

Lowy AM, Mansfield PF, Leach SD, Pazdur R, Dumas P, Ajani JA (1999) Response to neoadjuvant chemotherapy best predicts survival after curative resection of gastric cancer. Ann Surg 229:303–308

Lu JW, Gao CM, Wu JZ, Cao HX, Tajima K, Feng JF (2006) Polymorphism in the $3'$-untranslated region of the thymidylate synthase gene and sensitivity of stomach cancer to fluoropyrimidine-based chemotherapy. J Hum Genet 51:155–160

Macdonald JS (2009) Adopting postoperative chemoradiotherapy in resected gastric cancer. Gastrointest Cancer Res 3:245–246

Macdonald JS, Smalley SR, Benedetti J, Hundahl SA, Estes NC, Stemmermann GN, Haller DG, Ajani JA, Gunderson LL, Jessup JM, Martenson JA (2001) Chemoradiotherapy after surgery compared with surgery alone for adenocarcinoma of the stomach or gastroesophageal junction. N Engl J Med 345:725–730

Mandard AM, Dalibard F, Mandard JC, Marnay J, Henry-Amar M, Petiot JF, Roussel A, Jacob JH, Segol P, Samama G, et al. (1994) Pathologic assessment of tumor regression after preoperative chemoradiotherapy of esophageal carcinoma. Clinicopathologic correlations. Cancer 73:2680–2686

Messager M, Lefevre JH, Pichot-Delahaye V, Souadka A, Piessen G, Mariette C (2011) The impact of perioperative chemotherapy on survival in patients with gastric signet ring cell adenocarcinoma: a multicenter comparative study. Ann Surg 254:684–693 (discussion 693)

Metzger R, Leichman CG, Danenberg KD, Danenberg PV, Lenz HJ, Hayashi K, Groshen S, Salonga D, Cohen H, Laine L, Crookes P, Silberman H, Baranda J, Konda B, Leichman L (1998) ERCC1 mRNA levels complement thymidylate synthase mRNA levels in predicting response and survival for gastric cancer patients receiving combination cisplatin and fluorouracil chemotherapy. J Clin Oncol 16:309–316

Milano G, Etienne MC, Pierrefite V, Barberi-Heyob M, Deporte-Fety R, Renee N (1999) Dihydropyrimidine dehydrogenase deficiency and fluorouracil-related toxicity. Br J Cancer 79: 627–630

Moehler M, Mueller A, Hartmann JT, Ebert MP, Al-Batran SE, Reimer P, Weihrauch M, Lordick F, Trarbach T, Biesterfeld S, Kabisch M, Wachtlin D, Galle PR (2011) An open-label, multicentre biomarker-oriented AIO phase II trial of sunitinib for patients with chemo-refractory advanced gastric cancer. Eur J Cancer 47:1511–1520

Nagashima F, Boku N, Ohtsu A, Yoshida S, Hasebe T, Ochiai A, Sakata Y, Saito H, Miyata Y, Hyodo I, Ando M (2005) Biological markers as a predictor for response and prognosis of unresectable gastric cancer patients treated with irinotecan and cisplatin. Jpn J Clin Oncol 35:714–719

Nakata B, Chung KH, Ogawa M, Ogawa Y, Yanagawa K, Muguruma K, Inoue T, Yamashita Y, Onoda N, Maeda K, Sawada T, Sowa M (1998) p53 protein overexpression as a predictor of the response to chemotherapy in gastric cancer. Surg Today 28:595–598

Napieralski R, Ott K, Kremer M, Specht K, Vogelsang H, Becker K, Muller M, Lordick F, Fink U, Rudiger Siewert J, Hofler H, Keller G (2005) Combined GADD45A and thymidine phosphorylase expression levels predict response and survival of neoadjuvant-treated gastric cancer patients. Clin Cancer Res 11:3025–3031

Nishina T, Hyodo I, Miyaike J, Inaba T, Suzuki S, Shiratori Y (2004) The ratio of thymidine phosphorylase to dihydropyrimidine dehydrogenase in tumour tissues of patients with metastatic gastric cancer is predictive of the clinical response to $5'$-deoxy-5-fluorouridine. Eur J Cancer 40:1566–1571

Novotny AR, Schuhmacher C, Busch R, Kattan MW, Brennan MF, Siewert JR (2006) Predicting individual survival after gastric cancer resection: validation of a U.S.-derived nomogram at a single high-volume center in Europe. Ann Surg 243:74–81

Ohtsu A, Shah MA, Van Cutsem E, Rha SY, Sawaki A, Park SR, Lim HY, Yamada Y, Wu J, Langer B, Starnawski M, Kang YK (2011) Bevacizumab in combination with chemotherapy as first-line therapy in advanced gastric cancer: a randomized, double-blind, placebo-controlled phase III study. J Clin Oncol 29:3968–3976

Okada E, Murai Y, Matsui K, Isizawa S, Cheng C, Masuda M, Takano Y (2001) Survivin expression in tumor cell nuclei is predictive of a favorable prognosis in gastric cancer patients. Cancer Lett 163:109–116

Ott K, Fink U, Becker K, Stahl A, Dittler HJ, Busch R, Stein H, Lordick F, Link T, Schwaiger M, Siewert JR, Weber WA (2003) Prediction of response to preoperative chemotherapy in gastric carcinoma by metabolic imaging: results of a prospective trial. J Clin Oncol 21:4604–4610

Ott K, Vogelsang H, Mueller J, Becker K, Muller M, Fink U, Siewert JR, Hofler H, Keller G (2003) Chromosomal instability rather than p53 mutation is associated with response to neoadjuvant cisplatin-based chemotherapy in gastric carcinoma. Clin Cancer Res 9:2307–2315

Ott K, Vogelsang H, Marton N, Becker K, Lordick F, Kobl M, Schuhmacher C, Novotny A, Mueller J, Fink U, Ulm K, Siewert JR, Hofler H, Keller G (2006) The thymidylate synthase tandem repeat promoter polymorphism: A predictor for tumor-related survival in neoadjuvant treated locally advanced gastric cancer. Int J Cancer 119:2885–2894

Ott K, Weber WA, Lordick F, Becker K, Busch R, Herrmann K, Wieder H, Fink U, Schwaiger M, Siewert JR (2006) Metabolic imaging predicts response, survival, and recurrence in adenocarcinomas of the esophagogastric junction. J Clin Oncol 24:4692–4698

Ott K, Herrmann K, Lordick F, Wieder H, Weber WA, Becker K, Buck AK, Dobritz M, Fink U, Ulm K, Schuster T, Schwaiger M, Siewert JR, Krause BJ (2008) Early metabolic response evaluation by fluorine-18 fluorodeoxyglucose positron emission tomography allows in vivo testing of chemosensitivity in gastric cancer: long-term results of a prospective study. Clin Cancer Res 14:2012–2018

Ott K, Lordick F, Becker K, Ulm K, Siewert J, Hofler H, Keller G (2008) Glutathione-S-transferase P1, T1 and M1 genetic polymorphisms in neoadjuvant-treated locally advanced gastric cancer: GSTM1-present genotype is associated with better prognosis in completely resected patients. Int J Colorectal Dis 23:773–782

Ott K, Lordick F, Herrmann K, Krause BJ, Schuhmacher C, Siewert JR (2008) The new credo: induction chemotherapy in locally advanced gastric cancer: consequences for surgical strategies. Gastric Cancer 11:1–9

Ott K, Herrmann K, Schuster T, Langer R, Becker K, Wieder HA, Wester HJ, Siewert JR, zum Buschenfelde CM, Buck AK, Wilhelm D, Ebert MP, Peschel C, Schwaiger M, Lordick F, Krause BJ (2011) Molecular imaging of proliferation and glucose utilization: utility for monitoring response and prognosis after neoadjuvant therapy in locally advanced gastric cancer. Ann Surg Oncol 18:3316–3323

Piessen G, Messager M, Leteurtre E, Jean-Pierre T, Mariette C (2009) Signet ring cell histology is an independent predictor of poor prognosis in gastric adenocarcinoma regardless of tumoral clinical presentation. Ann Surg 250:878–887

Piessen G, Amielh D, Messager M, Vinatier E, Leteurtre E, Triboulet JP, Mariette C (2012) Is pretreatment endoscopic biopsy a good predictor of signet ring cell histology in gastric carcinoma? World J Surg 36:346–354

Pinto C, Di Fabio F, Siena S, Cascinu S, Rojas Llimpe FL, Ceccarelli C, Mutri V, Giannetta L, Giaquinta S, Funaioli C, Berardi R, Longobardi C, Piana E, Martoni AA (2007) Phase II study of cetuximab in combination with FOLFIRI in patients with untreated advanced gastric or gastroesophageal junction adenocarcinoma (FOLCETUX study). Ann Oncol 18:510–517

Pinto C, Di Fabio F, Barone C, Siena S, Falcone A, Cascinu S, Rojas Llimpe FL, Stella G, Schinzari G, Artale S, Mutri V, Giaquinta S, Giannetta L, Bardelli A, Martoni AA (2009) Phase II study of cetuximab in combination with cisplatin and docetaxel in patients with untreated advanced gastric or gastro-oesophageal junction adenocarcinoma (DOCETUX study). Br J Cancer 101:1261–1268

Sakuramoto S, Sasako M, Yamaguchi T, Kinoshita T, Fujii M, Nashimoto A, Furukawa H, Nakajima T, Ohashi Y, Imamura H, Higashino M, Yamamura Y, Kurita A, Arai K (2007) Adjuvant chemotherapy for gastric cancer with S-1, an oral fluoropyrimidine. N Engl J Med 357:1810–1820

Sarela AI, Miner TJ, Karpeh MS, Coit DG, Jaques DP, Brennan MF (2006) Clinical outcomes with laparoscopic stage M1, unresected gastric adenocarcinoma. Ann Surg 243:189–195

Shah MA, Coit YH et al. (2007) A phase II study of preoperative chemotherapy with irinotecan (CPT) and cisplatin (CIS) for gastric cancer (NCI 5917): FDG-PET/CT predicts patient outcome. J Clin Oncol 102(2):135–140

Shah MA, Ramanathan RK, Ilson DH, Levnor A, D'Adamo D, O'Reilly E, Tse A, Trocola R, Schwartz L, Capanu M, Schwartz GK, Kelsen DP (2006) Multicenter phase II study of irinotecan, cisplatin, and bevacizumab in patients with metastatic gastric or gastroesophageal junction adenocarcinoma. J Clin Oncol 24:5201–5206

Shah MA, Jhawer M, Ilson DH, Lefkowitz RA, Robinson E, Capanu M, Kelsen DP (2011) Phase II study of modified docetaxel, cisplatin, and fluorouracil with bevacizumab in patients with metastatic gastroesophageal adenocarcinoma. J Clin Oncol 29:868–874

Shoda H, Kakugawa Y, Saito D, Kozu T, Terauchi T, Daisaki H, Hamashima C, Muramatsu Y, Moriyama N, Saito H (2007) Evaluation of 18F-2-deoxy-2-fluoro-glucose positron emission tomography for gastric cancer screening in asymptomatic individuals undergoing endoscopy. Br J Cancer 97:1493–1498

Smith BR, Stabile BE (2009) Extreme aggressiveness and lethality of gastric adenocarcinoma in the very young. Arch Surg 144:506–510

Sun W, Powell M, O'Dwyer PJ, Catalano P, Ansari RH, Benson AB (2010) 3rd Phase II study of sorafenib in combination with docetaxel and cisplatin in the treatment of metastatic or advanced gastric and gastroesophageal junction adenocarcinoma: ECOG 5203. J Clin Oncol 28:2947–2951

Terashima M, Fujiwara H, Takagane A, Abe K, Araya M, Irinoda T, Yonezawa H, Nakaya T, Oyama K, Takahashi M, Saito K (2002) Role of thymidine phosphorylase and dihydropyrimidine dehydrogenase in tumour progression and sensitivity to doxifluridine in gastric cancer patients. Eur J Cancer 38:2375–2381

Terashima M, Fujiwara H, Takagane A, Abe K, Irinoda T, Nakaya T, Yonezawa H, Oyama K, Saito K, Kanzaki N, Ohtani S, Nemoto T, Hoshino Y, Kogure M, Gotoh M (2003) Prediction of sensitivity to fluoropyrimidines by metabolic and target enzyme activities in gastric cancer. Gastric Cancer 6(Suppl 1):71–81

Therasse P, Arbuck SG, Eisenhauer EA, Wanders J, Kaplan RS, Rubinstein L, Verweij J, Van Glabbeke M, van Oosterom AT, Christian MC, Gwyther SG (2000) New guidelines to evaluate the response to treatment in solid tumors. European Organization for Research and Treatment of Cancer, National Cancer Institute of the United States, National Cancer Institute of Canada. J Natl Cancer Inst 92:205–216

Vallbohmer D, Drebber U, Schneider PM, Baldus S, Bollschweiler E, Brabender J, Warnecke-Eberz U, Monig S, Holscher AH, Metzger R (2009) Survivin expression in gastric cancer: Association with histomorphological response to neoadjuvant therapy and prognosis. J Surg Oncol 99:409–413

Vallbohmer D, Holscher AH, Schneider PM, Schmidt M, Dietlein M, Bollschweiler E, Baldus S, Alakus H, Brabender J, Metzger R, Monig SP (2010) [18F]-fluorodeoxyglucose-positron emission tomography for the assessment of histopathologic response and prognosis after completion of neoadjuvant chemotherapy in gastric cancer. J Surg Oncol 102:135–140

Wang TT, Qian XP, Liu BR (2007) Survivin: potential role in diagnosis, prognosis and targeted therapy of gastric cancer. World J Gastroenterol 13:2784–2790

Warnecke-Eberz U, Hokita S, Xi H, Higashi H, Baldus SE, Metzger R, Brabender J, Bollschweiler E, Mueller RP, Dienes HP, Hoelscher AH, Schneider PM (2005) Overexpression of survivin mRNA is associated with a favorable prognosis following neoadjuvant radiochemotherapy in esophageal cancer. Oncol Rep 13:1241–1246

Watanabe H JJ, Sobin LH (1990) Histological typing of oesophageal and gastric tumors. WHO international classification of tumors. Springer, Berlin

Weber G, Nagai M, Natsumeda Y, Ichikawa S, Nakamura H, Eble JN, Jayaram HN, Zhen WN, Paulik E, Hoffman R et al. (1991) Regulation of de novo and salvage pathways in chemotherapy. Adv Enzyme Regul 31:45–67

Weber WA, Ott K, Becker K, Dittler HJ, Helmberger H, Avril NE, Meisetschlager G, Busch R, Siewert JR, Schwaiger M, Fink U (2001) Prediction of response to preoperative chemotherapy in adenocarcinomas of the esophagogastric junction by metabolic imaging. J Clin Oncol 19:3058–3065

Wells P, Aboagye E, Gunn RN, Osman S, Boddy AV, Taylor GA, Rafi I, Hughes AN, Calvert AH, Price PM, Newell DR (2003) 2-[11C]thymidine positron emission tomography as an indicator of thymidylate synthase inhibition in patients treated with AG337. J Natl Cancer Inst 95:675–682

Wieder HA, Geinitz H, Rosenberg R, Lordick F, Becker K, Stahl A, Rummeny E, Siewert JR, Schwaiger M, Stollfuss J (2007) PET imaging with [18F]3'-deoxy-3'-fluorothymidine for prediction of response to neoadjuvant treatment in patients with rectal cancer. Eur J Nucl Med Mol Imaging 34:878–883

Witton CJ, Reeves JR, Going JJ, Cooke TG, Bartlett JM (2003) Expression of the HER1-4 family of receptor tyrosine kinases in breast cancer. J Pathol 200:290–297

Ychou M, Boige V, Pignon JP, Conroy T, Bouche O, Lebreton G, Ducourtieux M, Bedenne L, Fabre JM, Saint-Aubert B, Geneve J, Lasser P, Rougier P (2011) Perioperative chemotherapy compared with surgery alone for resectable gastroesophageal adenocarcinoma: an FNCLCC and FFCD multicenter phase III trial. J Clin Oncol 29:1715–1721

Yeh KH, Shun CT, Chen CL, Lin JT, Lee WJ, Lee PH, Chen YC, Cheng AL (1998) High expression of thymidylate synthase is associated with the drug resistance of gastric carcinoma to high dose 5-fluorouracil-based systemic chemotherapy. Cancer 82:1626–1631

Yun M, Choi HS, Yoo E, Bong JK, Ryu YH, Lee JD (2005) The role of gastric distention in differentiating recurrent tumor from physiologic uptake in the remnant stomach on 18F-FDG PET. J Nucl Med 46:953–957

Yun M, Lim JS, Noh SH, Hyung WJ, Cheong JH, Bong JK, Cho A, Lee JD (2005) Lymph node staging of gastric cancer using (18)F-FDG PET: a comparison study with CT. J Nucl Med 46:1582–1588

Prediction of Response and Prognosis by a Score Including only Pretherapeutic Parameters in 410 Neoadjuvant Treated Gastric Cancer Patients

Lorenzen Sylvie, Blank Susanne and Ott Katja

Abstract

Introduction: Response to neoadjuvant chemotherapy (NAC) is an independent prognostic factor in locally advanced gastric cancer. However, no prospectively tested pretherapeutic parameters predicting response and/or survival in gastric cancer are available in clinical routine. *Patients and methods*: We evaluated the prognostic significance of various clinicopathologic parameters in 410 patients who were treated with NAC followed by gastrectomy. Clinical and histopathological response evaluation was performed using standardized criteria. A prognostic score was created on the basis of the variables identified in the multivariate analysis. *Results*: Multivariate analysis identified three pretherapeutic parameters as positive predictive factors for response and prognosis: tumor localization in the middle third of the stomach ($p = 0.001$), well differentiated tumors ($p = 0.001$) and intestinal tumor type according to Laurén's classification ($p = 0.03$). From the obtained data a prognostic index was constructed, dividing the patients into three risk groups: low (n = 73), intermediate (n = 274), and poor (n = 63). The three groups had significantly different clinical ($p = 0.007$) and histopathological response rates ($p = 0.001$) and survival times, with a median survival time that was not reached in the low-risk group, 39.2 months in the intermediate-risk group and 20.5 months in the poor-risk group. The corresponding 5-year survival rates were 65.3, 41.2, and 21.2 % ($p < 0.001$), respectively. *Conclusion*: A simple scoring system based

---

Original paper is published in Ann Surg Oncol. 2012 Mar 7. [Epub ahead of print]

L. Sylvie (✉)
National Center of Tumor Diseases, University of Heidelberg,
Im Neuenheimer Feld 460, 69120 Heidelberg, Germany
e-mail: sylvielorenzen@gmx.de

F. Otto and M. P. Lutz (eds.), *Early Gastrointestinal Cancers*,
Recent Results in Cancer Research 196, DOI: 10.1007/978-3-642-31629-6_18,
© Springer-Verlag Berlin Heidelberg 2012

on three clinicopathologic parameters, accurately predicts response and prognosis in neoadjuvant treated gastric cancer. This system provides additional useful information that could be applied to select gastric cancer patients pretherapeutically for different treatment approaches. Prospective testing of the score in an independent patient cohort is warranted.

Contents

1 Chapter 1 272
   1.1 Background.. 272
   1.2 Prognostic Biomarkers in Gastric Cancer 273
   1.3 Aims of the Study 274
2 Chapter 2 274
   2.1 Patients.. 274
   2.2 Clinical Staging 275
   2.3 Surgery.. 275
   2.4 Histopathological Work-up and Response Evaluation............................ 275
   2.5 Statistical Analysis 276
3 Chapter 3 276
   3.1 Results... 276
   3.2 Prognostic Index and Risk Groups... 280
4 Chapter 4 282
   4.1 Conclusions... 282
   4.2 Future Directions.. 286
References.. 287

1   Chapter 1

1.1   Background

Despite a continuous decline in incidence, gastric cancer remains a major health problem worldwide and is still the second leading course of cancer-related mortality in industrialized countries (Hohenberger and Gretschel 2003). Long-term survival after potentially curative gastrectomy for locally advanced gastric cancer remains poor with 5-year survival rates of 20–30 % (De Vita et al. 2007). In an attempt to improve outcomes, combined modality treatments using perioperative chemotherapy, radiotherapy, or chemoradiotherapy in combination with surgical resection have been evaluated (De Vita et al. 2007). Recent clinical studies have shown that pre-and perioperative chemotherapy are feasible and improve clinical outcome of patients with locally advanced gastric cancer (Cunningham et al. 2006; Ott et al. 2003a; Boige et al. 2007; Schuhmacher et al. 2010; Sakuramoto et al. 2007). However, response rates to chemotherapy are low and at the expense of significant toxicity, and the majority of patients still die of recurrent disease. Therefore, an early selection of patients who are not benefiting from neoadjuvant

Prediction of Response and Prognosis 271

therapy, and therefore avoid ineffective and toxic therapy in nonresponding patients with gastric cancer is of utmost interest.

The identification of pretherapeutic predictive markers for response and prognosis would therefore be invaluable in individualizing patient treatment. This would enable identifying patients pretherapeutically with medium-to-high risk of recurrence of who should be candidates for intensified neoadjuvant therapy and/or additional adjuvant treatment.

1.2 Prognostic Biomarkers in Gastric Cancer

In gastric cancer the response rates to cytotoxic therapy range between 20 and 60 % (Persiani et al. 2005; Lordick et al. 2004; Ajani et al. 1990). Several studies could demonstrate that clinically responding patients have a superior clinical outcome after surgical resection compared to clinically nonresponding patients (Ott et al. 2003a; Lowy et al. 1999; Rohatgi et al. 2006; Fink et al. 1995). Furthermore, available evidence suggests that a histopathological response to cytotoxic therapy is a prognostic marker in gastric carcinoma (Lowy et al. 1999; Becker et al. 2003; Fareed et al. 2010).

However, it has remained a challenge for decades to identify reliable biomarkers that may be able to predict who will respond and who will progress during cytotoxic chemotherapy, and only few studies on clinical or histopathological markers predicting response and prognosis in neoadjuvant treated gastric cancer exist so far (Persiani et al. 2005; Rohatgi et al. 2006; Ninomiya et al. 1999; Nagashima et al. 2005; Jhawer et al. 2009; Mansour et al. 2007). Prognostic factors following chemotherapy are pathological stage (Rohatgi et al. 2006), nodal status (Rohatgi et al. 2006; Mansour et al. 2007), perineural invasion (Jhawer et al. 2009; Mansour et al. 2007), vascular invasion (Mansour et al. 2007), complete resection (Persiani et al. 2005; Rohatgi et al. 2006; Fink et al. 1995), tumor differentiation (Ninomiya et al. 1999), and Laurén classification (Nagashima et al. 2005).

The focus of most published papers has been on postoperative prognostic factors (Mansour et al. 2007; Siewert et al. 1998; Alakus et al. 2010; Baiocchi et al. 2010; Bilici et al. 2010; Choi et al. 2010; Mikami et al. 2009; Marchet et al. 2007, 2008). In primary resected cancer, postoperative prognostic factors like the pTNM-stage, lymph node ratio, lymphangiosis, and perineural invasion are generally accepted (Mansour et al. 2007; Siewert et al. 1998; Alakus et al. 2010; Baiocchi et al. 2010; Bilici et al. 2010; Choi et al. 2010; Mikami et al. 2009; Marchet et al. 2007, 2008). Reports on simple preoperative evaluable factors have been rare (Baiocchi et al. 2010; Johnson et al. 1995; Park et al. 2010; Shin et al. 2010).

Tumor localization (Baiocchi et al. 2010; Johnson et al. 1995), Lauren classification (Baiocchi et al. 2010), tumor differentiation (Johnson et al. 1995), mucinous content (Choi et al. 2010; Ott et al. 2008a) as well as clinical stage (Park et al. 2010) have been identified as prognostic factors in patients who did not undergo preoperative chemotherapy for gastric cancer.

To our knowledge these factors have not yet been evaluated in neoadjuvantly treated patients so far.

Consequently, the identification of clinicopathologic parameters predicting response and/or survival and the implementation of a pretherapeutic score could allow for pretherapeutic stratification in patients with locally advanced gastric cancer.

1.3 Aims of the Study

The aims of this study were:
a) to evaluate the prognostic power of individual pretherapeutic parameters
b) to test the possible association of pretherapeutic factors with response and prognosis
c) to develop a simple and practical scoring system based on response and prognosis in a large series of neoadjuvantly treated gastric cancer patients with a long-term follow-up.

2 Chapter 2

2.1 Patients

This retrospective, exploratory study included 410 patients with histologically proven, locally advanced gastric cancer (clinical T3-T4, N0/+, M0), who underwent neoadjuvant chemotherapy (NAC) in consecutive Phase II trials followed by resection of the primary tumor between February 1987 and September 2005 at the Klinikum Rechts der Isar, Technische Universitaet Muenchen, Munich, Germany. The study protocol was approved by the Institutional Review Board of the Technische Universitaet Muenchen. Written informed consent according to the institutional guideline was obtained from all patients.

2.1.1 Chemotherapy
Patients underwent NAC, consisting of at least 6 weeks of either oxaliplatin 85 mg/m^2 or cisplatin 50 mg/m^2, given on days 1, 15, 29 (1 h infusion time) and folinic acid (500 mg/m^2 over 2 h) plus fluorouracil (2000 mg/m^2 over 24 h) on days 1, 8, 15, 22, 29, and 36, all repeated on day 49 (OLF/PLF regimen). Patients aged 60 years or younger with a good health status were additionally given Paclitaxel (80 mg/m^2 over 3 h) on days 0, 14, and 28. A minority of patients (15 %) received chemotherapy with doxorubicin 20 mg/m^2 on days 1 and 7, etoposide 120 mg/m^2 on days 4, 5, and 6, and cisplatin 40 mg/m^2 on days 2 and 7 as described previously (Kelsen et al. 1996). The dose of etoposide was reduced to 100 mg/m^2 in patients aged 60 years or more.

2.2 Clinical Staging

Clinical staging consisted of endoscopy including endoluminal ultrasound, CT scan of the abdomen and pelvis, and for proximal tumors, additionally a CT scan of the chest. Peritoneal carcinomatosis was excluded by diagnostic laparoscopy before NAC. Restaging by endoscopy, endoluminal ultrasound, and CT scan was performed in the last 3 days of every cycle of chemotherapy as described previously (Ott et al. 2003b). Assessment of response to neoadjuvant therapy was based on reduction of primary tumor size measured by upper GI series, upper endoscopy, and CT scan. Clinical response was defined as a reduction in bidimensional tumor diameter of >50 % on upper GI series compared to the pretherapeutic findings (Ott et al. 2003a, 2003b, 2008b, 2008c; Fink et al. 1995). Response to therapy was judged and agreed on by at least two observers who reviewed the data for each case. New lesions or more than a 25 % increase in primary tumor size were considered progressive disease.

2.3 Surgery

Tumor resection was attempted 2–3 weeks after chemotherapy was completed. In patients with proximal gastric cancer, a transhiatal extended gastrectomy and an extended D2 lymphadenectomy (resection of the lymph node groups 1 and 2 according to the Japanese Research Society for Gastric Cancer), including a left retroperitoneal lymphadenectomy were performed; in patients with proximal gastric cancer and invasion of the distal esophagus, in some cases, either an abdominothoracic approach (Ott et al. 2009) (Ivor Lewis procedure) or a transhiatal esophagectomy(Bader et al. 2008) was performed to achieve clear proximal resection margins. In those patients, an intraabdominal D2 lymphadenectomy was performed. For patients with tumor localization in the middle or distal third, a total gastrectomy with D2 lymphadenectomy was performed (Ott et al. 2003a, 2003b, 2008c). Only few patients with distal gastric cancer underwent a subtotal gastrectomy with D2 lymphadenectomy except lymphnode station 2.

2.4 Histopathological Work-Up and Response Evaluation

Histopathological evaluation was done by standardized protocols including the pTNM categories, grading, tumor localization, subtype according to Lauréns classification and resection margins, as demanded in the guidelines of the UICC (Greene et al. 2002).

The histopathologic response to NAC was classified on the basis of the percentage of residual tumor cells within the specimen.

Tumor regression was assessed semiquantitatively according to a previously published scoring system (Becker et al. 2003). All patients with <10 % residual tumor cells (regression score 1) were classified as histopathological responders. All other patients were classified as nonresponders.

Patients follow-up

The patients were followed in the outpatient clinic according to a standard protocol with visits every three months during the first year, then every six months during the second and third year, and once yearly thereafter.

At the time of analysis, the median follow-up for the 217 survivors was 35.5 months. Of the 194 deaths, 135 were related to recurrence of gastric cancer, 19 were due to tumor progression, 16 due to perioperative complications, and 24 were due to another disease or accident. The postoperative 30-and 90 days-mortality rates were 1 and 2.9 %, respectively.

2.5 Statistical Analysis

The Kaplan-Meier method was used for calculation of survival times and the comparison of the survival curves was carried out by the log-rank test. The association between the clinicopathologic variables and the clinical and histopathological response was computed with the χ^2-test and the Fisher's-exact test. Univariate analysis was used to evaluate prognostic factors, followed by multivariate analysis using stepwise Cox proportional hazard regression modeling. With the significant prognostic factors obtained in multivariate analysis, the hazard ratio (HR) was calculated for each patient. Every patient was then assigned a prognostic index value, calculated as follows: the value of each significant prognostic factor in the final model was summed up to obtain the prognostic index for each patient (tumor localization: proximal tumors = 2, tumors in the middle third = 1, distal or total tumors = 3; Type after Laurén: intestinal = 1, diffuse = 3, mixed = 2; Grading: low grade = 1, high grade = 2). The prognostic index was used to stratify patients into three risk groups: low (summation of single prognostic factors = 3 or 4), intermediate (summation of single prognostic factors = 5, 6, or 7), and high (summation of single prognostic factors = 8).

A two-sided significance test with a p value <0.05 was considered significant, all statistic calculations were done by SPSS 17.0 (SPSS Inc, Chicago, IL).

3 Chapter 3

3.1 Results

A total of 410 patients were included in the study. The patient's demographic, clinical, and tumor characteristics are listed in Table 1 and 2.

There were 298 men and 112 women, with a median age of 55.5 years (range 17.1–78.4).

Prediction of Response and Prognosis

Table 1 Patient's characteristics (preoperative)

Characteristics		Number of patients (%)
Age	Median (years)	55±11.4
	Range (years)	17.1–78.4
Sex	Female	112 (27.3)
	Male	298 (72.7)
Tumor localization	Proximal	263 (64.1)
	Middle	49 (12.0)
	Distal	83 (20.2)
	Total	15 (3.7)
Laurén classification	Intestinal	177 (43.2)
	Diffuse	134 (32.7)
	Mixed	83 (20.2)
	Unclassified	16 (3.9)
Grading	G1/2	77 (18.8)
	G3/4	333 (8.2)
CTx-duration	Complete	273 (66.6)
	>50 %	20 (4.9)
	50 %	49 (12.0)
	<50 %	57 (13.9)
CTx regimen	PLF	247 (60.2)
	OLF	12 (2.9)
	EAP	63 (15.4)
	E-PLF	14 (3.4)
	Paclitaxel+PLF	33 (8.0)
	Docetaxel+PLF	18 (4.4)
	Others	21 (4.6)
	RCTx	2 (0.5)

CTx chemotherapy; *PLF* cisplatin; folinic acid; fluorouracil; *OLF* oxaliplatin; folinic acid; fluorouracil; *EAP* etoposide, doxorubicin, cisplatin; *E-PLF* epirubicin+PLF; *RCTx* radiochemotherapy

Histologically, intestinal subtype according to Lauren classification was predominant (43 %) compared to diffuse tumors (33 %), mixed type (20 %), and tumors which could not be classified (4 %). Eighty one percent had a low-grade tumor compared to well- and medium-differentiated tumors (19 %). Concerning tumor localization, most patients had a proximal located cancer (64 %), compared to tumors located in the middle (12 %), and distal third (20 %). In 4 %, the tumor was located in the whole stomach.

Table 2 Patient's characteristics (postoperative)

Characteristics		Number of patients (%)
Type of surgery	GE	149 (36.3)
	THE	195 (47.6)
	EE transth.	22 (5.4)
	EE abdth.	16 (3.9)
	Subt. GE	8 (2.0)
	EE + GE	7 (1.7)
ypT-category	ypT0	17 (4.1)
	ypT1a	4 (1.9)
	ypT1b	24 (5.9)
	ypT2a	37 (9.0)
	ypT2b	187 (45.6)
	ypT3	107 (26.1)
	ypT4	32 (7.8)
ypN-category	ypN0	145 (35.4)
	ypN1	120 (29.3)
	ypN2	81 (19.8)
	ypN3	64 (3.9)
ypM-category	yc/pM0	300 (73.2)
	yc/pM1	109 (26.6)
R-category	R0	302 (73.7)
	R1	71 (17.3)
	R2	24 (5.9)
	Rx	12 (2.9)

GE gastrectomy; *subt.* subtotal; *THE* transhiatal extended gastrectomy; *EE* esophagectomy; *transth.* transthoracic; *abdth.* abdominothoracic

The median survival rate was 39.2 months (95 % CI 30.5; 47.9) with a 5-year survival rate of 42 %.

The clinical and histopathological response rates were 25 and 24 %, respectively. The median survival of patients who had a clinical response was not reached, with an estimated 2- and 5-year survival rate of 86.4 and 72.5 % respectively, compared to a median survival of 31.8 month, with an estimated 2- and 5-year survival rate of 56.3 and 34.3 % in clinical nonresponders. The median survival of patients who had a histopathologic response was not reached as well, and the estimated 2- and 5-year survival rates were 87.9 and 72.9 %, respectively. In contrast, histopathologic nonresponders had a median survival of 32.1 months

Table 3 Survival according to clinical parameters

Clinical characteristics	Number of patients (%)	Median (months)	5-year survival (%)	p value
Sex				
Female	112 (27.3)	40.4	44.5	0.477
Male	298 (72.7)	39.2	40.9	
Tumor localization				
Proximal	263 (64.1)	41.3	43.0	<0.001
Middle	49 (12.0)	77.8	54.2	
Distal	83 (20.2)	27.9	37.2	
Total	15 (3.7)	8.7	8.9	
Mucinous carcinoma				
Yes	74 (18.0)	38.1	39.2	0.736
No	312 (76.1)	41	42.4	
Grading				
Low grade (1/2)	77 (18.8)	Not reached	65.1	<0.001
High grade (3/4)	333 (8.2)	35.2	36.7	
Laurén				
Intestinal	177 (43.2)	50.5	46.9	<0.001
Diffuse	134 (32.7)	23.5	30.6	
Mixed	83 (20.2)	44	45.4	

with an estimated 2- and 5-year survival rate of 58.0 and 37.2 %, respectively. Differences in survival according to histopathologic regression grade were statistically significant ($p < 0.001$), as were differences in survival according to clinical response ($p < 0.001$).

Table 3 shows the survival according to the pretherapeutic clinicopathological variables that were tested: sex, Lauren's classification (Lauren 1965), tumor localization, mucinous content, and grading. The multivariate Cox stepwise proportional hazard model including preoperative prognostic factors identified tumor localization in the middle third (HR 0.53; 95 %CI 0.31–0.9; $p = 0.001$), intestinal tumor type according to Laurén's classification (HR 0.67; 95 %CI 0.45–1.0; $p = 0.03$), and well-differentiated tumors (HR 0.43; 95 %CI 0.26–0.71; $p = 0.001$), as independent predictors for survival (Table 4). Correlations with clinical and histopathological response are shown in Table 5. Tumor localization was the only factor associated with clinical response ($p = 0.001$), with a better response of the carcinomas in the proximal third of the stomach, whereas three parameters showed a significant correlation with histopathological response: tumor localization ($p = 0.023$), grading ($p = 0.018$), and Laurén classification

Table 4 Multivariate analysis including the pretherapeutic factors of sex, tumor localization, mucinous carcinoma, grading, and Laurén classification

Characteristic	HR	95 % CI	p value
Sex			
Female	0.97	0.68–1.37	0.967
Male	1.00		
Tumor localization			
Proximal	1.00		0.001
Middle	0.53	0.31–0.9	
Distal	0.93	0.61–1.39	
Total	2.50	1.32–4.78	
Mucinous carcinoma			
Yes	1.00		0.493
No	0.87	0.59–1.3	
Grading			
Low grade (1/2)	0.43	0.26–0.71	0.001
High grade (3/4)	1.00		
Laurén			
Intestinal	0.67	0.45–1.0	0.02
Diffuse	1.00		
Mixed	0.63	0.42–0.96	

($p = 0.007$). The survival curves according to those parameters are presented in Fig. 1a–c.

3.2 Prognostic Index and Risk Groups

A scoring system with an overall risk score ranging from 3 to 8 was developed as follows:

From the obtained data, each independent prognostic factor was assigned an index score, depending on its influence on OS: localization (middle vs proximal vs distal and total were assigned 1, or 2 or 3, respectively), grading (G1/2 vs G3/4 was assigned 1 or 2, respectively), Laurén's classification (intestinal vs diffuse and mixed was assigned 1 or 3, respectively). Patients with a prognostic index of ≤4 were categorized as low-risk group (n = 73; 17.8 %), those with a prognostic index ≥5 and ≤7 were categorized as intermediate-risk group (n = 274; 66.8 %), and those with a prognostic index of 8 were categorized as poor-risk group (n = 63; 15.4 %). The median survival for the low-risk group was not reached, whereas it was 39.2 and 20.5 months for the intermediate- and poor-risk group.

Prediction of Response and Prognosis

Table 5 Correlation between clinical factors and clinical and histopathological response

Clinical factor	Clinical response (%)	p value	Histopathological response (%)	p value
Sex				
Female	22.0	0.304	20.8	0.351
Male	27.3		25.6	
Tumor localization				
Proximal	32.2	0.001	29.2	0.023
Middle	15.2		15.2	
Distal	16.0		14.7	
Total	3.6		15.4	
Mucinous carcinoma				
Yes	18.3	0.171	21.4	0.643
No	26.7		24.4	
Grading				
Low grade (1/2)	34.2	0.075	35.8	0.018
High grade (3/4)	23.8		21.6	
Laurén				
Intestinal	29.8	0.288	32.9	0.007
Diffuse	20.5		17.4	
Mixed	27.3		18.4	

The 5-year survival rates were 65.3, 41.1, and 21.2 %, respectively. There was a significant difference in survival times among those three groups ($p < 0.001$) (Fig. 2). In addition, patients who were categorized as low-risk group had a higher chance of being clinical (34.2 %) and histopathological (35.6 %) responders compared to patients in the intermediate-risk group with a clinical and histopathological response rate of 24.8 and 20.8 %, respectively and patients categorized in the high-risk group with a clinical and histopathological response rate of only 11.2 % each. Consequently, the three risk groups were significantly associated with clinical response ($p = 0.007$) and histopathological response ($p = 0.001$).

Multivariate analysis including the univariate significant factors tumor localization, grading, Laurén classification, pretherapeutic score, chemotherapy regimen, lymphangiosis carcinomatosa, clinical response to chemotherapy, histopathological response, and lymph node regression revealed pretherapeutic score ($p = 0.028$), T-category ($p < 0.001$), N-category ($p < 0.001$), chemotherapy regimen ($p = 0,002$), R0 versus R1/2 ($p = 0.001$), and the clinical response to chemotherapy ($p = 0.044$) as independent prognostic factors (Table 6).

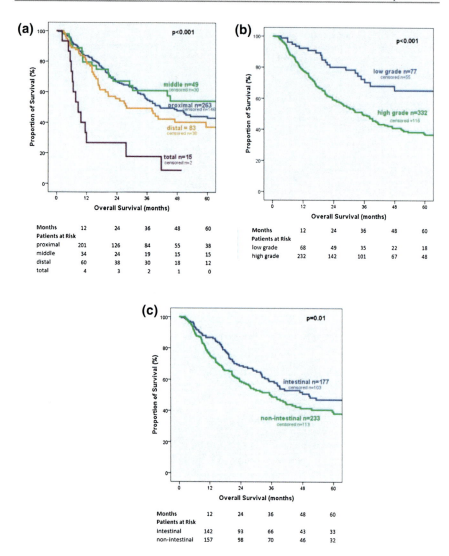

Fig. 1 a Survival according to tumor localization (n = 410). **b** Survival according to tumor differentiation (n = 410). **c** Survival according to Laurén's classification (n = 410)

4 Chapter 4

4.1 Conclusions

Traditionally, pathologic stage, composed of depth of tumor invasion, lymph node metastasis, and distant metastasis, is regarded as the most powerful indicator for the prognosis in the majority of malignant tumors. However, although this staging

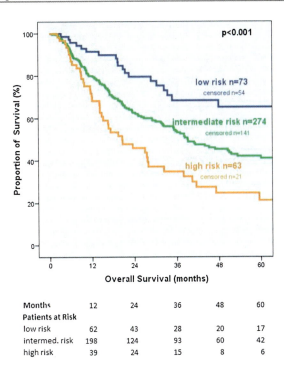

Fig. 2 Survival according to low-risk, intermediate-risk, and high-risk group (stratification by the pretherapeutic score) (n = 410)

system uses the most widely accepted prognostic factors, this tumor-node-metastasis system is only applicable in the postoperative setting and has no influence on preoperative treatment strategies.

We aimed to develop a stage-independent, simple, yet accurate model for prediction of response and prognosis on the basis of clinicopathologic characteristics that can be obtained easily before the onset of NAC in locally advanced gastric cancer patients. Therefore, the pooled data from 410 patients with neoadjuvant treated gastric cancer were analyzed in this single-institution retrospective exploratory study.

Three independent significant pretherapeutic parameters (tumor localization, grading, and Laurén classification) could be identified by multivariate analysis as highly significant predictive factors for response and survival. Our results clearly indicate that tumor location in the middle third of the stomach, intestinal tumor type according to Lauren's classification, and well-differentiated tumors correlated with a more favorable prognosis in locally advanced gastric cancer patients, as mentioned above. In addition, our series clearly suggests that each of these factors is an independent predictive marker for histopathological and clinical response to cytotoxic therapy, and therefore is a marker for patient's benefit. Both, histopathologic and clinical response to NAC was associated with a more than twofold increment in 5-year survival. This finding is in line with previous reports which could demonstrate that response to chemotherapy is predictive of patient's survival (Lowy et al. 1999; Becker et al. 2003).

Table 6 Multivariate analysis (n = 410)

Factor	HR	95 % CI	p value
Score			
3/4	0.40	0.18–0.81	0.028
5/6/7	0.67	0.45–1.01	
8	1.00		
T-category			
T0	0.08	0.01–0.6	<0.001
T1a	0.00[a]		
T1b	0.22	0.06–0.7	
T2a	0.11	0.04–0.32	
T2b	0.38	0.22–0.64	
T3	0.34	0.2–0.59	
T4	1.00		
N-category			
N0	0.25	0.15–0.44	<0.001
N1	0.42	0.26–0.68	
N2	0.38	0.24–0.62	
N3	1.00		
CTx regimen			
PLF or OLF or E-PLF	1.72	0.67–4.3	0.002
EAP	2.90	1.10–8.0	
Paclitaxel/docetaxel+PLF	0.77	0.25–2.4	
Others	1.00		
R-category			
R0	0.53	0.37–0.78	0.001
R1/2/x	1.00		
Clinical response			
Yes	0.61	0.37–0.99	0.044
No	1.00		

[a] No patient deceased during follow-up

CTx Chemotherapy; *PLF* cisplatin; folinic acid; fluorouracil; *OLF* oxaliplatin; folinic acid; fluorouracil; *EAP* etoposide; doxorubicin; cisplatin; *E-PLF* epirubicin+PLF; *RCTx* Radiochemotherapy

However, whether tumor localization, tumor grading, and tumor differentiation according to Lauren's classification are independent predictors of survival in primary resected gastric cancer, is controversially discussed in the literature (Park et al. 2010; Stemmermann and Brown 1974; Chiaravalli et al. 2001).

Therefore, it has been prospected that information for which these factors would be combined could compensate for the informative reliability of each factor and might provide physicians a quite useful information regarding the outcome of gastric cancer patients before onset of treatment.

By combining these three independent prognostic factors, we could develop three risk groups with significantly different response- and survival rates. In the low-risk group, every third patient is responding to chemotherapy, in the intermediate-risk group every fourth, and in the high-risk group only every tenth patient. Accordingly, patients in the low-, intermediate-, and poor-risk group showed highly significant survival differences with a median survival of not reached, 39.2 and 20.5 months, respectively ($p < 0.001$). Several alternative models designed to improve the accuracy of prognostic estimates of gastric cancer patients are published (Kattan et al. 2003; Inoue et al. 2002; Marubini et al. 1993; Kologlu et al. 2000). Nevertheless, to date none of them is routinely adopted in clinical setting.

This study developed a scoring system which incorporates in an easily applicable scale prognostic factors that are available for all patients in all centers before the onset of treatment.

A limitation of this prognostic system is that the developed score embraces only tumor-related factors and not patient- or treatment-related factors. Admittedly, patients-related factors such as age or sex were not correlated with response or prognosis in this study. The chemotherapy regimens applied were mostly cisplatin-based and early discontinuation did not influence prognosis either. Furthermore, these factors are not pretherapeutically available.

In contrast to other authors (Costa et al. 2006), male sex was not related to a worse prognosis in this series.

Other relevant aspects related to the patient, such as nutrition status, weight loss, and performance status were not taken into account. This can be mainly justified by the difficulty in objectively assessing the effect of these variables, although for gastric cancer, as well as for other cancers, these factors have been consistently recognized (Green et al. 2002; Harrison and Fielding 1995; Msika et al. 2000). We have to admit that neglecting clinical factors in a clinical staging system may lead to important problems, especially because different survival rates to a treatment may also be ascribed to the clinical picture and the functional condition of a patient. However, all patients included in the study had to have a Karnofsky index >80 and to be fit for cisplatin-containing chemotherapy followed by resection, so these concerns might be minimized (Ott et al. 2003a; Fink et al. 1995; Schuhmacher et al. 2001, 2010).

Furthermore, the scoring system does not embrace certain molecular markers which have been identified to hold prognostic significance in gastric cancer, such as p53 gene mutation, microsatellite DNA instability (Solcia et al. 2009) or tumor thymidylate synthase levels (Lenz et al. 1996; Fareed et al. 2009). However, despite the promising prognostic value of some molecular parameters, it will be critical to obtain a molecular analysis of a tumor biopsy before the onset of neoadjuvant treatment on gastric cancer in clinical routine so far.

The main advantage of the present investigation is that this scoring system adds feasibility and scientific background, and seems to be easily applicable in routine diagnostic practice. Since the use of preoperative therapy in gastric cancer continues to be actively investigated, we believe that this scoring system might become a useful stratification criterion in future clinical trials of pre- and perioperative treatment. However, further prospective clinical trials associating the clinical outcome with the above evaluated prognostic factors are warranted.

4.2   Future Directions

The current evidence for the role of biomarkers in predicting response to therapy in esophago–gastric cancer is evolving. In order to individualize treatment, minimize toxicity, and improve outcome for patients with gastric cancer, we need to develop strategies that allow identification of at-risk patients and tumors at an early stage and to identify prognostic and predictive biomarkers that are able to tailor patient's treatment.

In addition to clinical and histological features that have been found to predict tumor behavior, predictive biomarkers have been investigated at a genetic level (e.g. Polymorphisms), transcriptional level (mRNA expression), or at the protein level. Molecular findings that have been reported to be prognostically informative are e.g. high level instability of microsatellite DNA (MSI-H) (Yamamoto et al. 1999), p53 gene mutation (Shiao et al. 2000; Gibson et al. 2003), 18qLOH (Inoue et al. 2002), SMAD4, or 7 gene expression (Kim et al. 2004), c-erbB2 expression (Yonemura et al. 1991), E-cadherin gene mutation (Becker et al. 1994), and gene loss or gain by comparative genomic hybridization (Weiss et al. 2004). Other pathways involved in cellular responses to cytotoxic agents such as apoptosis (Letai 2008; Vallbohmer et al. 2009), hypoxia and angiogenesis (Boku et al. 2007), and signal transduction factors (Miyazono et al. 2004) have been investigated and are potential predictive markers (Fareed et al. 2009). Furthermore, the ultimate response to cytotoxic therapy in cancer might be dictated by genetic and epigenetic changes, and there is preliminary evidence that gene signatures may predict response in esophago–gastric cancer (Luthra et al. 2006, 2007). However, none of these findings has proven to be contributive and cost effective enough to enter routine diagnostic practice so far. Therefore, extensive evaluation of histologic and molecular determinants that can accurately predict response to specific therapies should be performed in prospective trials.

References

Ajani JA, Roth JA, Ryan B, McMurtrey M, Rich TA, Jackson DE, Abbruzzese JL, Levin B, DeCaro L, Mountain C (1990) Evaluation of pre- and postoperative chemotherapy for resectable adenocarcinoma of the esophagus or gastroesophageal junction. J Clin Oncol 8(7):1231–1238

Alakus H, Holscher AH, Grass G, Hartmann E, Schulte C, Drebber U, Baldus SE, Bollschweiler E, Metzger R, Monig SP (2010) Extracapsular lymph node spread: a new prognostic factor in gastric cancer. Cancer 116(2):309–315. doi:10.1002/cncr.24764

Bader FG, Lordick F, Fink U, Becker K, Hofler H, Busch R, Siewert JR, Ott K (2008) Paclitaxel in the neoadjuvant treatment for adeno carcinoma of the distal esophagus (AEG I). A comparison of two phase II trials with long-term follow-up. Onkologie 31 (7):366–372. doi:000135515[pii]10.1159/000135515

Baiocchi GL, Tiberio GA, Minicozzi AM, Morgagni P, Marrelli D, Bruno L, Rosa F, Marchet A, Coniglio A, Saragoni L, Veltri M, Pacelli F, Roviello F, Nitti D, Giulini SM, De Manzoni G (2010) A multicentric Western analysis of prognostic factors in advanced, node-negative gastric cancer patients. Ann Surg 252(1):70–73. doi:10.1097/SLA.0b013e3181e4585e

Becker KF, Atkinson MJ, Reich U, Becker I, Nekarda H, Siewert JR, Hofler H (1994) E-cadherin gene mutations provide clues to diffuse type gastric carcinomas. Cancer Res 54(14):3845–3852

Becker K, Mueller JD, Schulmacher C, Ott K, Fink U, Busch R, Bottcher K, Siewert JR, Hofler H (2003) Histomorphology and grading of regression in gastric carcinoma treated with neoadjuvant chemotherapy. Cancer 98(7):1521–1530. doi:10.1002/cncr.11660

Bilici A, Seker M, Ustaalioglu BB, Kefeli U, Yildirim E, Yavuzer D, Aydin FM, Salepci T, Oncel M, Gumus M (2010) Prognostic significance of perineural invasion in patients with gastric cancer who underwent curative resection. Ann Surg Oncol 17(8):2037–2044. doi: 10.1245/s10434-010-1027-y

Boige V, Pignon J, Saint-Aubert B, Lasser P, Conroy T, Bouché O, Segol P, Bedenne L, Rougier P, Ychou M (2007) Final results of a randomized trial comparing preoperative 5-fluorouracil (F)/cisplatin (P) to surgery alone in adenocarcinoma of stomach and lower esophagus (ASLE): FNLCC ACCORD07-FFCD 9703 trial. J Clin Oncol ASCO Annu Meet Proc [I] 25(18S):4510 (June 20 Supplement)

Boku N, Ohtsu A, Nagashima F, Shirao K, Koizumi W (2007) Relationship between expression of vascular endothelial growth factor in tumor tissue from gastric cancers and chemotherapy effects: comparison between S-1 alone and the combination of S-1 plus CDDP. Jpn J Clin Oncol 37(7):509–514. doi:hym05710.1093/jjco/hym057 [pii]

Chiaravalli AM, Cornaggia M, Furlan D, Capella C, Fiocca R, Tagliabue G, Klersy C, Solcia E (2001) The role of histological investigation in prognostic evaluation of advanced gastric cancer. Analysis of histological structure and molecular changes compared with invasive pattern and stage. Virchows Arch 439(2):158–169

Choi MG, Sung CO, Noh JH, Kim KM, Sohn TS, Kim S, Bae JM (2010) Mucinous gastric cancer presents with more advanced tumor stage and weaker beta-catenin expression than nonmucinous cancer. Ann Surg Oncol 17(11):3053–3058. doi:10.1245/s10434-010-1184-z

Costa ML, de Cassia Braga Ribeiro K, Machado MA, Costa AC, Montagnini AL (2006) Prognostic score in gastric cancer: the importance of a conjoint analysis of clinical, pathologic, and therapeutic factors. Ann Surg Oncol 13 (6):843–850. doi: 10.1245/ASO.2006.05.040

Cunningham D, Allum WH, Stenning SP, Thompson JN, Van de Velde CJ, Nicolson M, Scarffe JH, Lofts FJ, Falk SJ, Iveson TJ, Smith DB, Langley RE, Verma M, Weeden S, Chua YJ, Participants MT (2006) Perioperative chemotherapy versus surgery alone for resectable gastroesophageal cancer. N Engl J Med 355(1):11–20. doi:355/1/1110.1056/NEJMoa055531 [pii]

De Vita F, Giuliani F, Galizia G, Belli C, Aurilio G, Santabarbara G, Ciardiello F, Catalano G, Orditura M (2007) Neo-adjuvant and adjuvant chemotherapy of gastric cancer. Ann Oncol 18 (Suppl 6):vi120–123. doi:18/suppl_6/vi120[pii]10.1093/annonc/mdm239

Fareed KR, Kaye P, Soomro IN, Ilyas M, Martin S, Parsons SL, Madhusudan S (2009) Biomarkers of response to therapy in oesophago-gastric cancer. Gut 58(1):127–143. doi: 58/1/12710.1136/gut.2008.155861 [pii]

Fareed KR, Al-Attar A, Soomro IN, Kaye PV, Patel J, Lobo DN, Parsons SL, Madhusudan S (2010) Tumour regression and ERCC1 nuclear protein expression predict clinical outcome in patients with gastro-oesophageal cancer treated with neoadjuvant chemotherapy. Br J Cancer 102(11):1600–1607. doi:66056810.1038/sj.bjc.6605686 [pii]

Fink U, Schuhmacher C, Stein HJ, Busch R, Feussner H, Dittler HJ, Helmberger A, Bottcher K, Siewert JR (1995) Preoperative chemotherapy for stage III-IV gastric carcinoma: feasibility, response and outcome after complete resection. Br J Surg 82(9):1248–1252

Gibson MK, Abraham SC, Wu TT, Burtness B, Heitmiller RF, Heath E, Forastiere A (2003) Epidermal growth factor receptor, p53 mutation, and pathological response predict survival in patients with locally advanced esophageal cancer treated with preoperative chemoradiotherapy. Clin Cancer Res 9(17):6461–6468

Green D, Ponce de Leon S, Leon-Rodriguez E, Sosa-Sanchez R (2002) Adenocarcinoma of the stomach: univariate and multivariate analysis of factors associated with survival. Am J Clin Oncol 25(1):84–89

Greene FL, Fleming ID, Fritz A, Balch CM (2002) AJCC cancer staging manual, 6th edn. Springer, New York

Harrison JD, Fielding JW (1995) Prognostic factors for gastric cancer influencing clinical practice. World J Surg 19(4):496–500

Hohenberger P, Gretschel S (2003) Gastric cancer. Lancet 362(9380):305–315. doi: S014067360313975X [pii]

Inoue K, Nakane Y, Iiyama H, Sato M, Kanbara T, Nakai K, Okumura S, Yamamichi K, Hioki K (2002a) The superiority of ratio-based lymph node staging in gastric carcinoma. Ann Surg Oncol 9(1):27–34

Inoue H, Matsuyama A, Mimori K, Ueo H, Mori M (2002b) Prognostic score of gastric cancer determined by cDNA microarray. Clin Cancer Res 8(11):3475–3479

Jhawer M, Coit D, Brennan M, Qin LX, Gonen M, Klimstra D, Tang L, Kelsen DP, Shah MA (2009) Perineural invasion after preoperative chemotherapy predicts poor survival in patients with locally advanced gastric cancer: gene expression analysis with pathologic validation. Am J Clin Oncol 32(4):356–362. doi:10.1097/COC.0b013e31818c08e8

Johnson H, Belluco C, Masood S, Azama A, Kahn L, Wise L (1995) Preoperative factors of prognostic significance in gastric cancer. J Natl Med Assoc 87(6):423–426

Kattan MW, Karpeh MS, Mazumdar M, Brennan MF (2003) Postoperative nomogram for disease-specific survival after an R0 resection for gastric carcinoma. J Clin Oncol 21(19):3647–3650. doi:10.1200/JCO.2003.01.240-JCO.2003.01.240 [pii]

Kelsen D, Karpeh M, Schwartz G, Gerdes H, Lightdale C, Botet J, Lauers G, Klimstra D, Huang Y, Saltz L, Quan V, Brennan M (1996) Neoadjuvant therapy of high-risk gastric cancer: a phase II trial of preoperative FAMTX and postoperative intraperitoneal fluorouracil-cisplatin plus intravenous fluorouracil. J Clin Oncol 14(6):1818–1828

Kim YH, Lee HS, Lee HJ, Hur K, Kim WH, Bang YJ, Kim SJ, Lee KU, Choe KJ, Yang HK (2004) Prognostic significance of the expression of Smad4 and Smad7 in human gastric carcinomas. Ann Oncol 15(4):574–580

Kologlu M, Kama NA, Reis E, Doganay M, Atli M, Dolapci M (2000) A prognostic score for gastric cancer. Am J Surg 179(6):521–526. doi:S0002961000003858 [pii]

Lauren P (1965) The two histological main types of gastric carcinoma: diffuse and so-called intestinal-type carcinoma. An attempt at a histo-clinical classification. Acta Pathol Microb Scand 64:31–49

Lenz HJ, Leichman CG, Danenberg KD, Danenberg PV, Groshen S, Cohen H, Laine L, Crookes P, Silberman H, Baranda J, Garcia Y, Li J, Leichman L (1996) Thymidylate synthase mRNA level in adenocarcinoma of the stomach: a predictor for primary tumor response and overall survival. J Clin Oncol 14(1):176–182

Letai AG (2008) Diagnosing and exploiting cancer's addiction to blocks in apoptosis. Nat Rev Cancer 8(2):121–132. doi:nrc229710.1038/nrc2297 [pii]

Lordick F, Stein HJ, Peschel C, Siewert JR (2004) Neoadjuvant therapy for oesophagogastric cancer. Br J Surg 91(5):540–551. doi:10.1002/bjs.4575

Lowy AM, Mansfield PF, Leach SD, Pazdur R, Dumas P, Ajani JA (1999) Response to neoadjuvant chemotherapy best predicts survival after curative resection of gastric cancer. Ann Surg 229(3):303–308

Luthra R, Wu TT, Luthra MG, Izzo J, Lopez-Alvarez E, Zhang L, Bailey J, Lee JH, Bresalier R, Rashid A, Swisher SG, Ajani JA (2006) Gene expression profiling of localized esophageal carcinomas: association with pathologic response to preoperative chemoradiation. J Clin Oncol 24(2):259–267. doi:JCO.2005.03.368810.1200/JCO.2005.03.3688 [pii]

Luthra MG, Ajani JA, Izzo J, Ensor J, Wu TT, Rashid A, Zhang L, Phan A, Fukami N, Luthra R (2007) Decreased expression of gene cluster at chromosome 1q21 defines molecular subgroups of chemoradiotherapy response in esophageal cancers. Clin Cancer Res 13(3):912–919. doi:13/3/91210.1158/1078-0432.CCR-06-1577 [pii]

Mansour JC, Tang L, Shah M, Bentrem D, Klimstra DS, Gonen M, Kelsen DP, Brennan MF, Coit DG (2007) Does graded histologic response after neoadjuvant chemotherapy predict survival for completely resected gastric cancer? Ann Surg Oncol 14(12):3412–3418. doi:10.1245/s10434-007-9574-6

Marchet A, Mocellin S, Ambrosi A, Morgagni P, Garcea D, Marrelli D, Roviello F, de Manzoni G, Minicozzi A, Natalini G, De Santis F, Baiocchi L, Coniglio A, Nitti D (2007) The ratio between metastatic and examined lymph nodes (N ratio) is an independent prognostic factor in gastric cancer regardless of the type of lymphadenectomy: results from an Italian multicentric study in 1853 patients. Ann Surg 245(4):543–552. doi:10.1097/01.sla.0000250423.43436.e100000658-200704000-00009 [pii]

Marchet A, Mocellin S, Ambrosi A, de Manzoni G, Di Leo A, Marrelli D, Roviello F, Morgagni P, Saragoni L, Natalini G, De Santis F, Baiocchi L, Coniglio A, Nitti D (2008) The prognostic value of N-ratio in patients with gastric cancer: validation in a large, multicenter series. Eur J Surg Oncol 34(2):159–165. doi:S0748-7983(07)00207-710.1016/j.ejso.2007.04.018 [pii]

Marubini E, Bonfanti G, Bozzetti F, Boracchi P, Amadori D, Folli S, Nanni O, Gennari L (1993) A prognostic score for patients resected for gastric cancer. Eur J Cancer 29A(6):845–850

Mikami K, Maekawa T, Shinohara T, Hoshino S, Yamauchi Y, Noritomi T, Yamashita Y (2009) Predictive factors of early recurrent death after a curative resection of gastric cancer. Int Surg 94(2):144–148

Miyazono F, Metzger R, Warnecke-Eberz U, Baldus SE, Brabender J, Bollschweiler E, Doerfler W, Mueller RP, Dienes HP, Aikou T, Hoelscher AH, Schneider PM (2004) Quantitative c-erbB-2 but not c-erbB-1 mRNA expression is a promising marker to predict minor histopathologic response to neoadjuvant radiochemotherapy in oesophageal cancer. Br J Cancer 91(4):666–672. doi:10.1038/sj.bjc.66019766601976 [pii]

Msika S, Benhamiche AM, Jouve JL, Rat P, Faivre J (2000) Prognostic factors after curative resection for gastric cancer. A population-based study. Eur J Cancer 36(3):390–396. doi:S0959-8049(99)00308-1 [pii]

Nagashima F, Boku N, Ohtsu A, Yoshida S, Hasebe T, Ochiai A, Sakata Y, Saito H, Miyata Y, Hyodo I, Ando M (2005) Biological markers as a predictor for response and prognosis of unresectable gastric cancer patients treated with irinotecan and cisplatin. Jpn J Clin Oncol 35(12):714–719. doi:hyi19410.1093/jjco/hyi194 [pii]

Ninomiya Y, Yanagisawa A, Kato Y, Kitagawa T, Ishihara S, Nakajima T (1999) Histological indications of a favorable prognosis with far-advanced gastric carcinomas after preoperative chemotherapy. J Cancer Res Clin Oncol 125(12):699–706. doi:91250699.432 [pii]

Ott K, Sendler A, Becker K, Dittler HJ, Helmberger H, Busch R, Kollmannsberger C, Siewert JR, Fink U (2003a) Neoadjuvant chemotherapy with cisplatin, 5-FU, and leucovorin (PLF) in locally advanced gastric cancer: a prospective phase II study. Gastric Cancer 6(3):159–167. doi:10.1007/s10120-003-0245-4

Ott K, Fink U, Becker K, Stahl A, Dittler HJ, Busch R, Stein H, Lordick F, Link T, Schwaiger M, Siewert JR, Weber WA (2003b) Prediction of response to preoperative chemotherapy in gastric carcinoma by metabolic imaging: results of a prospective trial. J Clin Oncol 21(24):4604–4610. doi:10.1200/JCO.2003.06.574 JCO.2003.06.574 [pii]

Ott K, Lordick F, Herrmann K, Krause BJ, Schuhmacher C, Siewert JR (2008a) The new credo: induction chemotherapy in locally advanced gastric cancer: consequences for surgical strategies. Gastric Cancer 11(1):1–9. doi:10.1007/s10120-007-0448-1

Ott K, Lordick F, Becker K, Ulm K, Siewert J, Hofler H, Keller G (2008b) Glutathione-S-transferase P1, T1 and M1 genetic polymorphisms in neoadjuvant-treated locally advanced gastric cancer: GSTM1-present genotype is associated with better prognosis in completely resected patients. Int J Colorectal Dis 23(8):773–782. doi:10.1007/s00384-008-0490-4

Ott K, Herrmann K, Lordick F, Wieder H, Weber WA, Becker K, Buck AK, Dobritz M, Fink U, Ulm K, Schuster T, Schwaiger M, Siewert JR, Krause BJ (2008c) Early metabolic response evaluation by fluorine-18 fluorodeoxyglucose positron emission tomography allows in vivo testing of chemosensitivity in gastric cancer: long-term results of a prospective study. Clin Cancer Res 14(7):2012–2018. doi:14/7/2012[pii]10.1158/1078-0432.CCR-07-0934

Ott K, Bader FG, Lordick F, Feith M, Bartels H, Siewert JR (2009) Surgical factors influence the outcome after Ivor-Lewis esophagectomy with intrathoracic anastomosis for adenocarcinoma of the esophagogastric junction: a consecutive series of 240 patients at an experienced center. Ann Surg Oncol 16(4):1017–1025. doi:10.1245/s10434-009-0336-5

Park SR, Kim MJ, Ryu KW, Lee JH, Lee JS, Nam BH, Choi IJ, Kim YW (2010) Prognostic value of preoperative clinical staging assessed by computed tomography in resectable gastric cancer patients: a viewpoint in the era of preoperative treatment. Ann Surg 251(3):428–435. doi:10.1097/SLA.0b013e3181ca69a700000658-201003000-00008 [pii]

Persiani R, D'Ugo D, Rausei S, Sermoneta D, Barone C, Pozzo C, Ricci R, La Torre G, Picciocchi A (2005) Prognostic indicators in locally advanced gastric cancer (LAGC) treated with preoperative chemotherapy and D2-gastrectomy. J Surg Oncol 89 (4):227–236 discussion 237–228. doi:10.1002/jso.20207

Rohatgi PR, Mansfield PF, Crane CH, Wu TT, Sunder PK, Ross WA, Morris JS, Pisters PW, Feig BW, Gunderson LL, Ajani JA (2006) Surgical pathology stage by American Joint Commission on Cancer criteria predicts patient survival after preoperative chemoradiation for localized gastric carcinoma. Cancer 107(7):1475–1482. doi:10.1002/cncr.22180

Sakuramoto S, Sasako M, Yamaguchi T, Kinoshita T, Fujii M, Nashimoto A, Furukawa H, Nakajima T, Ohashi Y, Imamura H, Higashino M, Yamamura Y, Kurita A, Arai K (2007) Adjuvant chemotherapy for gastric cancer with S-1, an oral fluoropyrimidine. N Engl J Med 357(18):1810–1820. doi:357/18/1810.1056/NEJMoa072252 [pii]

Schuhmacher CP, Fink U, Becker K, Busch R, Dittler HJ, Mueller J, Siewert JR (2001) Neoadjuvant therapy for patients with locally advanced gastric carcinoma with etoposide, doxorubicin, and cisplatinum. Closing results after 5 years of follow-up. Cancer 91(5):918–927. doi:10.1002/1097-0142(20010301)91:5<918::AID-CNCR1081>3.0.CO;2-W[pii]

Schuhmacher C, Gretschel S, Lordick F, Reichardt P, Hohenberger W, Eisenberger CF, Haag C, Mauer ME, Hasan B, Welch J, Ott K, Hoelscher A, Schneider PM, Bechstein W, Wilke H, Lutz MP, Nordlinger B, Cutsem EV, Siewert JR, Schlag PM (2010a) Neoadjuvant chemotherapy compared with surgery alone for locally advanced cancer of the stomach and cardia: European organisation for research and treatment of cancer randomized trial 40954. J Clin Oncol 28(35):5210–5218. doi:JCO.2009.26.611410.1200/JCO.2009.26.6114 [pii]

Schuhmacher C, Gretschel S, Lordick F, Reichardt P, Hohenberger W, Eisenberger CF, Haag C, Mauer ME, Hasan B, Welch J, Ott K, Hoelscher A, Schneider PM, Bechstein W, Wilke H,

Lutz MP, Nordlinger B, Van Cutsem E, Siewert JR, Schlag PM (2010b) Neoadjuvant chemotherapy compared with surgery alone for locally advanced cancer of the stomach and cardia: European organisation for research and treatment of cancer randomized trial 40954. J Clin Oncol. doi:JCO.2009.26.611410.1200/JCO.2009.26.6114 [pii]

Shiao YH, Palli D, Caporaso NE, Alvord WG, Amorosi A, Nesi G, Saieva C, Masala G, Fraumeni JF Jr, Rice JM (2000) Genetic and immunohistochemical analyses of p53 independently predict regional metastasis of gastric cancers. Cancer Epidemiol Biomark Prev 9(6):631–633

Shin SH, Bae JM, Jung H, Choi MG, Lee JH, Noh JH, Sohn TS, Kim S (2010) Clinical significance of the discrepancy between preoperative and postoperative diagnoses in gastric cancer patients. J Surg Oncol 101(5):384–388. doi:10.1002/jso.21500

Siewert JR, Bottcher K, Stein HJ, Roder JD (1998) Relevant prognostic factors in gastric cancer: ten-year results of the German gastric cancer study. Ann Surg 228(4):449–461

Solcia E, Klersy C, Mastracci L, Alberizzi P, Candusso ME, Diegoli M, Tava F, Riboni R, Manca R, Luinetti O (2009) A combined histologic and molecular approach identifies three groups of gastric cancer with different prognosis. Virchows Arch 455(3):197–211. doi: 10.1007/s00428-009-0813-z

Stemmermann GN, Brown C (1974) A survival study of intestinal and diffuse types of gastric carcinoma. Cancer 33(4):1190–1195

Vallbohmer D, Drebber U, Schneider PM, Baldus S, Bollschweiler E, Brabender J, Warnecke-Eberz U, Monig S, Holscher AH, Metzger R (2009) Survivin expression in gastric cancer: Association with histomorphological response to neoadjuvant therapy and prognosis. J Surg Oncol 99(7):409–413. doi:10.1002/jso.21271

Weiss MM, Kuipers EJ, Postma C, Snijders AM, Pinkel D, Meuwissen SG, Albertson D, Meijer GA (2004) Genomic alterations in primary gastric adenocarcinomas correlate with clinicopathological characteristics and survival. Cell Oncol 26(5–6):307–317

Yamamoto H, Perez-Piteira J, Yoshida T, Terada M, Itoh F, Imai K, Perucho M (1999) Gastric cancers of the microsatellite mutator phenotype display characteristic genetic and clinical features. Gastroenterology 116(6):1348–1357. doi:S0016508599005491 [pii]

Yonemura Y, Ninomiya I, Ohoyama S, Kimura H, Yamaguchi A, Fushida S, Kosaka T, Miwa K, Miyazaki I, Endou Y (1991) Expression of c-erbB-2 oncoprotein in gastric carcinoma. Immunoreactivity for c-erbB-2 protein is an independent indicator of poor short-term prognosis in patients with gastric carcinoma. Cancer 67(11):2914–2918

Adjuvant Chemotherapy: An Option for Asian Patients Only?

Yung-Jue Bang

Abstract

Survival rates following curative resection for gastric cancer are higher in East Asia than in Europe and the US. The aggressive surgical approach adopted in East Asia may explain these observations. In Japan and Korea, gastrectomy with extended lymphadenectomy (D2 gastrectomy) has been standard of care for many years, whereas gastrectomy with lymphadenectomy of the perigastric lymph nodes (D1 surgery) has been favored in Europe and the US until recently. D2 surgery is now recommended globally based on the 15-year findings from the large Dutch D1D2 study, which showed a reduction in cancer-related deaths with D2 versus D1 surgery. Improved outcomes are now being reported in the US and Europe as D2 surgery becomes more widely used. In addition to surgery, systemic therapy is also required to control recurrences, although the preferred regimen differs by region. Given that some of the studies on which these preferences are based predate the widespread acceptance of D2 surgery, the optimal regimen should be considered carefully. Recent studies from East Asia support the use of adjuvant chemotherapy after D2 surgery. Adjuvant chemotherapy should also be considered a valid approach in other regions now that the benefits of D2 surgery have been demonstrated unequivocally.

Abbreviations

ACTS-GC   Adjuvant Chemotherapy Trial of TS-1 for Gastric Cancer
ARTIST   Adjuvant Chemoradiation Therapy in Stomach Cancer

Y.-J. Bang (✉)
Department of Internal Medicine, Seoul National University College of Medicine,
101 Daehak-ro, Jongno-gu, Seoul 110-744, Republic of Korea
e-mail: bangyj@snu.ac.kr

F. Otto and M. P. Lutz (eds.), *Early Gastrointestinal Cancers*,
Recent Results in Cancer Research 196, DOI: 10.1007/978-3-642-31629-6_19,
© Springer-Verlag Berlin Heidelberg 2012

CLASSIC	Capecitabine and Oxaliplatin Adjuvant Study in Stomach Cancer
GASTRIC	Global Advanced/Adjuvant Stomach Tumor Research International Collaboration
MAGIC	Medical Research Council Adjuvant Gastric Infusional Chemotherapy
XELOX	Capecitabine plus oxaliplatin

Contents

1 Introduction 294
2 Surgery 295
   2.1 Extent of Lymphadenectomy 295
   2.2 Epidemiology 298
   2.3 Maruyama Index 298
3 Post/Perioperative Therapy 299
   3.1 Adjuvant Chemotherapy 299
   3.2 Postoperative Chemoradiotherapy 303
   3.3 Perioperative Chemotherapy 304
4 Conclusions 305
References 306

1 Introduction

Surgery alone was the internationally accepted standard of care for patients with potentially resectable gastric cancer until 2001. Landmark trials from the US, UK, and Japan then emerged to show that surgery combined with perioperative or postoperative systemic therapy improves the prognosis of this patient group (Macdonald et al. 2001; Cunningham et al. 2006; Sakuramoto et al. 2007). It is now acknowledged globally that multimodal therapy should be used in patients with resectable gastric cancer (Cunningham and Chua 2007), although the preferred type of regimen differs by region.

The purpose of the present paper is to discuss the key studies to emerge over the last 15 years regarding operable gastric cancer with regard to the type of surgery performed and the systemic treatment given. It is hoped that this discussion will provide insight into the relevance and generalizability of recent trials performed in East Asia regarding adjuvant therapy following D2 surgery. Gastric cancer, including cancer of the gastroesophageal junction, will be considered in this discussion, but not esophageal cancer.

2 Surgery

Surgical resection is the cornerstone of treatment for patients with localized gastric cancer. While the generally accepted therapeutic goal is to achieve a micro- and macro-scopically complete resection (R0), data from large randomized clinical trials performed over the last decade reveal marked differences in outcomes. To illustrate this point, the 5-year overall survival rates after curative gastrectomy were 23 % in the Medical Research Council Adjuvant Gastric Infusional Chemotherapy (MAGIC) trial performed predominantly at UK centers (Cunningham et al. 2006), 28 % in the Intergroup 0116 trial performed in the US (Macdonald 2011) compared with 61 % in the Adjuvant Chemotherapy Trial of TS-1 for Gastric Cancer (ACTS-GC) trial performed in Japan (Sakuramoto et al. 2007).

There are two possible explanations for the observed differences between regions. First, the outcomes may be a result of different surgical techniques, or second, because there are differences in the disease biology of the various gastric cancer populations.

2.1 Extent of Lymphadenectomy

The number of pathologically positive lymph nodes is an important prognostic indicator in patients with gastric cancer (Kodera et al. 1998; Adachi et al. 1994). It follows that surgeons should perform adequate lymphadenectomy in order to achieve the best outcomes. In Japan, Korea, and some specialized centers in the West, gastrectomy with extended lymph node dissection (D2 gastrectomy) has been performed regularly as a standard procedure for many years (Sasako et al. 2010; Japanese Gastric Cancer Society 2004). However, the preferred surgery in most European and US centers is generally gastrectomy plus lymphadenectomy of the perigastric lymph nodes (D1 gastrectomy). The aggressive approach adopted in Japan and Korea may explain, in part, the improved survival outcomes observed in trials conducted in East Asia compared with other regions.

2.1.1 D1 versus D2 surgery

The possible benefits of extended lymph node dissection have been tested in four randomized controlled trials (Cuschieri et al. 1996; Bonenkamp et al. 1999; Wu et al. 2006; Deguili et al. 2010), which compared D1 with D2 gastrectomy in patients with operable gastric cancer. The findings from all four trials are summarized in Table 1.

The largest of these were studies conducted by the UK Medical Research Council (MRC ST01) (Cuschieri et al. 1996) and the Dutch Gastric Cancer Group (Dutch D1D2) (Bonenkamp et al. 1999) in the 1990s. After 5 years of follow-up, both trials did not report any significant benefit in overall survival between D1 and D2 surgery (Table 1) (Cuschieri et al. 1996; Bonenkamp et al. 1999). The conclusion drawn from both studies was that there was generally no support for the use of D2 surgery in patients with gastric cancer in Western countries.

Table 1 Randomized controlled trials (>200 patients) comparing D1 versus D2 or D3 resection in patients with gastric cancer

Reference [trial]	n	Surgery	Postoperative morbidity (%)	Mortality (%)	5-year overall survival rate (%)
Cuschieri et al. 1996, 1999 [MRC ST01]	200	D1	28*	6.5**	35
	200	D2	46	13	33
Bonenkamp et al. 1999; Songun et al. 2010 [Dutch D1D2]	380	D1	25*	4[†]	34 (48)[a‡]
	331	D2	43	10	33 (37)[a]
Wu et al. 2006	110	D1	–	0	54**
	111	D3[b]	–	0	60
Degiuli et al. 2010 [IGCSG-R01]	133	D1	12	3.0	NA
	134	D2	18	2.2	NA

$*p < 0.001$; $**p = 0.04$; [†] $p = 0.004$; [‡] $p = 0.01$ between groups
[a] 15-year gastric cancer-related death rate
[b] Surgery described as D3 in the published paper, but is D2 surgery according to the current Japanese guidelines
NA not available

The negative results of these major trials have been the subject of much discussion. In both studies, postoperative morbidity (43 and 46 %) and operative mortality rates (10 and 13 %) after D2 surgery were high (Cuschieri et al. 1996; Bonenkamp et al. 1999). Several possible reasons have been cited for this. In both studies, splenopancreatectomies were performed routinely as part of D2 surgery. Splenectomy was subsequently identified as a major risk factor for mortality and morbidity in the Dutch trial (Sasako 1997). It is possible that the operative mortality caused by splenectomy in both trials obscured a potential benefit of D2 surgery.

It is also recognized that D2 surgery has a protracted learning curve of about 15–25 procedures (Parikh et al. 1996), before surgeons reach a plateau in terms of surgical technique. Many of the hospitals in the Dutch trial were low-volume institutions in which only a few resections were performed each year. Further, accrual in both studies was slow. In the MRC ST01 trial, there were 400 patients and 32 surgeons involved over 7 years (i.e. <2 patients per surgeon per year), and in the Dutch trial there were 711 patients from 80 centers over 4 years (<3 patients per center per year) (Cuschieri et al. 1996; Bonenkamp et al. 1999). It is likely that many surgeons had limited experience in maintaining the quality of surgery and managing the complications associated with D2 surgery, and that the study results were reported before many surgeons had reached the plateau of their learning curve for D2 surgery (Saka et al. 2011).

The Dutch trial included several quality control measures, including training surgeons in the D2 technique by an experienced Japanese surgeon (Bonenkamp et al. 1999). Despite these efforts, both non-compliance (not removing all lymph node stations) and contamination (removing more lymph nodes than indicated) occurred (Bunt et al. 1994) and are likely to have confounded the interpretation of the study outcomes. It was estimated that non-compliance occurred in 17–73 % of D1 patients and 7–55 % of D2 patients depending on the lymph node station, and that contamination occurred in an estimated 0–64 % of D1 patients and 1–42 % of D2 patients depending on the lymph node station (Bunt et al. 1994).

Several decades of debate about the relevance of D2 resection to Western centers ended recently when the 15-year follow-up data of the Dutch D1D2 study demonstrated a survival benefit with extended D2 lymphadenectomy (Songun et al. 2010). The gastric cancer-related death rate was found to be significantly lower in the D2 group than in the D1 group (37 versus 48 %; $p = 0.01$), whereas, deaths due to other causes were similar in both groups (35 versus 31 %; $p = 0.12$). These findings were supported by a smaller Taiwanese study which also demonstrated a survival benefit for D3[1] versus D1 dissection (Wu et al. 2006). In the intention-to-treat population ($n = 221$), 5-year overall survival was 59·5 % for the D3 group and 53·6 % for the D1 group (difference between groups 5·9 %, log-rank $p = 0.041$).

These positive findings have since led to a firm recommendation for the use of D2 gastrectomy in Europe (Okines et al. 2010; Allum et al. 2011) and the US (NCCN 2011) for patients with operable gastric cancer.

2.1.2 D2 lymphadenectomy today

Over the last decade, D2 resection has become more widely used in Europe and the US. Further, there is evidence to suggest that there have been steady improvements in postoperative outcomes versus the European trials performed in the 1990s.

Recent reports from Europe and the US describe postoperative morbidity rates of 18–29 % (Kulig et al. 2007; Degiuli et al. 2010; Díaz de Liaño et al. 2008) which are lower than the rates of 43–46 % reported in the Dutch D1D2 and MRC ST01 trials (Cuschieri et al. 1996; Bonenkamp et al. 1999), and mortality rates of 2–5 % (Díaz de Liaño et al. 2009; Kulig et al. 2007; Degiuli et al. 2010; Martin et al. 2002; Mansfield 2004) compared with rates of 10–13 % in the Dutch D1D2 and MRC-ST01 trials (Cuschieri et al. 1996; Bonenkamp et al. 1999). Improved 5-year rates of overall survival of 52 and 65 % have also been reported (Díaz de Liaño et al. 2009; Schuhmacher et al. 2010) compared with 33 % in both of the European trials (Cuschieri et al. 1996; Bonenkamp et al. 1999).

Collectively, these data suggest that D2 gastrectomy is associated with improved overall survival in Western countries (Songun et al. 2010). The morbidity and mortality rates reported in recent trials and patient series indicate that the procedure is safe when performed by experienced surgeons at specialized centers, although rates are still not as low as those achieved in East Asia.

---

[1] The surgery is described as D3 in the published paper, but is D2 surgery according to the current Japanese guidelines.

2.2 Epidemiology

As well as the type of surgery performed, it has been suggested that differences in the clinicopathological features and the epidemiology of gastric cancer may be responsible for the differing outcomes between regions.

A comparison of pathological characteristics between patients with gastric cancer from a Korean institution ($n = 1646$) and a US institution ($n = 711$) showed that there were significant differences between the two populations (Strong et al. 2010). The Korean population had fewer gastroesophageal junction (<1 %) and proximal (9 %) tumors compared with the US cohort (18 and 21 %, respectively; $p < 0.0001$ for overall distribution). In terms of tumor histology according to the Lauren classification, diffuse type tumors were more common in the Korean cohort (38 versus 29 % in US cohort), whereas intestinal type tumors were more common in US patients (59 versus 44 % in Korean cohort; $p < 0.0001$ for overall distribution) (Strong et al. 2010). A recent analysis of prognosis according to gastric tumor type (Shah et al. 2012) suggests that diffuse type gastric cancer is associated with a poor prognosis regardless of region. Further, patients with proximal tumors from European or American centers have a better prognosis than other subtypes of gastric cancer (Shah et al. 2012). These observations suggest that differences in tumor characteristics between populations are unlikely to explain observed differences in outcomes between East Asian and Western countries.

Disease stage also differed significantly between the two cohorts, with Korean patients tending to have earlier stage disease than US patients ($p < 0.0001$ for overall distribution) (Strong et al. 2010). However, the median number of positive lymph nodes, a strong negative prognostic factor, was similar in both cohorts [5 (range 1–53) for Korean patients versus 4 (range 1–63) for US patients; $p = 0.16$]. Macdonald (2011) in a recent editorial also reported similar observations from an informal analysis of the INT-0116, MAGIC, and ACTS-GC study populations and concluded that, overall, there were no marked prognostic disparities between study populations.

It is likely that the reasons for the differences in outcomes between regions are multifactorial and complex, and are as yet incompletely understood. The inclusion of biomarker programs in ongoing large-scale trials may help to better understand the molecular make-up of gastric carcinomas and identify more precisely potential differences between populations.

2.3 Maruyama Index

Understanding the patterns of spread and sites of disease recurrence after R0 resection in patients with gastric cancer may help to direct therapy for individual patients. In the late 1980s, Maruyama and colleagues developed a computer program to estimate the probability of locoregional relapse based on data from 2000 surgically resected patients treated at the National Cancer Center Hospital in

Tokyo. The program included data on tumor size, macroscopic appearance, depth of infiltration, location, grade, and type. The model predictions were found to be highly accurate in Japanese (Kampschöer et al. 1989), German (Bollschweiler et al. 1992), and Italian gastric cancer patient populations (Guadagni et al. 2000).

In the United States, Hundahl et al. (2002) retrospectively applied the model to the Intergroup 0116 trial data to evaluate the adequacy of lymphadenectomy relative to the likely extent of nodal disease. For the purposes of the analysis, the authors developed the "Maruyama index of undetected disease" defined as the sum of the Maruyama program predictions for Japanese-defined node stations left in situ by the surgeon. The median Maruyama index in the study population was high (70; range, 0–429), which is consistent with the poor outcomes observed in this study. Further, the Maruyama index was found to be a strong and independent predictor of survival after adjustment for T stage and number of positive nodes ($p = 0.0049$). The prognostic value of the Maruyama index was further investigated by Peeters et al. (2005) who reanalyzed the Dutch D1D2 trial data in a blinded fashion. The median Maruyama index was lower in this study population (26), and an index of <5 was found to be a strong independent predictor of overall survival ($p = 0.016$) and relapse risk ($p = 0.010$).

The Maruyama index allows surgeons to plan the extent of lymphadenectomy for an individual patient before or during surgery, rather than performing a fixed D level lymphadenectomy. The extent of lymphadenectomy can then be customized for each patient to improve regional control and survival.

3   Post/Perioperative Therapy

Surgery is essential to achieve a cure for stage II and III gastric cancer, but it is often not sufficient. The failure pattern for patients with resected gastric cancer includes a substantial risk of regional recurrence and spread of metastatic disease to distant sites. This has led to extensive investigation of the use of post- or perioperative systemic therapy in patients with resected gastric cancer.

There are three possible approaches:
1. Postoperative or adjuvant chemotherapy;
2. Postoperative radiotherapy/chemoradiotherapy;
3. Perioperative chemotherapy.

Each of these approaches has been investigated in large randomized controlled trials, the findings of which are summarized in Table 2.

3.1   Adjuvant Chemotherapy

To date, two large randomized controlled trials have investigated adjuvant chemotherapy after D2 surgery. The first, ACTS-GC, compared adjuvant S-1 therapy after D2 surgery with surgery alone in 1059 patients with stage II or III gastric

Table 2 Randomized controlled trials comparing perioperative or postoperative (radio) chemotherapy plus surgery versus surgery alone in patients with operable gastroesophageal cancer

Trial (reference)	No. of patients	Type of surgery	Treatment groups	Follow-up	Hazard ratio [95 % confidence intervals]*		
					Disease-free survival	Relapse-free survival	Overall survival
Postoperative (adjuvant) chemotherapy							
ACTS-GC (Sakuramoto et al. 2007)	1059	D2	S-1 + surgery vs surgery alone	3 years	–	0.62 [0.50–0.77] ($p < 0.001$)	0.68 [0.52–0.87] ($p = 0.003$)
(Sasako et al. 2011)				5 years	–	0.65 [0.54-0.79]	**0.67 [0.54–0.83]**
CLASSIC (Bang et al. 2012)	1035	D2	XELOX + surgery vs surgery alone	3 years	**0.56 [0.44–0.72]** ($p < 0.0001$)	–	0.72 [0.52–1.00] ($p = 0.493$)
Postoperative chemoradiotherapy							
Intergroup-0116 (Macdonald et al. 2001)	556	D2 [10 %] D1 [36 %] D0 [54 %]	5-FU/LV + radiotherapy + surgery vs surgery alone	3 years	–	1.52 [1.23–1.80] ($p < 0.001$)	**1.35 [1.09–1.66]** ($p = 0.005$)
ARTIST (Lee et al. 2012)	458	D2	XP → X-radiotherapy → XP + surgery vs XP + surgery	3 years	$P = \mathbf{0.086}^{\dagger}$	–	–
Perioperative chemotherapy							
MAGIC (Cunningham et al. 2006)	503	D2 [68 %]	Perioperative ECF + surgery vs surgery alone	4 years	–	0.66 [0.53–0.81]‡ ($p < 0.001$)	**0.75 [0.60–0.93]** ($p = 0.009$)

(continued)

Table 2 (continued)

Trial (reference)	No. of patients	Type of surgery	Treatment groups	Follow-up	Hazard ratio [95 % confidence intervals]*		
					Disease-free survival	Relapse-free survival	Overall survival
(Ychou et al. 2011)	224	D2 recommended	Perioperative FP + surgery vs surgery alone	5 years	0.65 [0.48–0.89] ($p = 0.003$)	–	**0.69 [0.50–0.95]** ($p = 0.02$)

*Hazard ratio expressed as (neo)adjuvant regimen + surgery vs surgery alone, with the exception of the Intergroup 0116 trial which was expressed as surgery alone vs chemoradiotherapy plus surgery; † No hazard ratio presented in published paper; ‡ Progression-free survival

Note **Bold text** denotes primary study endpoint

5-FU/LV 5-fluorouracil/leucovorin; *ACTS-GC* adjuvant chemotherapy trial of TS-1 for gastric cancer; *ARTIST* adjuvant chemoradiation therapy in stomach cancer; *CLASSIC* capecitabine, and oxaliplatin adjuvant study in stomach cancer; *ECF* epirubicin plus cisplatin plus 5-fluorouracil; *FP* 5-fluorouracil plus cisplatin; *MAGIC* Medical Research Council adjuvant gastric infusional chemotherapy; *XELOX* capecitabine plus oxaliplatin; *XP* capecitabine plus cisplatin

cancer (Sakuramoto et al. 2007). The adjuvant regimen comprised the oral flu-oropyrimidine S-1 (tegafur, gimeracil, and oteracil) 80 mg/m^2/day given for 4 weeks of a 6-week cycle for 12 months. The primary study endpoint was overall survival. After a median follow-up of 2.9 years, the hazard ratio for death for S-1 adjuvant therapy versus surgery alone was 0.68 (95 % CI 0.52–0.87; $p = 0.003$) and for relapse-free survival was 0.62 (95 % CI 0.50–0.77; $p < 0.001$). After 5 years, the hazard ratio for death was 0.67 (95 % CI 0.54– 0.83) and for relapse-free survival was 0.65 (95 % CI 0.54–0.79) (Sasako et al. 2011). However, a subgroup analysis indicated that S-1 was most effective for stage II disease (hazard ratio 0.57, 95 % CI 0.41–0.80 for relapse-free survival)[2]; the effect size was smaller in patients with stage IIIa (hazard ratio 0.63, 95 % CI 0.45–0.89), stage IIIb disease (hazard ratio 0.71, 95 % CI 0.45–1.14), and stage IV disease (hazard ratio 0.83, 95 % CI 0.49–1.43) (Sasako et al. 2011).

The Capecitabine and Oxaliplatin Adjuvant Study in Stomach Cancer (CLASSIC) trial investigated the combination of the oral fluoropyrimidine cape-citabine plus oxaliplatin (XELOX) as adjuvant therapy after D2 surgery versus surgery alone in patients with stage II or III gastric cancer (Bang et al. 2012). The XELOX regimen consisted of oxaliplatin 130 mg/m^2 given on day 1 followed by capecitabine 1,000 mg/m^2 twice daily for 14 days every 3 weeks for 6 months. The primary study endpoint was 3-year disease-free survival, defined as time from randomization to the time of recurrence of the original gastric cancer, development of a new gastric cancer or death. After a median follow-up of 34 months, the hazard ratio for disease-free survival was 0.56 (95 % CI 0.44–0.72; $p < 0.0001$). For overall survival, the hazard ratio was 0.72 (95 % CI 0.52–1.00; $p = 0.49$), although these findings were only preliminary and patient follow-up is ongoing. Unlike fluoropyrimidine monotherapy, XELOX was effective for all disease stages with hazard ratios for disease-free survival of 0.55 (95 % CI 0.36–0.84), 0.57 (95 % CI 0.39–0.82), and 0.57 (95 % CI 0.35–0.95) for patient subgroups with stage II, IIIa, and IIIb disease, respectively.

As both ACTS-GC and CLASSIC were conducted in East Asia, the general-izability of these findings to other countries has been questioned. However, the relevance of adjuvant therapy to other regions has been demonstrated by the Global Advanced/Adjuvant Stomach Tumor Research International Collaboration (GASTRIC) Group meta-analysis which analyzed individual patient data ($n = 3838$) from 17 randomized trials, 13 of which were from Europe or the US. The studies tested included a range of different adjuvant regimens and all studies involved curative resection, but there were no restrictions regarding the type of the surgery performed. Overall, there was a modest but significant benefit associated with the use of adjuvant chemotherapy after resection of gastric cancers in terms of overall survival (hazard ratio 0.82, 95 % CI 0.76–0.90; $p < 0.001$) with absolute benefits of 5.8 % at 5 years and 7.4 % at 10 years in favor of adjuvant therapy (GASTRIC 2010). When analyzed by region, the hazard ratios for overall survival

---

[2] Classification according to International Union Against Cancer (UICC) TMN classification of malignant tumors.

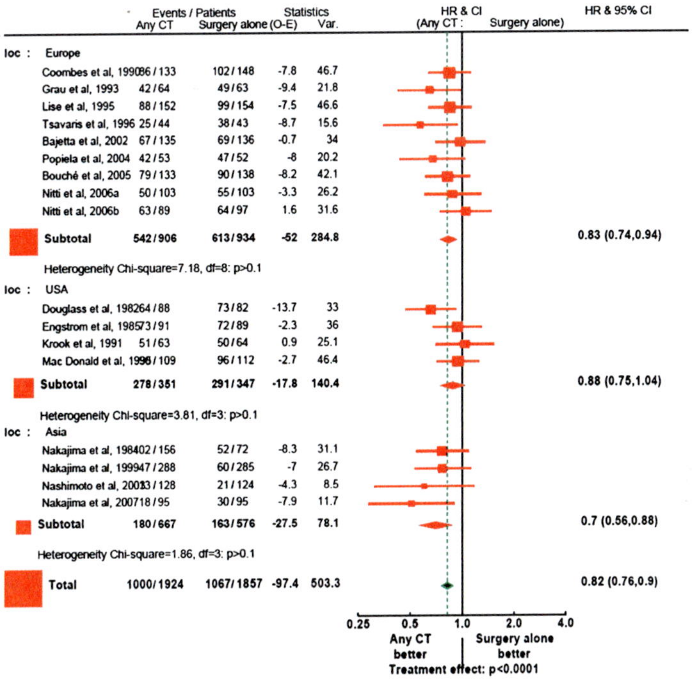

CT; Chemotherapy. O and E respectively denote the number of observed and expected events under the hypothesis of absence of treatment effect at all timespoints. Var is the variance of the statistics, which also measures the weight of each trial. Hazard ratio (HR) and their associated 95% confidence intervals (CI) are provided. P values are p-for-effect modification testing for heterogeneity within or across the group of regimens. Size of the data markers is proportional to the sample size of the trial populations.

Fig. 1 Meta-analysis of randomized controlled trials of adjuvant chemotherapy plus surgery versus surgery alone for overall survival grouped according to the region where the trial was conducted (GASTRIC 2010). Copyright © (2010) American Medical Association. All rights reserved. Reprinted, with permission, from GASTRIC 2010

were 0.83 (95 % CI 0.74–0.94) for studies performed in Europe, 0.88 (95 % CI 0.75–1.04) for studies performed in the US and 0.70 (95 % 0.56–0.88) for studies performed in Asia (Fig. 1).

3.2 Postoperative Chemoradiotherapy

The first major study to investigate the value of multimodal therapy was the US Intergroup 0116 trial (MacDonald et al. 2001) which compared a regimen of 5-fluorouracil/leucovorin plus radiotherapy following surgery compared with surgery alone. The aim of postoperative chemoradiotherapy in the Intergroup 0116 trial was to reduce local and regional relapse after surgery. After a median follow-up of 5 years, the median duration of overall survival was 36 months in the chemoradiotherapy group and 27 months in the surgery-alone group, giving a hazard ratio of 1.35 for death (95 % CI 1.09–1.66; $p = 0.005$). While these data provided clear support for the concept of postoperative chemoradiotherapy, D2 surgery was performed in only 10 % of the study population and it has been suggested that the addition of radiotherapy compensated for suboptimal surgery. The local relapse rate was 29 % in the surgery-alone arm, and was reduced to 19 % with postoperative chemoradiotherapy. Local relapse after D2 surgery is low and is further reduced by adjuvant chemotherapy. For example, in the ACTS-GC study, local relapses were observed in 1.3 % of patients in the adjuvant chemotherapy group and 2.8 % of patients in the surgery-alone group [hazard ratio 0.42, 95 % CI 0.16–1.00; $p = 0.05$] and relapses in lymph nodes occurred in 5.1 and 8.7 % of patients, respectively [hazard ratio 0.54, 95 % CI 0.33–0.87; $p = 0.01$] (Sakuramoto et al. 2007). This raises questions as to whether or not radiotherapy is necessary when D2 surgery is performed.

This question was addressed recently in the Adjuvant Chemoradiation Therapy in Stomach Cancer (ARTIST) trial, which compared postoperative chemotherapy with chemotherapy plus radiotherapy in patients with D2-resected gastric cancer (Lee et al. 2012). The chemotherapy regimen was capecitabine plus cisplatin (XP) for six 3 weekly cycles, and the comparator regimen comprised XP (two 3-week cycles) followed by capecitabine plus radiotherapy (5 weeks continuously) followed by XP (two 3-week cycles). After a median follow-up of 55 months, the estimated 3-year disease-free survival rates were 78 % in the radiotherapy-containing arm and 74 % in the chemotherapy arm ($p = 0.086$), suggesting that postoperative radiotherapy may not be necessary after D2 resection. In a subgroup analysis, the addition of radiotherapy significantly prolonged disease-free survival in a subset of patients with pathologic lymph-node positive disease ($n = 396$; $p = 0.0365$).

3.3 Perioperative Chemotherapy

Perioperative chemotherapy was investigated by the UK Medical Research Council in the MAGIC trial (Cunningham et al. 2006). In this study, patients with operable gastroesophageal cancer were assigned to preoperative (3 cycles) and postoperative (3 cycles) chemotherapy with 5-fluorouracil, cisplatin plus epirubicin versus surgery alone. D2 resection was performed in 68 % of the study population (Cunningham and Chua 2007). Perioperative chemotherapy was associated with improved outcomes; the 5-year rates of overall survival were 36 % in the perioperative chemotherapy group versus 23 % in the surgery-alone group (hazard ratio 0.75; 95 % CI 0.60–0.93; $p = 0.0009$). These findings are supported by a smaller French phase III study which compared perioperative 5-fluorouracil plus cisplatin versus surgery alone in patients with gastroesophageal cancer (Ychou et al. 2011). The 5-year overall survival rate was 38 % in the perioperative chemotherapy group versus 24 % in the surgery-alone group (hazard ratio 0.69; 95 % CI 0.50 to 0.95; $p = 0.02$).

It is important to note that these trials showed the benefit of perioperative chemotherapy over surgery alone, rather than versus postoperative chemotherapy. It should also be noted that both studies included patients with lower esophageal cancer (approximately 11 % of both study populations) which confounds the interpretation of these studies, as the staging and types of surgery for this cancer differ from those used for gastric cancer. In the MAGIC trial, it is also possible that the effect in the surgery-alone group was underestimated since many patients in this arm did not receive chemotherapy for metastatic disease (Cunningham et al. 2006) which is now recognized as standard of care for metastatic or recurrent gastric cancer.

4 Conclusions

Gastrectomy with extended lymphadenectomy (D2 surgery) is now recommended as standard of care for patients with operable gastric cancer in Asia, the US, and Europe (Japanese Gastric Cancer Society 2004; Okines et al. 2010; Allum et al. 2011; NCCN 2012; Sasako et al. 2010). Although data from phase III studies performed in Europe in the 1990s suggested that D2 gastrectomy was associated with high rates of morbidity and mortality, greatly improved outcomes have been reported in recent clinical studies and patient series from high-volume institutions in the US and Europe supporting the safety of this type of surgery.

Adjuvant chemotherapy with a fluoropyrimidine with or without oxaliplatin improves patient outcomes following D2 surgery. The relevance of adjuvant chemotherapy after less than D2 surgery, and in regions other than East Asia, is supported by the GASTRIC meta-analysis, which reported a modest but significant benefit when data from 17 randomized studies were considered. An intensified regimen (i.e. fluoropyrimidine plus oxaliplatin) improves outcomes in patients with stage II or III disease after D2 surgery, whereas fluoropyrimidine monotherapy has a smaller effect in patients with stage III disease and may not be optimal in this patient subgroup.

While adjuvant chemotherapy is favored in East Asia, perioperative chemotherapy has been adopted as standard of care in many parts of Europe and postoperative chemoradiotherapy tends to be favored in the US (Okines et al. 2010). The trials on which the European and US preferences are based predate the widespread acceptance and use of D2 surgery. This raises questions about the relevance of these regimens, particularly postoperative radiotherapy, after D2 surgery. A large randomized international trial of perioperative versus adjuvant chemotherapy after D2 surgery (possibly with a 2×2 factorial design to test the addition of epirubicin to a fluoropyrimidine/oxaliplatin couplet) in patients with stage II and III gastric cancer is warranted.

In conclusion, when the evidence from recent randomized clinical trials is considered collectively, adjuvant therapy should be considered as a valid approach for Western patients following D2 surgery.

Acknowledgments Support for third-party writing assistance for this manuscript was provided by Roche Korea.

References

Adachi Y, Kamakura T, Mori M et al (1994) Prognostic significance of the number of positive lymph nodes in gastric carcinoma. Br J Surg 81:414

Allum WH, Blazeby JM, Griffin SM et al (2011) Guidelines for the management of oesophageal and gastric cancer. Gut 60:1449–1472

Bang YJ, Kim YW, Yang HK et al (2012) Adjuvant capecitabine and oxaliplatin for gastric cancer after D2 gastrectomy (CLASSIC): a phase 3 open-label, randomised controlled trial. Lancet 379:315–321

Bollschweiler E, Boettcher K, Hoelscher AH et al (1992) Preoperative assessment of lymph node metastases in patients with gastric cancer: evaluation of the Maruyama computer program. Br J Surg 79:156–160

Bonenkamp JJ, Hermans J, Sasako M et al (1999) Extended lymph-node dissection for gastric cancer. N Engl J Med 340:908–914

Bunt TM, Bonenkamp HJ, Hermans J et al (1994) Factors influencing noncompliance and contamination in a randomized trial of "Western" (r1) versus "Japanese" (r2) type surgery in gastric cancer. Cancer 73:1544–1551

Cunningham D, Allum WH, Stenning SP et al (2006) Perioperative chemotherapy versus surgery alone for resectable gastroesophageal cancer. N Engl J Med 355:11–20

Cunningham D, Chua YJ (2007) East meets west in the treatment of gastric cancer. N Engl J Med 357:1863–1865

Cuschieri A, Fayers P, Fielding J et al (1996) Postoperative morbidity and mortality after D1 and D2 resections for gastric cancer: preliminary results of the MRC randomised controlled surgical trial. The Surgical Cooperative Group. Lancet 347:995–999

Cuschieri A, Weeden S, Fielding J et al (1999) Patient survival after D1 and D2 resections for gastric cancer: long-term results of the MRC randomized surgical trial. Surgical co-operative group. Br J Cancer 79:1522–1530

Degiuli M, Sasako M, Ponti A et al (2010) Morbidity and mortality in the Italian gastric cancer study group randomized clinical trial of D1 versus D2 resection for gastric cancer. Br J Surg 97:643–649

Díaz de Liaño A, Yarnoz C et al (2008) Rationale for gastrectomy with D2 lymphadenectomy in the treatment of gastric cancer. Gastric Cancer 11:96–102

Díaz de Liaño A, Yárnoz C, Artieda C et al (2009) Results of R0 surgery with D2 lymphadenectomy for the treatment of localised gastric cancer. Clin Transl Oncol 11:178–182

GASTRIC (Global Advanced/Adjuvant Stomach Tumor Research International Collaboration) Group, Paoletti X, Oba K et al (2010) Benefit of adjuvant chemotherapy for resectable gastric cancer: a meta-analysis. JAMA 303:1729–1737

Guadagni S, de Manzoni G, Catarci M et al (2000) Evaluation of the Maruyama computer program accuracy for preoperative estimation of lymph node metastases from gastric cancer. World J Surg 24:1550–1558

Hundahl SA, Macdonald JS, Benedetti J et al (2002) Surgical treatment variation in a prospective, randomized trial of chemoradiotherapy in gastric cancer: the effect of under treatment. Ann Surg Oncol 9:278–286

Japanese Gastric Cancer Society (2004) Guidelines for Diagnosis and Treatment of Carcinoma of the Stomach. http://www.jgca.jp/PDFfiles/Guidelines2004_eng.pdf Accessed 2 Mar 2010

Kampschöer GH, Maruyama K, van de Velde CJ et al (1989) Computer analysis in making preoperative decisions: a rational approach to lymph node dissection in gastric cancer patients. Br J Surg 76:905–908

Kodera Y, Yamamura Y, Shimizu Y et al (1998) The number of metastatic lymph nodes: a promising prognostic determinant for gastric carcinoma in the latest edition of the TNM classification. J Am Coll Surg 187:597

Kulig J, Popiela T, Kolodziejczyk P et al (2007) Standard D2 versus extended D2 (D2+) lymphadenectomy for gastric cancer: an interim safety analysis of a multicenter, randomized, clinical trial. Am J Surg 193:10–15

Lee J, Lim do H, Kim S et al (2012) Phase III trial comparing capecitabine plus cisplatin versus capecitabine plus cisplatin with concurrent capecitabine radiotherapy in completely resected gastric cancer with D2 lymph node dissection: the ARTIST trial. J Clin Oncol 30:268–273

Macdonald JS (2011) Gastric cancer: Nagoya is not New York. J Clin Oncol 29:4348–4350

Macdonald JS, Smalley SR, Benedetti J et al (2001) Chemoradiotherapy after surgery compared with surgery alone for adenocarcinoma of the stomach or gastroesophageal junction. N Engl J Med 345:725–730

Mansfield PF (2004) Lymphadenectomy for gastric cancer. J Clin Oncol 22:2759–2761

Martin RC 2nd, Jaques DP, Brennan MF et al (2002) Achieving RO resection for locally advanced gastric cancer: is it worth the risk of multiorgan resection? J Am Coll Surg 194:568–577

NCCN. (2012) NCCN Clinical Practice Guidelines in Oncology. Gastric Cancer (including cancer in the proximal 5 cm of the stomach). Version 2.2012. http://www.nccn.org/professionals/physician_gls/pdf/gastric.pdf Accessed 2 Mar 2010

Okines A, Verheij M, Allum W et al (2010) Gastric cancer: ESMO Clinical Practice Guidelines for diagnosis, treatment and follow-up. Ann Oncol 21(5):50–54

Parikh D, Johnson M, Chagla L et al (1996) D2 gastrectomy: lessons from a prospective audit of the learning curve. Br J Surg 83:1595–1599

Peeters KC, Hundahl SA, Kranenbarg EK et al (2005) Low Maruyama index surgery for gastric cancer: blinded reanalysis of the Dutch D1–D2 trial. World J Surg 29:1576–1584

Saka M, Morita S, Fukagawa T et al (2011) Present and future status of gastric cancer surgery. Jpn J Clin Oncol 41:307–313

Sakuramoto S, Sasako M, Yamaguchi T et al (2007) Adjuvant chemotherapy for gastric cancer with S-1, an oral fluoropyrimidine. N Engl J Med 357:1810–1820

Sasako M (1997) Risk factors for surgical treatment in the Dutch gastric cancer trial. Br J Surg 84:1567–1571

Sasako M, Inoue M, Lin JT et al (2010) Gastric cancer working group report. Jpn J Clin Oncol 40(1):28–37

Sasako M, Sakuramoto S, Katai H et al (2011) Five-year outcomes of a randomized phase III trial comparing adjuvant chemotherapy with S-1 versus surgery alone in stage II or III gastric cancer. J Clin Oncol 29:4387–4393

Schuhmacher C, Gretschel S, Lordick F et al (2010) Neoadjuvant chemotherapy compared with surgery alone for locally advanced cancer of the stomach and cardia: European Organisation for Research and Treatment of Cancer randomized trial 40954. J Clin Oncol 28:5210–5218

Shah MA, Van Cutsem E, Kang YK, et al. (2012) Survival analysis according to disease subtype in AVAGAST: First-line capecitabine and cisplatin plus bevacizumab (bev) or placebo in patients (pts) with advanced gastric cancer. J Clin Oncol 30: (suppl 4; abstr 5)

Songun I, Putter H, Kranenbarg EM et al (2010) Surgical treatment of gastric cancer: 15 year follow-up results of the randomised nationwide Dutch D1D2 trial. Lancet Oncol 11:439–449

Strong VE, Song KY, Park CH et al (2010) Comparison of gastric cancer survival following R0 resection in the United States and Korea using an internationally validated nomogram. Ann Surg 251:640–646

Wu CW, Hsiung CA, Lo SS et al (2006) Nodal dissection for patients with gastric cancer: a randomised controlled trial. Lancet Oncol 7:309–315

Ychou M, Boige V, Pignon JP et al (2011) Perioperative chemotherapy compared with surgery alone for resectable gastroesophageal adenocarcinoma: an FNCLCC and FFCD multicenter phase III trial. J Clin Oncol 29:1715–1721

Selecting the Best Treatment for an Individual Patient

Alessandro Bittoni, Luca Faloppi, Riccardo Giampieri and Stefano Cascinu

Abstract

Several factors concur in determining outcome for locally advanced gastric cancer patients. Shockingly, geographic origin of the patient seems to play a major role. In Eastern countries, the high level of surgery that can be expected grants a high percentage of success in a strategy that employs surgery as immediate treatment followed by adjuvant chemotherapy, mainly based on oral fluoropyrimidines (S-1 or Capecitabine), with satisfactory results. In Western countries, the expertise of the surgeon maintains its role as predictor of high likelihood of cure. Indeed, patients treated with standard D2 lymph node dissection have a significantly better survival than those who do not obtain the same kind of treatment. For patients who underwent a suboptimal resection (less than a D1) the classical indication is for a combined adjuvant chemoradiotherapy. In patients who obtain a good surgical outcome, the benefit of the addition of adjuvant chemotherapy is still debatable: the gain in survival seems to be small (around 8 % at 5 years) and with noticeable toxicities (usually with dismal compliance for patients treated). On this basis, neoadjuvant treatment is a promising option even if there is a general lack of conclusive data regarding which is the best regimen to

A. Bittoni · L. Faloppi · R. Giampieri · S. Cascinu (✉)
Clinica di Oncologia Medica, AOU "Ospedali Riuniti"
Università Politecnica delle Marche, via Conca, 60020 Ancona, Italy
e-mail: cascinu@yahoo.com

A. Bittoni
e-mail: alebitto@tiscali.it

L. Faloppi
e-mail: lucafaloppi@libero.it

R. Giampieri
e-mail: kakeru@libero.it

F. Otto and M. P. Lutz (eds.), *Early Gastrointestinal Cancers*,
Recent Results in Cancer Research 196, DOI: 10.1007/978-3-642-31629-6_20,
© Springer-Verlag Berlin Heidelberg 2012

use. Even with the limitation of a small number of studies (with difficulties in enrollment), neoadjuvant chemotherapy is usually feasible, allows for a greater chance of receiving chemotherapy at all, and opens the possibility of a downstaging and downsizing of the tumor, allowing an easier surgery. Regarding this strategy preliminary results have also been presented about the addition of monoclonal antibodies. For example, in the TOGA trial, a significant benefit in terms of overall survival, response rate, and progression free survival was observed also for patients with locally advanced gastric cancer and not just for the metastatic ones. In the AVAGAST trial also, the addition of Bevacizumab failed to determine a significant improvement in the primary outcome, overall survival, for patients treated with the combination, but in the subgroup analysis, patients with locally advanced gastric cancer had a significantly better overall survival and response rate. This data was the basis for the newest neoadjuvant trial, of Cunningham et al., the MAGIC2 trial, with the peri-operative use of ECX+Bevacizumab. Finally, an increasing interest in the use of hyperthermic intraperitoneal chemotherapy in other types of solid tumors (including those of the gastrointestinal tract such as colon cancer) has led to evaluate this treatment modality in gastric cancer patients with peritoneal involvement. It should be noted that it is still to be considered an experimental approach, even though it would be intriguing to evaluate if a particular subset of patients, those who are more likely to develop peritoneal metastasis, may benefit from this technique in the adjuvant setting. It should be considered that other than histologic subtype (diffuse vs intestinal) there seems to be a series of polymorphisms of genes usually involved in cell interaction and migration that can explain a different metastatic pattern in resected patients. Further research on these determinants of metastatic spread could be used to select those patients who may benefit from HIPEC and those who may benefit from standard adjuvant or that gain no benefit at all.

Contents

1   Introduction.. 310
2   Treatment of Early Gastric Cancer... 311
    2.1   Adjuvant Setting... 311
    2.2   Peri-Operative Setting 313
3   Pharmacogenomics 316
    3.1   Adjuvant Setting... 316
    3.2   Peri-Operative Setting 317
4   Conclusions... 318
References... 318

1   Introduction

Despite the observation that gastric cancer incidence in Western countries is decreasing, this disease is still one of the major cause of cancer-related death worldwide. Surgical resection represent the cornerstone of any curative treatment

Selecting the Best Treatment for an Individual Patient

at early stages but, especially in Western countries, most of tumors are diagnosed at an advanced stage. Multidisciplinary approaches involving surgery, chemotherapy and radiation therapy can improve patients' prognosis in these settings (Cunningham et al. 2006a, b; Macdonald et al. 2001). Specifically, chemotherapy may play a key role both before and after surgery in operable gastric cancer, improving disease-free survival and overall survival, or as a palliative treatment for recurrent or advanced disease. Many antitumoral agents have shown to be effective against gastric cancer in clinical trials, including fluorouracil, cisplatin, irinotecan, anthracyclines and taxanes, but response rates are variable, with a not negligible proportion of patients undergoing toxic and costly chemotherapeutic regimens without a survival benefit.

In the last few years, several studies tried to explore the molecular biology and pathogenesis of gastric cancer, which emerged as a biologically heterogeneous disease. Findings from these studies lead to the identification of many molecular markers that may play a crucial role as prognostic or predictive indicators, hypothetically improving prognostic stratification selection of the appropriate therapeutic strategy. In particular, it has been demonstrated that some of these factors could correlate with response to specific antineoplastic drugs theoretically allowing a tailored treatment based on molecular features of single patient's gastric cancer. In this review, we will present current treatment options for early gastric cancer and discuss the role of molecular markers that may play a crucial role as prognostic or predictive indicators, hypothetically improving prognostic stratification selection of the appropriate therapeutic strategy.

2 Treatment of Early Gastric Cancer

Although recent advances in the treatment of gastric cancer, surgery still remains the mainstay of any curative treatment for these patients with radical gastrectomy including a D2 radical lymphadenectomy representing the procedure of choice. However, patients with locally advanced disease show high rates of locoregional or distant recurrence even after potentially curative resections. In this setting, adjuvant and neoadjuvant treatments showed to improve significantly patients' clinical outcome.

2.1 Adjuvant Setting

The role of adjuvant chemotherapy in gastric cancer has been extensively studied in the past three decades, often with disappointing results. Meta-analyses of clinical trials in this setting have shown only a small benefit deriving from adjuvant chemotherapy on overall survival, with a risk of death reduction ranging from 12 to 18 % (Hermans et al. 1993; Earle and Maroun 1999; Mari et al. 2000; Panzini et al. 2002). However, methodological limits prevented clinicians from drawing definitive conclusions, specially because small clinical trials using older platinum-free regimens were included. Subsequently, four clinical trials evaluated the role of cisplatin-based chemotherapy regimens in the adjuvant treatment of gastric cancer, unfortunately with no better results. In the study by GOIRC (Gruppo Oncologico Italiano di Ricerca Clinica), 258 patients with adenocarcinoma of the stomach, were randomized to receive surgery alone or surgery followed by four cycles of PELF (cisplatin, epirubicin, leucovorin and 5-FU). In this study, adjuvant chemotherapy did not improve disease-free survival (HR of recurrence = 0.92, 95 % CI = 0.66–1.27) or overall survival (HR of death = 0.90, 95 % CI = 0.64–1.26) (di Costanzo et al. 2008). The French Federation Francophone de Cancerologie Digestive (FFCD) study, randomized 260 gastric cancer patients to post-operative chemotherapy, with 5-FU and cisplatin, or surgery alone. Also this study failed to demonstrate a benefit in terms of survival for adjuvant chemotherapy (Bouche' et al. 2005). Similar results were obtained from an ITMO (Italian Trials in Medical Oncology) group study comparing surgery alone with adjuvant EAP (etoposide, adryamicin, cisplatin) chemotherapy (Bajetta et al. 2002) and from a GISCAD study comparing post-operative chemotherapy with 5-FU versus weekly PELF regimen (Cascinu et al. 2007). In 2009 ASCO (America Society of Clinical Oncology) conference, a further meta-analysis investigating the role of adjuvant chemotherapy in gastric cancer has been presented (Buyse and Pignon 2009). This study included 32 randomized clinical trials, for a total of 3710 evaluable patients, across Europe, the USA, and Asia. Global result suggested a moderate but significant survival benefit for adjuvant chemotherapy in resected gastric cancer, with an hazard ratio of 0.83 (95 % CI = 0.76–0.91) and a 17 % reduction in risk of death. Subgroup analyses showed a correlation between disease stage and treatment effect. In fact, patients with higher stages derived higher benefit from adjuvant chemotherapy (HR for death of 0.77 and 0.66 for stage III and IV, respectively) when compared with patients with earlier stages (HR 0.88 and 0.79 for stage I and II). In addition, Asian patients were confirmed to have a much better survival than other patients although no significant interactions between geographic area and chemotherapy effect was demonstrated.

The high rates of locoregional relapse observed in resected gastric cancer patients, led investigators to evaluate the association of radiotherapy to post-operative chemotherapy, with the aim to improve patients outcome. The efficacy of adjuvant chemoradiotherapy after gastric cancer resection was evaluated in a large phase III trial, the INT-0116, which randomized 556 patients who underwent surgery for gastric or esophageal-gastric cancer junction to post-operative chemoradiation or observation (Macdonald et al. 2001). In this study, the use of adjuvant chemoradiotherapy compared to surgery alone resulted in a statistically significant improvement in median overall survival (36 vs. 27 months, HR = 1.31, 95 % CI = 1.08–1.61) and disease-free survival (30 vs. 19 months, HR = 1.52, 95 % CI = 1.25–1.85). The treatment was particularly effective in improving local control, lowering the incidence of local relapse (from 29 to 19 %). An update of INT-0116 trial results was recently presented (Macdonald et al. 2009). After a median follow up that has reached 11 years, benefit in

Selecting the Best Treatment for an Individual Patient 311

OS and DFS for chemoradiation have remained essentially unchanged and no significant late effect of treatment has emerged. Hovewer, quality of surgical treatment in the study should be considered poor, with only 10 % of patients receiving D2 lymph node resection and more than half (54 %) receiving D0 resection. We can then postulate that adjuvant chemoradiotherapy in this group of patients may have been beneficial as a "salvage local treatment, compensating for an inadequate surgery that exposed patients to a particularly relevant risk of local recurrence (Scartozzi et al. 2005).

2.2 Peri-Operative Setting

2.2.1 Peri-Operative Chemotherapy

Two recent trials showed that peri-operative treatment could improve clinical outcome in resectable gastric cancer patients. The MAGIC (Medical Council Adjuvant Gastric Infusional Chemotherapy) trial randomized 504 patients with resectable stomach, lower esophagus, or gastroesophageal junction adenocarcinoma to receive surgery alone or peri-operative chemotherapy with three cycles of epirubicin/cisplatin/5-FU (ECF) given pre-operatively and post-operatively (Cunningham et al. 2006a, b). Patients receiving peri-operative chemotherapy had a significantly better OS, with a 36 % survival rate at 5 years compared to 23 % in patients treated with surgery alone (Table 1). Peri-operative chemotherapy showed significant results also in tumor downsizing and R0 resection rate. Interestingly, a subgroup analysis showed that the greatest benefit from the treatment was obtained in gastroesophageal junction patients, a subtype of tumors that is increasing in incidence in Western countries. These results were confirmed by a French trial (ACCORD07-FFCD 9703) that evaluated a chemotherapy regimen containing 5-FU and cisplatin (Boige et al. 2007). A total of 224 patients were randomized to surgery alone or surgery and peri-operative chemotherapy (two to three neoadjuvant cycles and three to four post-operative cycles). Peri-operative chemotherapy improved R0 resection rates (84 versus 73 %, $P = 0.04$), 5-year DFS (34 versus 21 %), and OS (38 versus 24 %) rates. The magnitude of these benefits was similar to that observed in the MAGIC trials. Interestingly, in both studies, about 85 % of patients completed the neoadjuvant part of treatment while less than 50 % received the planned adjuvant part of systemic therapy, maybe due to decreased tolerance to chemotherapy observed after gastrectomy. This latter observation was confirmed by a phase III trial that compared neoadjuvant versus adjuvant docetaxel-based chemotherapy in 69 resectable gastric cancer patients (Roth et al. 2007). In the neoadjuvant arm, 75 % of patients completed the treatment plan, including four TCF (docetaxel, cisplatin, fluorouracil) cycles, while in the adjuvant arm, 66 % of patients started the treatment and only 34 % completed the four cycles. In a further trial by Schuhmacher et al. (Schuhmacher et al. 2009), 144 patients, 40 % of the 360 planned patient population, were randomized to receive surgery alone or pre-operative chemotherapy with two cycles of cisplatin and 5-FU. The study demonstrated an increase in R0 resection for

Table 1 Peri-operative treatment trials in gastric cancer

Trial	Number of patients	Chemotherapy regimen	Hazard ratio for disease-free survival	Hazard ratio for overall survival	5-year overall survival rate (%)
MAGIC	504	ECF	0.66 (0.53–0.81)	0.75 (0.60–0.93)	36 versus 23
FFCD 9703	224	5FU, CDDP	0.63 (0.46–0.86)	0.69 (0.50–0.95)	38 versus 24
EORTC 40954	144	5FU, CDDP	0.66 (0.42–1.03)	0.84 (0.52–1.35)	–
SAKK/ EIO	69	TCF	–	–	–

the chemotherapy arm versus the surgery-only arm (81.9 versus 66.7 %, $P = 0.036$) and showed a trend for a benefit in DFS (HR $= 0.66$, 95 CI $= 0.42 - 1.03$, $P = 0.065$) but failed to reach the primary end point, and no significant differences in OS were observed between the two groups of patients (HR $= 0.84$, 95 CI $= 0.52 - 1.35$, $P = 0.466$).

The MAGIC and FFCD-9703 trials are the first studies to demonstrate survival advantage with peri-operative chemotherapy in gastric and esophagogastric junction (EGJ) cancer. Based on these data, peri-operative chemotherapy with ECF or 5-FU and cisplatin should be considered for stage II to IV M0 gastric cancer patients. More recently, a trial by Stahl et al. (2009), evaluated the addition of radiotherapy to neoadjuvant chemotherapy. The study was restricted to patients with locally advanced adenocarcinomas of the EGJ and compared pre-operative chemotherapy alone with pre-operative chemotherapy followed by chemoradiotherapy, with cisplatin and etoposide associated with radiation treatment. The trial was prematurely closed due to low accrual and total of 126 patients were enrolled (the planned target accrual was of 354 patients). Primary endpoint of the study was overall survival.

Although the R0 resection rate in operated patients was increased from 79 to 88 % by chemoradiotherapy, the intent-to-treat probability of complete resection was not different between treatment arms. Pathological complete response (pCR) rate and the rate of tumor-free lymph nodes were significantly increased by chemoradiotherapy compared with chemotherapy alone. Interestingly, tumor-free lymph nodes after pre-operative therapy resulted in a survival benefit in subgroup analysis. The authors of the study applied a relatively low radiation dose of 30 Gy to keep low the risk of radiation therapy-related complications after surgery. Nevertheless, the addition of radiotherapy determined a significant increase in toxicity, with a more than doubled post-operative mortality (10.2 vs. 3.8 %). The 3-year survival rate appeared higher in the chemoradiotherapy arm than in the chemotherapy arm (47.7 vs. 27.7 %) but the benefit was not statistically significant ($P = 0.07$) and the study failed to reach his primary endpoint. Even if negative,

Selecting the Best Treatment for an Individual Patient 313

the study's results provided evidence that pre-operative chemoradiotherapy may improve survival and could be further investigated.

2.2.2 Peri-Operative Target Therapy

Following successful results in other solid tumors, targeted agents are currently being evaluated in esophagogastric cancer. Recently, positive results from the randomized phase III ToGA (Trastuzumab for Gastric Cancer) study have changed the treatment paradigm for patients with human epidermal growth factor receptor 2-positive advanced gastric cancer, for whom treatment with a platinum and fluoropyrimidine doublet plus trastuzumab can be considered the new standard of care (Bang et al. 2010). Clinial trials evaluating the efficacy of trastuzumab in the adjuvant or peri-operative treatment of gastric cancer are required before the introduction of trastuzumab also in this setting. Indeed, experience in other tumor types has taught us that the efficacy of targeted agents in the advanced disease setting does not always translate to the operable disease setting, as shown by the recent negative trial of bevacizumab in the adjuvant treatment of colon cancer.

The second targeted agent to undergo phase III evaluation in advanced esophagogastric cancer was an antiangiogenic agent, bevacizumab. Angiogenesis is an essential event for small, established tumors to grow beyond a critical size of a few millimeters. It is thought that without the necessary microenvironment for neovascularization, tumor growth is arrested. The international, randomized phase III AVAGAST (Avastin for advanced gastric cancer) study randomized 774 patients with advanced gastric or EGJ adenocarcinoma to a cisplatin–fluoropyrimidine doublet with bevacizumab or placebo in just 14 months. Although bevacizumab showed efficacy in this disease in terms of a higher RR and longer median PFS interval, the study failed to meet the primary endpoint of a statistically significant longer OS duration. Possible regional variation in efficacy was reported in a subgroup analysis, with an apparent benefit noted in patients treated in pan-America but no benefit in those treated in Asia (Kang et al. 2010). The evaluation of bevacizumab in localized esophagogastric cancer is ongoing in phase II and phase III studies, and only safety data are available. In a phase II study on esophageal cancer, of 14 evaluable patients treated with bevacizumab (7.5 mg/kg every 3 weeks) in combination with weekly irinotecan and cisplatin chemoradiation, 10 underwent surgery, in whom there were no unexpected surgical or wound-healing problems, but anastomotic leaks were reported in two patients (20 %) (Ilson et al. 2009). In contrast, in the phase II/III ST03 study of peri-operative epirubicin, cisplatin, and capecitabine with or without bevacizumab (7.5 mg/kg every 3 weeks), preliminary safety data from the first 104 patients randomized showed no difference in the incidence of wound-healing complications or anastomotic leaks and similar rates of thromboembolic events (Okines et al. 2010). The phase III part of the study is still ongoing and efficacy data are pending. Despite intensive preclinical and clinical research, no biomarkers for bevacizumab efficacy are yet available. However, several candidates predictive factors for response have been identified in clinical trials of bevacizumab in different diseases, including: VEGF expression, VEGF polymorphisms, circulating endothelial cells (CECs), and circulating endothelial progenitors cells (CEPS) (Okines et al. 2011). Also hypertension during the treatment has been suggested as a clinical biomarker of response (Scartozzi et al. 2009).

3 Pharmacogenomics

The 5-FU represents the cornerstone of chemotherapy treatment in gastric cancer. The 5-FU metabolic pathway is mainly dependant on the activity of several intracellular enzymes. Among them, four in particular, thymidylate synthase (TS), dihydropyrimidine dehydrogenase (DPD), thymidylate kinase (TK), and thymidylate phosphorylase (TP) are considered as the key points in determining sensitivity or resistance to this drug. These four enzymes are needed to metabolize the drug in its active form (TP, TK) or to drop the concentration of the active drug in the cell (DPD) or either as the target of the active from of the drug (TS). Another interesting enzyme, often considered to be relevant in changing susceptibility to 5-FU based treatment is orotate phosphoribosyltransferase (OPRT), responsible for converting the drug to a form ultimately able to block RNA synthesis. Several different studies have tried to investigate the relationship between the presence of mutations in these enzymes and a reduced/improved activity of treatment based on 5-FU or its derivatives. In this part of the review we will focus on the, often contradictory, results of these studies.

3.1 Adjuvant Setting

In a study by Suh et al. (2005) the role of 3R allele gene as prognostic factor has been evaluated. The assessment was performed on tumor samples of 121 patients resected for stage II or III colon cancer and treated with adjuvant 5-FU according to Mayo clinic regimen. In particular, 3R/3R patients had a significantly worse 5-year actuarial survival when compared with either 2R/3R patients or 2R/2R (58 vs. 80 %, $P = 0.048$). In stage II patients, this difference suggested a trend toward a worse survival, but it was not statistically significant ($P = 0.1678$). In stage III patients, the difference was greater and statistically significant (41 vs. 77 %, $P = 0.0414$).

In a study of Gosens et al. (2008) 38 patients treated with adjuvant 5FU based chemotherapy for resected N+ colon adenocarcinoma were tested for TS genotyping also in tumor tissue. Findings from this study suggested a statistical significant difference in terms of overall survival between the two groups (i.e. high and low TS expression), but only when testing those patients who did not relapse during adjuvant treatment (34 patients). Patients with the low TS expression genotype had a minor recurrence rate than the patients with high TS genotype ($p = 0.038$). Cancer specific survival rate resulted also significantly improved for patients with low TS genotype versus those with the high TS genotype

($p = 0.021$). Authors also compared genotyping analysis results with standard histological parameters such as T or N status and concluded that TS genotyping could have a better gain in terms of prognostic value than histological features.

Fernandez-Contreraz et al. (2006) reached completely different results in a similar study. In detail, when analyzing whether the genotype subset (2R/2R versus 2R/3R versus 3R/3R) was related to disease-free survival in the 201 patients treated with adjuvant 5-FU post surgical intervention for colon or rectal cancer, no significant difference between the various groups (with estimated 5-year disease-free survival rate among the groups respectively of 18.0 months vs. 20.5 months vs. 18.6 months, $P = 0.997$) was evident. The analysis conducted on tumor samples, accordingly to high and low TS expression genotypes also did not show any statistical significant difference ($P = 0.731$), thus discouraging its role as prognostic factor.

Similar conclusions, even if using a different method of evaluation, were reached by Gusella et al. (2009). The authors analyzed blood samples of 122 patients treated with 5-FU in order to determine whether the VNTR or the G/C SNP had a correlation with both PFS and OS. The odds-ratio for PFS between those harboring the guanine in place of cytosine nucleotide polymorphism versus wild type status was 0.99 (CI: 0.48–2.047, $P = 0.98$). The OR between the high TS expression genotype versus the low expression group was 0.86 (and also not statistical significant, with a CI between 0.41 and 1.77, $P = 0.68$). Authors concluded that traditional predictive/prognostic factors such as clinico-pathological features, were still major determinants in the outcome prediction of 5-FU based chemotherapy.

3.2 Peri-Operative Setting

In a recent study of Paez et al. (2010), blood samples were collected from 51 patients before chemoradiation therapy for advanced rectal cancer. An interesting correlation between the 3R/3R genotype was observed in terms of higher response rate, than both the 2R/3R genotype and the 2R/2R genotype also (pCR rates of 61 % for the 3R/3R genotype vs. 22 % of the 2R/3R and 2R/2R subtype, $P = 0.013$), thus suggesting a role as predictive factor. Alas, the same study showed also that the expression of 3R/3R genotype was linked to a better overall survival regardless of treatment, thus suggesting a possible prognostic role ($P < 0.05$).

Conversely, another study of Villafranca et al. (2001), performed on tissue obtained via tissue biopsies of 65 rectal cancer patients who were scheduled to receive chemoradiation found a significant relationship between the expression of 3R/3R status and lack of response. In particular, patients' homozygote for 3R had a lower probability (22 %) of response than patients' heterozygote or 2R homozygote (60 %) ($P = 0.002$). Among the 9 patients who achieved a complete response, only 1 had the 3R homozygote status, whereas the remaining 8 had either a 2R/3R or 2R/2R even though the difference was not statistically significant

$(P = 0.06)$. Authors also observed that, in regards to disease-free survival, patients with a 3R/3R polymorphism had a lower 3-year DFS (41 %) when compared with the other (81 %) even tough the result was not statistically significant $(P = 0.17)$. These data coupled together lead to consider this marker as a predictive factor in rectal cancer patients undergoing pre-operative chemoradiation.

4   Conclusions

Although recent research advances, global results for medical treatment of gastric cancer patients are still disappointing. Peri-operative chemotherapy represents a crucial option for locally advanced resectable gastric carcinoma. Indeed, several different trials showed a clinical advantage in terms of not just an improvement for the subsequent surgical approach but also for overall survival for the peri-operative treatment. In EGJ adenocarcinoma, the addition of radiotherapy to chemotherapy is an interesting hypothesis that is still to be validated. Further focus on the standard chemotherapy research should be more directed toward minimizing toxicities and improving compliance for the drugs that we have at our disposition. More data are expected in the next few years that hopefully may further improve treatment options for gastric cancer patients. Along with new effective therapeutic opportunities, a better clinical and molecularly driven patient selection will represent the cornerstone of the global care for these patients.

References

Bajetta E, Buzzoni R, Mariani L et al (2002) Adjuvant chemotherapy in gastric cancer: 5-year results of a randomized study by the Italian trials in medical oncology (ITMO) group. Ann Oncol 13:299–307

Bang YJ, Van Cutsem E, Feyereislova A et al (2010) Trastuzumab in combination with chemotherapy versus chemotherapy alone for treatment of HER2-positive advanced gastric or gastro-oesophageal junction cancer (ToGA): a phase 3, open-label, randomised controlled trial. Lancet 376:687–697

Boige V, Pignon J, Saint-Aubert B et al (2007) Final results of randomized trial comparing preoperative 5-fluorouracil (F)/cisplatin (P) to surgery alone in adenocarcinoma of the stomach and lower esophagus (ASLE): FNLCC ACCORD07-FFCD 9703 trial. J Clin Oncol 25(18S):4510

Bouche' O, Ychou M, Burtin P et al (2005) Adjuvant chemotherapy with 5-fluorouracil and cisplatin compared with surgery alone for gastric cancer: 7-year results of the FFCD randomized phase III trial (8801). Ann Oncol 16:1488–1497

Buyse ME, Pignon J (2009) Meta-analyses of randomized trials assessing the interest of postoperative adjuvant chemotherapy and prognostic factors in gastric cancer. J Clin Oncol 27:15s (suppl; abstr 4539)

Cascinu S, La bianca R, Barone C et al (2007) Adjuvant treatment of high-risk, radically resected gastric cancer patients with 5-fluorouracil, leucovorin, cisplatin, and epidoxorubicin in a randomized controlled trial. J Natl Cancer Inst 99:601–607

Cunningham D, Allum W, Stenning S et al (2006a) Perioperative chemotherapy versus surgery alone for resectable gastroesophageal cancer. N Engl J Med 355:11–20

Cunningham D, Allum WH, Stenning SP et al (2006b) MAGIC trial participants. Perioperative chemotherapy versus surgery alone for resectable gastroesophageal cancer. N Engl J Med 355:11–20

Di Costanzo F, Gasperoni S, Manzione L et al (2008) Adjuvant chemotherapy in completely resected gastric cancer: a randomized phase III trial conducted by GOIRC. J Natl Cancer Inst 100:388–398

Earle CC, Maroun JA (1999) Adjuvant chemotherapy after resection for gastric cancer in non-Asian patients. Revisiting a meta-analysis of randomized trials. Eur J Cancer 35:1059–1064

Fernandez-Contreras ME, Sanchez-Prudencio S et al (2006) Thymidylate synthase expression pattern, expression level and single nucleotide polymorphism are predictors for disease-free survival in patients of colorectal cancer treated with 5-fluorouracil. Int J Oncol 28(5):1303–1310

Gosens MJ, Moerland E et al (2008) Thymidylate synthase genotyping is more predictive for therapy response than immunohistochemistry in patients with colon cancer. Int J Cancer 123:1941–1949

Gusella M, Frigo AC, Bolzonella C et al (2009) Predictors of survival and toxicity in patients on adjuvant therapy with 5-fluorouracil for colorectal cancer. Br J Cancer 100(10):1549–1557. Epub 2009 Apr 21

Hermans J, Bonekamp JJ, Bon MC et al (1993) Adjuvant therapy after resection for gastric cancer: meta-analysis of randomized trials. J Clin Oncol 11:1441–1447

Ilson D, Bains M, Rizk N et al (2009) Phase II trial of preoperative bevacizumab (Bev), irinotecan (I), cisplatin (C), and radiation (RT) in esophageal adenocarcinoma: preliminary safety analysis. J Clin Oncol 27(15 Suppl):4573

Kang Y, Ohtsu A, Van Cutsem E et al (2010) AVAGAST: a randomized, double- blind, placebo-controlled, phase III study of first-line capecitabine and cisplatin plus bevacizumab or placebo in patients with advanced gastric cancer (AGC) [abstract LBA4007]. J Clin Oncol 28(18 Suppl):950S

Macdonald JS, Smalley SR, Benedetti J et al (2001) Chemoradiotherapy after surgery compared with surgery alone for adenocarcinoma of the stomach or gastroesophageal junction. N Engl J Med 345:725–730

Macdonald JS, Benedetti J, Smalley S et al (2009) Chemoradiation of resected gastric cancer: a 10-year follow-up of the phase III trial INT0116 (SWOG 9008). J Clin Oncol 27:15s (suppl; abstr 4515)

Mari M, Floriani I, Tinazzi A et al (2000) Efficacy of adjuvant chemotherapy after curative resection for gastric cancer: a meta-analysis for published randomised trials. A study of the GISCAD (Gruppo Italiano per lo Studio dei Carcinomi dell'Apparato Digerente). Ann Oncol 11:837–843

Okines AF, Langley R, Cafferty FH et al (2010) Preliminary safety data from a randomized trial of perioperative epirubicin, cisplatin plus capecitabine (ECX) with or without bevacizumab (B) in patients (pts) with gastric or oesophagogastric junction (OGJ) adenocarcinoma. J Clin Oncol 28(15 Suppl):4019

Okines AF, Reynolds AR, Cunningham D (2011) Targeting angiogenesis in esophagogastric adenocarcinoma. Oncologist 16(6):844–858. Epub 2011 May 31. Review

Paez D, Pare L, et al (2010) Thymidylate synthase germline polymorphisms in rectal cancer patients treated with neoadjuvant chemoradiotherapy based on 5-fluorouracil. J Cancer Sci 101(9):2048–2053. doi: 10.1111/j.1349-7006.2010.01621.x

Panzini I, Gianni L, Fattori PP et al (2002) Adjuvant chemotherapy in gastric cancer: a meta-analysis of randomized trials and a comparison with previous metaanalyses. Tumori 88:21–27

Roth et al (2007) Comparative evaluation in tolerance of neoadjuvant versus adjuvant docetaxel based chemotherapy in resectable gastric cancer in a randomized trial of the Swiss group for clinical cancer research (SAKK) and the European institute of oncology (EIO). World Congress on Gastrointestinal Cancer

Scartozzi M, Galizia E, Graziano F et al (2005) Over-D1 dissection may question the value of radiotherapy as a part o fan adjuvant programme in high-risk radically resecate gastric cancer patients. Br J Cancer 92:1051–1054

Scartozzi M, Galizia E, Chiorrini S et al (2009) Arterial hypertension correlates with clinical outcome in colorectal cancer patients treated with first-line bevacizumab. Ann Oncol 20:227–230

Schuhmacher C, Schlag P, Lordick F et al (2009) Neoadjuvant chemotherapy versus surgery alone for locally advanced adenocarcinoma of the stomach and cardia: Randomized EORTC phase III trial #40954. J Clin Oncol 27:15s (suppl; abstr 4510)

Stahl M, Walz KM, Stuschke M et al (2009) Phase III comparison of preoperative chemotherapy compared with chemoradiotherapy in patients with locally advanced adenocarcinoma of the esophagogastric junction. J Clin Oncol 27:851–856

Suh KW, Kim JH et al (2005) Thymidylate Synthase Gene Polymorphism as a Prognostic Factor for Colon Cancer. J Gastrointest Surg 9:336–342

Villafranca E, Okruzhnov Y et al (2001) Polymorphisms of the repeated sequences in the enhancer region of the thymidylate synthase gene promoter may predict downstaging after preoperative chemoradiation in rectal cancer. J Clin Oncol 19:1779–1786

Printed by Publishers' Graphics LLC